Praise for
Living Well on the Spectrum

"As an Aspie, I found this an excellent and readable guide. The book gives readers a better understanding of their social, intellectual, and physical strengths and weaknesses, and provides strategies for improving communication and social skills. It includes helpful techniques for choosing goals and setting course toward them. Kudos to Dr. Gaus for creating this manual—I hope it will be much read."
        —*Eric Schissel, Ithaca, New York*

"A marvelous book with extremely helpful and practical advice. This book will be of tremendous help to individuals with AS/HFA."
        —*Fred R. Volkmar, MD, coauthor of* A Practical Guide to Autism

"Dr. Gaus presents her ideas clearly and effectively and makes terrific use of practical examples. She offers great ideas to help those on the spectrum decrease stress and maximize their progress toward life goals by understanding, fully utilizing, and celebrating their special qualities."
        —*Gary B. Mesibov, PhD, coauthor of* Understanding Asperger
        Syndrome and High-Functioning Autism

"Valerie Gaus offers readers on the autism spectrum a positive, powerful plan for living life to the fullest. Presenting autism as a different rather than a disordered way of being, Dr. Gaus personally guides readers toward self-discovery and then shows practical ways to address challenges. As a person on the spectrum, I find Dr. Gaus's examples, ideas, and approaches ring true with my own life experiences. . . . More than just a 'must read'; this book is a 'must experience' for everyone on the autism spectrum, as well as those who support them."
        —*from the Foreword by Stephen Shore, author of* Beyond the Wall:
        Personal Experiences with Autism and Asperger Syndrome

Living Well on the Spectrum

Living Well on the Spectrum

How to Use Your Strengths to Meet the Challenges of Asperger Syndrome/ High-Functioning Autism

Valerie L. Gaus, PhD

Foreword by Stephen Shore

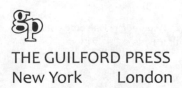

THE GUILFORD PRESS
New York   London

© 2011 The Guilford Press
A Division of Guilford Publications, Inc.
370 Seventh Avenue, Suite 1200, New York, NY 10001
www.guilford.com

Printed in the United States of America

This book is printed on acid-free paper.

Last digit is print number: 9   8   7

Library of Congress Cataloging-in-Publication Data

Gaus, Valerie L.
    Living well on the spectrum : how to use your strengths to meet the challenges of Asperger
  syndrome/high-functioning autism / Valerie L. Gaus.
          p.   cm.
    Includes bibliographical references and index.
    ISBN 978-1-60623-634-5 (pbk.)
    1. Asperger's syndrome—Psychological aspects.   2. Asperger's syndrome—Social
  aspects.   3. Asperger's syndrome—Patients—Life skills guides.   I. Title.
    RC553.A88G384 2011
    616.85′8832—dc22
                                          2010045211

For Gabriel, my sunshine

Contents

Foreword

From the opening page of *Living Well on the Spectrum*, where she hooks the reader in with a "yes, that's me!" example, Valerie Gaus offers readers on the autism spectrum a positive, powerful plan for living life to the fullest. Presenting autism as a different rather than a disordered way of being, Dr. Gaus personally guides readers toward self-discovery and then shows practical ways to address challenges. As a person on the spectrum, I find Dr. Gaus's examples, ideas, and approaches ring true with my own life experiences as well as what I know from my friends with autism.

Through many means—including the author's discussion of how people on the spectrum often interpret the cognitive, social, sensory, emotional, and other aspects of the world around us—this book will help readers develop a true and deeper self-understanding. Moreover, the book emphasizes the importance of viewing differences not as vulnerabilities but as strengths. Time and time again, Dr. Gaus shows how differences in the ways that persons with autism think, socialize, sense the world, and perceive thought and emotion are brought to bear as powerful strengths. For example, the characteristic of dichotomous thinking is reframed as *realism*. Or speaking honestly without filtering can now be thought of as *authenticity*. Even the tendency toward having less communication between the thinking and emotional parts of the brain is reconsidered as *courage* or *optimism*.

The point that "even neurotypicals have stress in their lives" is well taken, as is Dr. Gaus's realization that people on the autism spectrum often have more stress due to having fewer tools for understanding and resolving the very issues that may cause it. Dr. Gaus makes us aware that those on the autism spectrum are actually just like everyone else, but perhaps just more so. This particular point is something I wish I had known as I struggled through so many of the challenges addressed here.

Accessing the positive aspects of the autism spectrum is very empowering, but it also requires hard work. Fortunately, Dr. Gaus shows us the way by taking the understanding gained in the first part of the book about the many strengths that come from being on the autism spectrum and applying an eight-step approach to arrive at effective solutions to the most common problems we face. Whether these are difficulties related to relationships, life transitions, employment, or just day-to-day getting along, Dr. Gaus shows people with autism how their differences in thinking, social interaction, emotional processing, and sensory characteristics can be used as powerful levers for effective and positive change.

Living Well on the Spectrum is more than just a "must read"; this book is a "must experience" for everyone on the autism spectrum, as well as those who support them. This is a book that I am grateful to have—my only wish being that I had had it years ago. It is a resource that will help me, and others, lead a fulfilling and productive life and reach our greatest potential through better understanding of ourselves in the world.

STEPHEN SHORE, EdD
Adelphi University

Acknowledgments

Many authors would agree with me when I say that this is the most difficult section of a book to write. Putting together this type of book is like assembling a massive quilt made up of the ideas and experiences of so many people that it is hard to trace the exact origin of each segment. It is here that I must try to give full recognition to each contributor, all the while knowing I will not do everyone justice.

Without a doubt the most important pieces of fabric in this quilt came from my patients. Although I cannot name them, they have been my primary teachers on the subject of this book. The story of each of their lives provided inspiration to me as a psychologist and as a person, to look for ways to capitalize on strengths and gifts when facing obstacles and adversity. In the midst of writing the manuscript, I had the good fortune and lucky timing to be invited to a preview screening of the HBO movie *Temple Grandin*, an event that was attended by Dr. Grandin, her family, and many of the movie's creators. The director, Mick Jackson, was among those who made opening remarks, and during his speech he shared an anecdote in which a misinformed (and/or unkind) acquaintance of his had suggested he was making a movie about "the disease of the month," which was autism. His response was, quite simply, "This movie is not about a disease; it is about a gift." That quote kept coming to my mind after that evening because it so well captured how I feel about my work with my patients and the message I hope to convey here. This is not to minimize the great struggles and painful experiences that are too often part of life on the spectrum, but to emphasize that the characteristics of autism do not *only* bring those things. My patients have all demonstrated to me how their unique characteristics have been assets, giving them tools not only to use in the face of difficulty but also to enrich the lives of others.

I owe thanks to several people who were so generous with their time, reading portions of the manuscript and giving thoughtful feedback through various stages of the project. Gary Mesibov was instrumental in helping me formulate the initial outline of the book, while Eustacia Cutler, by sharing her thoughts with me, gave me inspiration during that early phase. Pat Schissel, Eric Schissel, and Bernice Polinsky provided much needed feedback on the entire first draft. Speech–language pathologists Lara Scher and Karen Gambino were kind enough to make suggestions about the sections related to language and communication. I owe a huge debt to Candice Baugh, who not only reviewed the whole first draft, but put in many hours compiling the resource list at the end of the book. Stephen Shore set aside a lot of his time despite his busy travel schedule to review and provide detailed comments on the manuscript, and ultimately blessed the book with a foreword. This was especially meaningful because he has been an important influence on me as a colleague as well as a role model to others for taking a positive approach to living on the spectrum.

Operating as a sole therapist in a private practice can mean countless hours working in isolation. Add writing to the mix, and things can get downright lonesome. Luckily, I rarely feel alone because I am privileged to have a network of colleagues who share with me various goals and activities. All of these people have been crucial in shaping my ideas about the autism spectrum and have each encouraged me as I put together this book. Some were mentioned above, and other key players are Michael John Carley, Lynda Geller, Peter Gerhardt, Jane Perr, and Dave Roll. My peer supervision group has been an invaluable source of support, thanks to Maria Scalley-Gagnon, Halley Ceglia, Arlene Yarwood, Kristen Memoli-Ruthkowski, Shana Nichols, Faith Kappenberg, and, already mentioned, Candice Baugh.

The time I have spent consulting at the Vincent Smith School in Port Washington, New York, has been an important influence on my thoughts about positive psychology as it pertains to people with learning differences. As a small special-needs school serving students with a variety of learning disabilities (including students on the spectrum), Vincent Smith provides a nurturing and stimulating environment for young people in grades 4–12. The school's students are either preteens or teens, struggling with those all-too-difficult ages when social and emotional growth can be so painful. Living up to their motto—"It's OK to learn differently"—the school allows students to understand their own individual profiles of strengths and needs and gives them the skills to communicate effectively about them. I have had the pleasure of participating in the Vincent Smith's schoolwide positive behavioral support and self-advocacy programs, where I learned how crucial it is for people with learning differences to start young on their journey toward being self-sufficient and self-respecting adults. I am forever indebted to Ronnie McCue, Arlene Wishnew, and Ellen Forrest, who are not only the key leaders of the Vincent Smith community, fearless and tireless in their efforts to give the students their best, but have also been my very good friends.

Other great friends are found in my "dinner group." Mary Brady, Pam Wolff, Eddie Velasquez, Kathleen Ziccardi, and Arnetta McKenna have been there for me during the best and worst times of my life these past few years. There were many moments when I would have found it hard to keep going if not for their steadfast support.

I cannot possibly measure the value of the people at The Guilford Press who supported this project from start to finish. Obviously there would be no book without them, but my gratitude goes beyond that. Kitty Moore and Chris Benton were there when this idea was nothing more than some thoughts shared in conversation. They listened and were willing to take on something that, at least at the time, seemed unconventional. I truly benefited from their team approach because they were always available, no matter when I needed help, to give me guidance and direction. I sometimes forgot that we were each working in a different city. Kitty maintained the clarity of our vision and the needs of our readers, keeping the project on track with unwavering humor and good cheer. Chris artfully shifted back and forth between mentoring me about writing for a broad audience and deferring to me on issues that were particularly sensitive for our intended readers. It was an absolute privilege to work with these two wise women. I also want to thank Anna Brackett, Editorial Project Manager, for her eye for detail and ability to pull everything together at the end. Finally, much appreciation goes to Art Director Paul Gordon for designing such a beautiful cover.

Last but not least, I owe the most to my family. My parents, June and Ray Gaus, always encouraged me to work hard but also let me define success in my own terms, one of the key elements of the positive psychology that is the cornerstone for this book. Their unconditional love, which has been a constant in my life, gave me the type of springboard for which there is no substitute. My big brother, Greg, approaches his life with such courage and humor; while he is not on the spectrum, he has provided a living example for the ideas I express in this book. I also thank his wife, Rachel, for her encouragement and input on parts of the book. I appreciate my older son, Sean, who was away at college during the bulk of my manuscript preparation, but would never forget to regularly check in on my progress. My little son, Gabriel, conceived long after the genesis of this book but delivered long before the final product, was an unexpected and delightful companion on this journey. A daily dose of his sunshine was very sustaining indeed. Special thanks go to his nanny, Cordelia Blackett, a beautiful person who gave him an endless supply of genuine love and laughter while his daddy was at work and his mommy disappeared for days at a time to finish this project.

The person who contributed the most to me for this book was my husband, Lider Raynor. Although he was a veteran author's spouse, this being my second book, we did not have a young baby to take care of the first time around. As during the first time, he tolerated months of my middle-of-the-night writing sessions and my complete neglect of household responsibilities. Also as before, he cooked for me every night, sometimes bringing a meal to my desk and reminding me to eat. And as if that were not enough, he also took on the role of single parent without hesitation, while also continuing to work full time running his own business. As a very loving and involved father since Gabriel's birth, it was natural for him to take on virtually all of the parenting responsibilities until the book was done. Because of my husband's willingness to sacrifice, my son suffered nothing. Knowing Gabriel was in good hands allowed me to work more freely. Without that support, I would never have been able to complete this project. Thank you, Lider!

Introduction

How to Get the Most Out of This Book

Do you feel exhausted before you even start your work or school day because it takes all of your energy just to get yourself out of the house?

Does the idea of attending a family gathering or social event leave you feeling completely stressed out?

Do you ever feel like you will never complete all the tasks you are responsible for during your day?

If you have been diagnosed on the autism spectrum, you know very well how hard it can be just to get through the day. Mundane tasks that come easily to other people may leave you completely drained, seriously interfering with your quality of life and happiness. As a clinical psychologist, I have been working with adults with milder forms of autism for over 15 years, with a focus on people with Asperger syndrome (AS) or "high-functioning" autism (HFA). My patients have described to me countless times what a struggle it is to get along in a world designed by people who think so differently from them. Their family members have also offered vivid descriptions of the strains and pressures of daily life on the spectrum.

Fortunately, I have also heard inspiring stories about people on the spectrum who have used their differences to their advantage. I have seen many individuals benefit from a better understanding of how their brain works, how AS or HFA may increase stress, and what they can do to gain more control over their lives. Together, my patients and I have formulated numerous practical strategies that can be used from day to day to minimize stress, maximize progress toward life goals, and increase their overall sense of well-being. In this book I share the approaches that I have found to be supported by both the behavioral science literature and favorable responses from my patients.

Success: Your Way

I believe you can improve the quality of your life by knowing yourself better, as well as where you are different from and similar to people not on the spectrum. The more you know yourself, the more you can capitalize on the differences that are strengths while accepting and compensating for differences that have limited you.

This book is designed to help you make the lifestyle changes you need to make to feel more satisfied and less stressed from day to day. To do this, you need to have some idea of the lifestyle you wish to have. Everyone has some kind of goal— something he or she wants to achieve. Can you name a goal you have for your lifestyle? What are you trying to achieve? You don't have to be able to answer this question in full right now. This book will take you through the process of figuring out what you want and what you can do to get it. A key part of this process will be determining what is standing in the way of reaching your goals. I'll help you figure out which obstacles are related to your AS/HFA characteristics and how you can apply positive solutions to address them.

This approach is based on the assumption that life goals and lifestyle choices are very individualized; what is good for one person may not be good for another. In working with my patients, I have found their problems often stem from their attempts to fit into a mold shaped by others. The characteristics of AS and HFA can play a major role in keeping you from your goals—but not because the traits are all bad or are defects. Rather, your brain works so differently from the brains of people who are not on the spectrum that you may find yourself at odds with so-called typical people and the environments designed by them.

As the cliché says, you cannot fit a square peg into a round hole. *But I have learned from my patients that it is possible for a square peg to find a square hole.* The square peg does not have to try to turn into a round peg. In other words, you do not have to change into someone you are not to experience happiness and satisfaction in your life. As a person on the spectrum you can find and shape places to better fit yourself, but you do have to know what you need in your environment if you are to do this successfully. You have to know yourself well and what "makes you tick" before you can really design your lifestyle to best meet your needs. This book will help you do that.

How Positive Psychology Can Help

In the behavioral science and clinical community, "positive psychology" is a growing field that focuses on enhancing the mental and physical health of human beings by highlighting and strengthening assets. Researchers and clinicians work to understand the characteristics that are associated with happiness as well as the factors linked with resilience and surviving adverse circumstances. While these efforts have been helpful to the general population for a number of years, only recently have experts begun to study how building strengths and coping skills may be helpful to people diagnosed on the autism spectrum. One important part of this movement has been a focus on defining autism characteristics as *differences,* not *defects.* In line with this type of thinking, I take the position that autism is *not a disease* but gives a person a unique way of processing information about the world and the people in it. Taking this approach has been very useful to me and my patients because, while this unique way of perceiving the world does indeed cause some of the problems that bring adults into my office, it also gives them strengths and talents. If I were to follow a *disease* model of autism, I would have to try to "eliminate the autism." But to do so would be to sacrifice the assets that patients have *because* of the autism. The positive psychology approach allows me and my patients to *use* some the autistic characteristics as tools and assets in the therapy.

This entire book is based on the principles of positive psychology. Even though the field is relatively new, emerging around 1998, it is large and includes many different types of scholars and scientists. I will describe it more fully in Chapter 1, but for now you could think of positive psychology as the psychology of human strengths. Essentially, positive psychology encourages you to think of yourself in terms of strengths you can capitalize on instead of solely in terms of deficits or weaknesses that you should try to "fix." A good example is the concept of intelligence. Positive psychology redefines intelligence more broadly than it was generally defined in the past, as a set of skills a person needs to succeed in life. These skills involve being able to:

- define success in your own terms, which may or may not correspond to societal or conventional definitions of success
- adapt to, modify, and choose the environments you are in
- do all of the above by capitalizing on your strengths and correcting or compensating for your weaknesses

While this definition was not designed specifically for people on the spectrum, it "hits the nail on the head" for this book by offering people with AS and HFA the freedom to be themselves and to be successful. This book is full of exercises designed to help you develop the skills on that list. You will be encouraged to define your own goals and to become more knowledgeable about your specific strengths and weaknesses and then use that information to adapt to, choose, and shape your surroundings.

The Changing Face of Autism

Never before has the topic of autism received as much attention as it does today. Discussions about "autism spectrum disorders" are widespread through every medium in public, scientific, and clinical forums. Once considered a rare disorder of which the average person would never be aware, *autism* is now a household word. Mention it at any gathering and someone will tell you of a personal experience with the syndrome. Despite the universal familiarity with the term, there is anything but a collective understanding of what it means, whom it applies to, and how it should be addressed in our society. You will find vastly different opinions among and between groups of people who have autism, who are caring for those with autism, who are scientists studying autism, and who are professionals serving people with autism. At the time of this writing there is ongoing controversy about:

- which terms should be used to refer to autism
- what causes autism
- whether it is a disease that needs to be cured or a set of unique characteristics that should be embraced
- whether it is a single disorder or a collection of related syndromes
- who should pay for educational and clinical services meant to improve the lives of people affected by autism

These are complex issues that do not have simple answers, and I am confident that these debates will continue for many years to come. One thing that can be stated without much argument, however, is that the number of people being diagnosed with autism spectrum disorders (ASDs) has risen dramatically over the past 20 years. In a December 2009 report, the Centers for Disease Control estimated that approximately 1% (1 in 110) of children in the United States have an ASD. While most research has focused on children, autism is a lifelong condition that does not disappear in adulthood. I am assuming, therefore, that if 1% of U.S. children have an ASD, there's a good chance that 1% of U.S. adults have an ASD. A recent study conducted on adults in Great Britain supports that idea; the investigators found that approximately 1% (1 in 100) of adults sampled in that country are living with an ASD.

What about you? You may have been diagnosed as a child, you could have been diagnosed more recently, or perhaps professional evaluators have not rendered a conclusive diagnosis of your problems. Regardless of when or how you were diagnosed, you can read and benefit from this book if you have the characteristics associated with ASDs.

Autism spectrum disorders are a group of syndromes that have been documented by scientists and mental health professionals since the 1940s. Over the past 60 years, there have been many shifts and changes in the way the symptoms are classified and labeled, which sometimes makes it difficult to attach an accurate label to every individual who has these symptoms. Some core features, however, have remained consistent throughout autism's documented history. Professionals who may disagree on the details of classification would all agree that people with ASDs struggle to some degree with *social interaction*, *language and/or communication*, and *restricted or repetitive behavior patterns*. When you think about how such difficulties might come into play during any ordinary day, it's no surprise that you might feel stressed out, frustrated, or tired.

Perhaps the most dramatic shift in the definition of autism, and the one with the greatest relevance to you, came only in the mid-1990s, when the majority of the mental health community began to recognize that autism symptoms can vary widely in severity. This realization was triggered by the publication in 1994 of the fourth edition of *The Diagnostic and Statistical Manual of Mental Disorders* (known as DSM-IV), the source that most North American mental health professionals rely on for diagnostic criteria. While the previous edition of that manual divided the autism-related disorders (or pervasive developmental disorders) into only two categories, DSM-IV classified them as five separate disorders. Most significant to this discussion was the recognition of Asperger's disorder, which is described as similar to autistic disorder but occurring in people without intellectual or language impairments. In addition, while the manual did not have any category called "high-functioning autism," that term has been used informally by professionals to bring attention to the diagnosis of Autistic Disorder when it occurs in someone whose intellectual and language functioning is less affected. This is why autism has come to be referred to as a *spectrum* of disorders; autism can affect a highly intelligent and verbally skilled person, or a nonverbal person with profound intellectual disability, or anyone else in between those two extremes.

When the controversial fifth edition of *The Diagnostic and Statistical Manual of Mental Disorders* (DSM-5) was published in May 2013, there was an attempt to improve the description of the syndrome by using the spectrum concept, but the changes were so significant that it has caused confusion and concerns for some people, perhaps even you. The five distinct pervasive developmental disorders defined in DSM-IV were collapsed into a single disorder that is called simply *autism spectrum disorder* and described on a dimension rather than in categories. The term "Asperger's disorder" is no longer used in that system, which could be unsettling for people who were diagnosed with that not so long ago. Most people meeting criteria for Asperger's would now be diagnosed with a milder form of "autism spectrum disorder," and would not be left with no diagnosis.

Even when labels change, the people they describe do not, in terms of the issues and challenges they face every day. Regardless of the diagnosis you may have been assigned recently or in the distant past, you are dealing with your own specific problems and goals, and this book will be useful now and in the years ahead. You may continue to hear, however, about the changes in the autism nomenclature used by mental health professionals and others around you, and you should know what the implications of such changes may be for you personally:

- Your mental-health and medical providers may have changed the term they use when they document your diagnosis.
- You might use different terminology if you choose to share your diagnosis with some people in your life.
- Your health insurance provider may or may not change the types of services covered under the newer diagnostic system.
- Your eligibility for support services may be affected, depending on how your particular state responds to the newer diagnostic criteria (e.g., even with the previous system, some states recognized Asperger's disorder as a developmental disability eligible for certain services, and other states did not).

To be sure my terminology is clear in the context of all the shifts and changes described above, following are the terms that you will see in this book, in **bold** type, with equivalent terms (historical and current) next to them.

- **Autism spectrum disorders (ASDs):** the collection of syndromes previously called pervasive developmental disorders (PDD), including the earlier termed autistic disorder, Asperger syndrome, and pervasive developmental disorder-not otherwise specified (PDD-NOS)
- **Asperger syndrome (AS):** Asperger's disorder as defined above
- **High-functioning autism (HFA):** ASD as seen in a person with average or above average intelligence and verbal ability
- **Neurotypical:** Typical person or any person who does *not* have an ASD

How to Use This Book

The following chapters will give you tools and step-by-step instructions so that you can:

- understand the specific ways your brain works differently
- identify which brain differences are causing the greatest difficulty, and in which areas of daily life
- remedy problematic differences that can be improved
- accept and compensate for problematic differences that cannot be changed
- strengthen the positive differences that can enhance your quality of life and promote happiness

The strategies and information in this book are presented in a variety of forms and grouped in ways that will allow you to pick and choose what is most relevant to your life. You can read the text alone now and later come back to certain information that you'll find in boxes and sidebars as you need it or find yourself interested. You can fill in the worksheets and question boxes directly on the book pages or photocopy the forms to fill them in separately, as many times as you need them. You'll discover that you can use the strategies and other ideas in a wide range of living situations (independent living as a single or with a committed partner, living with parents or siblings, living with peers in a supervised group setting) and vocational situations (working full-time, unemployed and seeking work, employed with supports, attending college or a vocational training program). These approaches apply to the struggles that can be associated with all stages of adult life, ranging from late adolescence (e.g., dealing with the stress of transitioning to adulthood) all the way to late middle age (e.g., preparing for retirement, facing loss of loved ones). Whether you plan to use the book independently or with the help of someone else, you might want to share it with close family members or any of the healthcare professionals or teachers you're working with so they can support your efforts to use the strategies.

The book is divided into two sections. Part I (Chapters 1–5) introduces the many areas of functioning in which you may struggle with a diminished quality of life. You'll know you're hardly alone when you read Chapter 1, which describes in depth "a day in the life" of an adult on the spectrum. Next comes a "crash course" in the thinking, social, emotional, and sensory differences you've been experiencing. Finally, I'll help you learn a lot about yourself and accept these differences so you can build resilience and acquire coping skills.

Part II begins with a detailed explanation of the problem-solving process (Chapter 6). Then, in Chapters 7–13, you'll read about the seven most common arenas of struggle for people on the spectrum and how to apply the eight steps of problem solving to your own issues. Each of those chapters is organized the same way and can be a stand-alone resource for you. Once you have completed Part I and Chapter 6, you can skip to any of the other chapters in Part II in whatever order works best for you without reading all of them. Some people, for example, may have no interest in the chapter on school-related stress or marital problems. Or you may need help in a particular area right now and another one in the future.

The final chapter in Part II (Chapter 14) is devoted to helping you pull together all of the relevant information you have gleaned from the book to define success your way. There you will find guidelines for getting the help you might need from others to support your personal solution package. I hope you'll call all of your many strengths into play to make your life as happy and satisfying as it can be.

Part I

Life on the Spectrum

A Typical Day in Your Life

Problems and Solutions

In today's society, everybody appears to be on the go much of the time, trying to juggle many things at once. Any person can feel pressured under these circumstances, but people on the spectrum may feel even more overwhelmed by the demands of daily adult life than typical people. In fact, when people on the spectrum come to my office for help, they often report a lot of stress in their lives. They describe how getting through the day, trying to complete the simplest things, seems so difficult and taxing. Even when a day is considered successful, they feel completely exhausted by the end, as if a supposedly simple set of tasks had drained all of their resources.

In this chapter I will help you identify the key parts of your life where you are feeling the most pressure or disappointment. First I will walk you through your own typical day to help you pinpoint the trouble spots. Then I will introduce several other people on the spectrum whose struggles may be familiar to you. Reading about these common problems may remind you of some that you experience but didn't identify at first. Then you will learn more about how the growing field of positive psychology, mentioned in the Introduction, can offer solutions to these problems and how this approach will drive all of the strategies and suggestions I offer throughout this book. The chapter ends with a description of self-help techniques that you can use to solve a wide variety of problems, discussed in full in the chapters ahead.

A Typical Day on the Spectrum

No two days are exactly alike, but I am going to ask you specific questions about each part of your *average* day. If it is hard for you to imagine your typical day, just pick one specific day from the past week, such as yesterday or last Friday, and use that as your example.

First think about your morning. Are there things that happen in the morning that cause you discomfort in any way? Here are some questions to help you assess for trouble spots during that period of the day. Jot down your answers in the blank lines if you find this useful.

- What time do you wake up and how do you wake up? _____
- Do you use an alarm? _____
- Does someone in your family wake you up? _____
- Do you feel rested when you wake up? _____
- Are you able to get up when you want to? _____
- Are you getting up to go someplace (work, school), or do you typically stay home in the morning? _____
- Do you have enough time to prepare if you are leaving? _____
- Do you have breakfast? _____
- Do you eat alone or with someone? _____
- Do you get along with the people in your household in the morning? _____
- Do you have difficulty leaving on time? _____
- Are you able to find everything you need, or do you struggle with things being misplaced (clothes, books, keys)? _____
- How do you get where you are going (car, public transportation)? _____ _____
- Do you have any difficulty with your transportation? _____
- Are you frustrated or bored because you have no place to go (e.g., unemployed)? _____
- Are you nervous or scared about leaving the house? _____
- If you have work or school, what is it like once you arrive at your destination? _____
- Do you arrive on time, or are you late? _____
- Do you greet other people when you arrive? _____
- How do you get along with your coworkers or fellow students/trainees? _____

Then move to midday as you picture your typical routine. The following questions can help you consider sources of stress during this time of the day.

■ If you work or go to school, what is it like settling in for the day? _____
_____

■ Are you able to be productive with your work? _____

■ Do have difficulty getting your work started? _____

■ Are you able to follow the instructions given to you by your boss or instructors? _____

■ Do you feel pressured by the work? _____

■ Do you enjoy what you are doing? _____

■ Are you able to use your talents in your work, or are you underutilized?
_____

■ Do you have time for a lunch break? _____

■ What do you do for lunch? _____

■ Do you eat alone or with others? _____

■ Are you reluctant to talk to others? _____

■ Do you try to talk to people but find you are not making connections?
_____

■ If you are not employed or in school, how do you spend the middle part of
your day? _____

■ Do you have meaningful activities or things to do that you enjoy? _____
_____

■ Are you bored, depressed, or frustrated because you are at home? _____
_____

■ Do you feel cooped up at home and wish to be out more than you are? ____
_____

■ Are you satisfied with the amount of contact you have with other people, or
do you feel lonely? _____

Now think about the afternoon and how it usually goes for you.

■ As the day moves through the afternoon, do you tend to become more or
less productive? _____

■ If you are at work, does the end of the workday bring more pressure? _____
_____

■ Do you have difficulty stopping your work when it is time to go home? ____
_____

■ Do you feel overwhelmed when the day draws to a close because you did not
get done what you had hoped to? _____

■ If you are a student, is the afternoon a better or worse time to be in class or study? _____

■ If you have been home all day, do you find more activities to do in the later part of the day, or do you continue to feel bored or frustrated? _____

■ Do you have any difficulty while running errands, such as going to the bank or post office? _____

■ If you commute home from work or school at this time of day, do you have any difficulty with travel, either by car or by public transportation? _____ _____

As the day turns into evening, how do things shift or change for you?

■ If you are arriving home from work or school, what is the transition back to your home like? _____

■ Who is there to greet you, if anyone? _____

■ If you do live with someone, what is interacting with this person like at this time of day? _____

■ If you have been home all day and others in your household are arriving home in the evening, what is it like getting along with them at this time? _____

■ Do you eat dinner? _____

■ Whom do you eat with, and what is it like getting along with them? _____ _____

■ Is mealtime with your family stressful? _____

■ If you eat alone, do you prepare a meal yourself or eat take-out? _____ _____

■ Do you feel lonely? _____

■ Do you have household chores to do in the evening? _____

■ Do you find your household responsibilities overwhelming at this time? _____

■ Do you look through your mail, and if so, do you find anything about that stressful? _____

■ Do you have any time for recreational or leisure activities in the evening? _____

■ Do you get bored in the evening? _____

■ Do you feel more or less energetic in the evening than at other times of day? _____

When the evening turns into late night, or a time that many people go to bed, what do you find yourself doing?

- Do you go to bed early or like to stay up late? _____

- If you are a "night owl," do other people in your household complain about this? _____

- Do you have difficulty falling asleep? _____

- Do you spend more time than you meant to watching TV or using the computer because you get caught up in it? _____

- Do you feel more depressed or anxious late at night than during the day?
  _____

And finally, during the overnight hours:

- Do you get enough sleep? _____

- Do you fall asleep but then wake up frequently throughout the night? _____
  _____

- Do you wake up much earlier than you'd like?_____

Are you starting to get a picture of the best and worst times of your day? To clarify the picture of your day further, fill out Worksheets 1 and 2. If you need an example of what to write down on your worksheets, look at the ones filled out by Blanca, the first person you will meet in the next section. I will ask you to refer to your worksheets later in the book as you do other exercises in the process of improving your satisfaction with your day-to-day life.

Common Trouble Spots

The preceding lists and worksheets may have helped you start to piece together a picture of your own typical day. The following "snapshots" from the typical days of others on the spectrum may help you fill in any gaps. These descriptions illustrate the most stressful point in each person's day and serve as examples of the most common trouble spots to be addressed in this book. The people in the following scenarios are all quite different, but they do have one thing in common: each person has been diagnosed with AS or HFA.

Blanca is 23 years old and single. She lives with her parents and her younger brother. Her most difficult time of the day is the morning. Her day begins when the alarm clock rings at 7:00 A.M. She gets out of bed immediately because she has been lying awake since 5:00 A.M. even though she goes to bed at midnight. She has morning class at the university, where she is working toward a master's degree in marine biology. She has about an hour before she has to leave to make the 30-minute drive to campus. As she gets ready, she feels very anxious, because she often forgets things she needs for her day.

My Favorite Time

Draw hands on the clock below to indicate your favorite time of the day. Underline AM or PM.

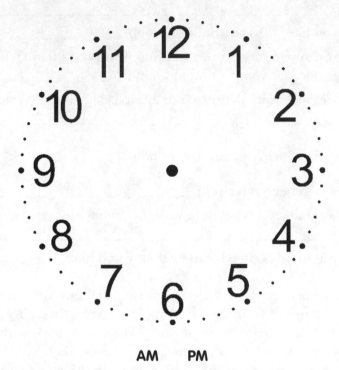

AM   PM

What is it about this time of day that you look forward to?

_____

_____

_____

_____

She struggles as she packs her book bag because she has difficulty finding things in her messy room. She also has trouble concentrating in the morning because she feels tired from lack of sleep.

Henry *is age 29 and lives with his father in the house in which he grew up. He holds a bachelor's degree in English and has been unemployed for 6 years. He spends most days home alone while his father works. He tries to look for a job by exploring adver-*

tisements on the Internet. The most stressful time of day for him is the late afternoon, because he begins to feel pressured by the fact that he has not gotten much done. He anticipates the argument that he and his father will have when his father gets home from work. Dad often asks him what he did all day and criticizes him for not having found work.

Arnold *is an 18-year-old college freshman living in a dorm with two roommates. He dreads the evenings, because his roommates invite a lot of people in to hang out. He*

My Worst Time

Draw hands on the clock below to indicate your *least* favorite time of the day. Underline AM or PM.

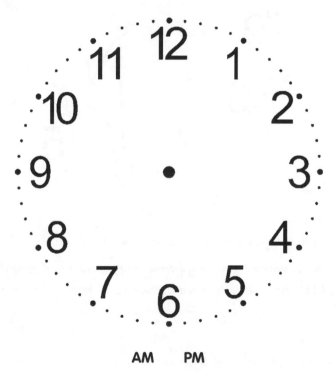

AM   PM

What is it about this time of day that you find stressful or unpleasant?

_____

_____

_____

_____

Example from Blanca
WORKSHEET 1

My Favorite Time

Draw hands on the clock below to indicate your favorite time of the day. Underline AM or PM.

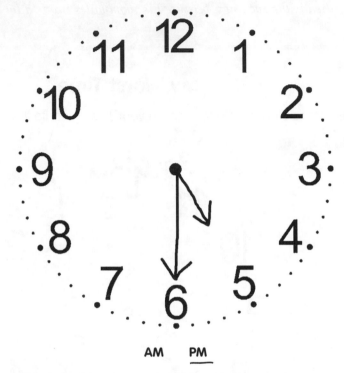

AM   **PM**

What is it about this time of day that you look forward to?

I look forward to coming home from school and spending time with my little brother. We have dinner together and he is funny.

wants to make friends, but he is very shy. He has always tried to "disappear" when around kids his own age, a habit that protected him from the bullies in middle school. Now he wants to be more sociable, but he doesn't know how to start conversations and even when he thinks of something to say, he is too scared to try. For the most part, his roommates and their friends ignore him.

Jake is single, 20, and living with his parents. He recently dropped out of community college after only two semesters and now works part-time in the dairy department of a grocery store. The most difficult times of day for him are when he has to drive himself to or from work. He got his driver's license just before starting college and did so very reluctantly. He is anxious on any road other than his own suburban residential street, and his anxiety increases with the number of other cars on the road. He will not drive on highways at all. The 10-mile commute to work is extremely unpleasant for him, and when the anxiety is particularly high, he calls in sick. Though he does not feel comfortable admitting this to his parents, his fear of driving contributed to his decision to drop out of school.

Noel, *age 37, owns his own house and lives in it by himself. He works full time as a computer programmer. The most difficult time of day for him is the evening, when he goes home to his empty house. Weekend evenings are even worse than weekdays because he feels very lonely. He wants very much to get married and have children, but he has had very little success with dating. He has joined several online dating services through the years, but he has gone on only two dates. Each time, he felt very uncom-fortable making conversation with his dates, and neither woman was willing to go on*

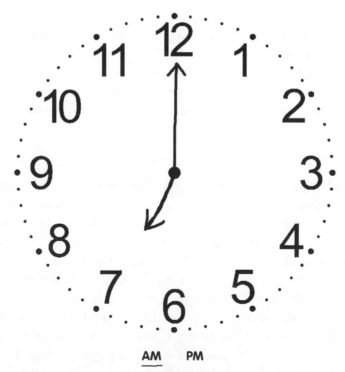

Example from Blanca

WORKSHEET 2

My Worst Time

Draw hands on the clock below to indicate your *least* favorite time of the day. Underline AM or PM.

<u>AM</u>   PM

What is it about this time of day that you find stressful or unpleasant?

I hate getting ready for school in the morning. I can't find half the stuff I need and I am always running late.

a second date. He is frustrated because he thinks he is doing something wrong, but he does not know what it is.

Meredith *is 46, single, and shares an apartment with a roommate. She has a law degree but has never worked as a lawyer. She currently has a part-time job at a nursery/home garden center. She has diabetes, and the most stressful time of her day is the morning, when she must take her first glucose reading and give herself a shot of insulin. The tasks involved in taking care of this chronic medical condition have overwhelmed her for all of her adult life. She often thinks that she would have been able to handle a career in law if she did not have to devote so much time to managing her health.*

Even though none of these people is exactly like you, you might find yourself struggling in similar ways. You may have noticed that being on the spectrum can create dissatisfaction or difficulty in any area of life:

- Home life
- Community life
- Work life
- Social life
- Educational life
- Health

In the following pages you'll have a chance to look at your own experiences in each of these arenas of daily life to get an idea of where you struggle most. This self-knowledge will help you figure out which chapters in Part II may be most helpful to you. Each of them covers one of these areas of life in more depth, offering more answers about the causes and solutions for these difficulties.

Home Life

Think about your life at home. Maybe you live in a house or an apartment. You could live in an urban area or a suburb or a rural area. Perhaps you live alone, or you live with one person or several people, related to you or not. No matter what your situation, your home is the "headquarters" for every other part of life discussed in this book. At the very best, your home can be your sanctuary, providing a place to rest, relax, and take a break from the pressures of the outside world. A positive home life can give you the strength to take on the challenges you face whenever you venture into the outside world. But a home of any kind also imposes responsibilities—from doing chores to maintaining relationships to adhering to the household rules and routines—and these demands can sometimes get difficult to manage. Unfortunately when home *becomes* a source of stress, it can have a negative impact on almost every other area of your life. After all, home is usually where you begin each day. That is why your home life is discussed first here.

Blanca's story illustrated problems with getting the day started at home as she struggled with getting enough sleep and organizing her space. **Henry's** problem at home involved his relationship with his father. Charles also struggles with a relationship problem at home:

> **Charles,** age 52, lives with his wife and 11-year-old son. He has a full-time job as a high school social studies teacher. The most stressful time of day for him is late afternoon, when he gets home from work. His son usually arrives home at the same time, but his wife doesn't get there for 2 more hours. Charles is always happy to see his son, but he also feels really tense from his own day at work and overwhelmed by the things his son needs at that time. His son talks a lot and very loudly and asks him a lot of questions. After being with his own students all day, Charles does not feel like talking to anyone. Sometimes he snaps at his son, and then he feels guilty.

Some other common problems reported by adults on the spectrum are described below. Check the box next to any of the comments that make you think about yourself.

Problems with managing personal responsibilities:

☐ "I can't keep my space organized."

☐ "I am always losing things."

☐ "I have trouble keeping up with the cleaning."

☐ "I have trouble managing my time."

☐ "I procrastinate on tasks I have to do around the house."

☐ "I can't fall asleep at night, and I stay up later than I want to."

☐ "I can't wake up when I am supposed to—I sleep through my alarm."

☐ "I have difficulty sleeping and wake up a lot during the night and early morning."

☐ "I have trouble paying my bills on time."

☐ "I have too much debt."

☐ "I don't know how to handle household repairs when they are needed."

☐ "I can't seem to prepare food on my own."

Problems with the people I live with:

☐ "My parents don't give me enough privacy."

☐ "My roommate makes too much noise."

☐ "My sister is always picking on me."

☐ "My family has guests too often—I don't like to mingle so often."

☐ "I have a lot of arguments with my mother [or father]."

☐ "People in my house get mad at me a lot because I procrastinate."

☐ "People in my house get annoyed about my sleeping habits."

☐ "My roommate is constantly hounding me to clean."

☐ "My grandmother is always watching TV when I want to see my own show."

☐ "My spouse/partner does not understand that I need time alone."

If you checked off several of these comments, be sure to read Chapter 7. There you will find worksheets and tools that will help you solve these types of problems in your own home life.

Work Life

Now think about your work life. Do you have a job? If not, unemployment and all the problems that come with it may give you a lot to worry about. If you do, you might not be completely satisfied with your job. Unfortunately, too many adults on the autism spectrum are unemployed or "underemployed," which means working at jobs that don't take advantage of their training, experience, or talent in a given field or specialty. Research in the science of happiness (subjective well-being) has repeatedly shown a strong correlation between job satisfaction and overall life satisfaction; that is, the higher one's job satisfaction, the higher the overall satisfaction with life is likely to be and vice versa. So problems in this area of life are likely to be associated with poor quality of life in other areas as well.

Henry, for example, is having problems at home, in terms of personal contentment and also his relationship with his father, that can be traced to his being unemployed. But many adults on the spectrum who do have a job are struggling with different aspects of work life, such as Margaret.

> *Margaret, at age 61, is divorced and living by herself. She has two grown children who are each married and living on their own. She is an endocrinologist and works with several other physicians in a group medical practice. The most difficult time of day for her is lunchtime at work. There is a lunch room for staff to use during their breaks. Margaret would prefer to eat alone, but there is a shortage of office space, so she is forced to use the lunch room. There are almost always one or two people in the lunch room. She tries to be polite to them, but she has never felt comfortable making "small talk." She is not quite sure what to say and often does not find any pleasure in discussing the topics that come up in that setting. She has gotten feedback from the office manager that she is not well liked by the staff.*

Listed below are some other complaints that I have heard from my clients about work-related problems. Check the box next to those that seem like they might apply to you.

Problems getting or keeping a satisfying job:

☐ "I can't seem to find a job."

☐ "I get so overwhelmed by the job search that I often avoid it altogether."

☐ "I want to look for a job, but I don't know where to begin."

☐ "I get so nervous on job interviews, and I never get called back."

☐ "I often go on interviews that I think went well, but then I never hear back from the employer. I don't know what is going wrong."

☐ "I can only find low-level jobs where I can't use my talents."

☐ "I always do well at a new job, but eventually things fall apart and I get fired."

☐ "I get bored really easily, and I have quit a lot of jobs in my life."

☐ "I've given up on trying to work—I have stopped searching for jobs, but I worry because I don't have enough money to live on."

Problems getting work done on the job:

☐ "I can't seem to get everything done."

☐ "I procrastinate."

☐ "I never seem to have enough time."

☐ "I make so many mistakes, over and over again."

☐ "I can't get any work done when I am constantly interrupted."

☐ "My desk is always a mess, and I can't find what I need."

☐ "I have to have my work materials arranged a certain way, or I get thrown off."

☐ "The schedule is too strenuous for me."

☐ "I can't concentrate because my workspace is too noisy."

☐ "I can't concentrate because the lighting bothers me."

☐ "I hate telephone work; I have trouble following what the other person is saying."

Problems with work relationships:

☐ "I am always getting criticized."

☐ "I am worried I am displeasing my supervisor."

☐ "I never get promoted, even though I deserve it."

☐ "I get upset when customers or clients ask questions that I can't answer."

☐ "I have a lot of arguments with the people I work with."

☐ "I have gotten into arguments with customers."

☐ "I can't seem to connect with my coworkers."

☐ "I have been told I am not a good team player."

☐ "I am always getting irritated with my coworkers or supervisors."

☐ "I have trouble sharing workspace because other people keep moving my stuff."

☐ "I am afraid to ask my supervisor questions; he/she always looks too busy."

☐ "My supervisor gets annoyed when I ask too many questions."

If you're struggling with one or more of these issues, be sure to read Chapter 8, where you will be given some strategies to try out to improve your occupational life.

Educational Life

If you're not currently a student, this section doesn't pertain to you, though you might have use for it in the future should you return to school. If you're a high school senior, a college student, a graduate student, or a trainee in a vocational preparation program, you'll want to read this section now. People with AS and HFA, by definition, are intelligent people. Some have intelligence measured in the superior range of functioning. If you are in this group, you're in an odd predicament: you and others may expect you to perform academically without difficulty, and yet the differences in the way your brain operates can cause you to struggle. The fact that you are reading this book indicates you are likely a bright person who *is* trying *very hard* to make things better. Still, like some of my patients, you might end up feeling misunderstood. Well-meaning supporters may say things like "But you're so smart—you should be able to handle this" or "You always got A's in high school; how come you're failing at college?" or "You're just not trying hard enough—just apply yourself and you can do it."

Blanca's home-related problems (sleep and organization) also affected her school life. Difficulty with gathering her things in the morning often made her late or unprepared for class. *Arnold,* the young man living in a dorm, was struggling with some of the interpersonal aspects of school life, such as making friends. Below are some other school problems reported by people on the spectrum. Check off those you can identify with.

Problems performing the work:

☐ "I can't seem to get everything done."

☐ "I always run out of time."

☐ "I start things at the last minute—I procrastinate too much."

☐ "I find myself worrying about my grades all the time."

☐ "The schedule is too strenuous for me."

☐ "I can't stand sitting in the classroom."

☐ "Sometimes I get so overwhelmed, but I have no clue where to get help."

☐ "I would rather fail than go get help at the center for students with disabilities."

- ☐ "I will stop going to class if I begin to struggle with a course."
- ☐ "I have too many 'withdrawals' or Fs on my transcript."
- ☐ "I get bored easily with the work."
- ☐ "I can't concentrate in the classroom if there is background noise."
- ☐ "I can't concentrate in the classroom if the lighting bothers me."
- ☐ "I can't seem to find a good space to study where I don't get distracted."
- ☐ "I can't study when I keep getting interrupted."

Problems with relationships at school:

- ☐ "I can't seem to get to know the other students."
- ☐ "Other students bother me."
- ☐ "I try to make friends, but other students are already in their own groups."
- ☐ "I always end up in conflict with my professors or instructors."
- ☐ "My professors or instructors get annoyed by the questions I ask in class."
- ☐ "Other students get annoyed by the things I say in class discussions."
- ☐ "I have been told I am too loud."
- ☐ "I am afraid the professor or instructor will think I am stupid if I go for extra help."
- ☐ "Other students taunt or tease me."
- ☐ "I am in classes/groups with other students who have obvious disabilities, and that makes me feel uncomfortable."

If any of these examples sounded remotely like problems you are having at school or in your vocational program, be sure to read Chapter 9, which will show you how to approach this part of your life in a new way.

Community Life

Earlier I discussed the importance of having a satisfying home life, but some people on the spectrum spend too much time at home, trying to avoid the stress of being outside the house. Many of my patients are very uncomfortable participating in community life but also frustrated because they would like to be involved in more activities. For them, home may come to feel more like a prison than a sanctuary.

Take *Jake*, whose life became restricted by his problems with trouble with driving. Another example of someone struggling with community life can be found in the story of Richard.

Richard is a 25-year-old college graduate with a degree in English literature. He lives with his mother and has been unemployed since he graduated from college 3 years ago. The most stressful time of day for him is the morning, after his mother leaves for work. He feels bored and lonely. He has been working with a state-funded vocational rehabilitation counselor toward finding a job and has become more hopeful about working. Outside of attending these sessions, he does not leave his house by himself. He is very anxious about talking to anyone he does not know. He would like to be able to run his own errands, such as to the bank or post office, join a gym, and use his local library, but he is afraid to address the personnel in any of those places. Simply thinking about doing any of these things by himself makes him highly anxious, because he has always relied on his mother to speak for him. Now, however, he is highly motivated to become more independent, because he does not enjoy sitting in the house all day while his mother works.

Below are additional comments made by people on the spectrum about community life. Check off any that you may have experienced.

Problems getting around and managing tasks:

- ☐ "I have had a lot of car accidents."
- ☐ "I am too nervous to drive."
- ☐ "I never seem to carry enough money with me."
- ☐ "I am bothered by the lighting in some stores."
- ☐ "I am afraid of elevators or escalators."
- ☐ "I always seem to be dropping everything [my money, shopping items]."
- ☐ "I lose things a lot [wallet, purse, keys]."
- ☐ "I can't seem to figure out the bus/train schedule."
- ☐ "I like to stick to routes that I know; otherwise I get lost."
- ☐ "I get lost a lot, even going to places I have been before."
- ☐ "I fumble when I try to buy my ticket using the automatic machine."
- ☐ "I am bothered by the lighting in my gym."
- ☐ "I love to swim, but I can't deal with the noisy community pool."
- ☐ "I get too impatient while sitting through long religious services."
- ☐ "There is too much background noise/echo in my church or temple."

Problems with people in the community:

- ☐ "I feel nervous when I have to go to any public place."
- ☐ "I get furious with other drivers."
- ☐ "Public transportation [train/bus] is too crowded for me."
- ☐ "I can't stand to have strangers bumping into me, even if by accident."
- ☐ "I have had arguments with conductors on the train."
- ☐ "I have had arguments with bus drivers."
- ☐ "I am afraid to ask for directions."

☐ "I have been told that my clothes are not right for the weather (I either wear too little for the cold or too much for the heat)."

☐ "I get thrown off if the bank teller asks me something I was not expecting."

☐ "I get upset if a clerk seems rude."

☐ "I don't like to ask for help when I can't find something at the library."

☐ "I am always afraid the cashier is giving me the wrong change."

☐ "I am afraid to ask for assistance or direction from store employees."

☐ "I practically panic if a salesperson approaches me when I am browsing."

☐ "I feel really uncomfortable talking to people at my church or temple."

☐ "I feel really uncomfortable talking to people at my fitness center or gym."

☐ "I get very nervous when I walk my dog and a stranger tries to talk to me."

☐ "I have problems getting along with my sports teammates [e.g., bowling, softball, basketball]."

☐ "I belong to a club related to my hobby, but I don't enjoy it when people talk about anything other than the hobby."

If you have any of these problems or similar ones, be sure to read Chapter 10. There you will find a collection of strategies to help you make the most of your community and to help you stop missing out on things you want to do.

Social Life: Friendships

One of the biggest problems that people on the spectrum face is dissatisfaction with the social aspects of life. Difficulty with social interactions is part of the definition of AS and HFA. Your social life involves your relationships with others. I've covered family members in the home life section; here we'll start with friendships.

Arnold, the young college student mentioned earlier, is having problems *making* friends. The story of Fred gives us an example of a person having difficulty *keeping* friends.

Fred is 31 and lives alone in a studio apartment. He works full time at a bank, processing loan applications. His most stressful time is on Friday nights, when he goes out with his best friend to a local sports bar. The two men have been friends since high school and have been meeting every Friday night at the same bar for years. Fred sticks with this friend because they both love sports. However, they get into an argument every week because his friend has different opinions, and it makes Fred very angry. There have been times when his friend has brought other friends along, but the others end up getting frustrated with Fred and don't come back. Fred has been told that he yells too much and is too aggressive when he states his opinions. Lately his own friend has been threatening to quit their Friday night get-togethers because of the way Fred acts.

Here are some additional problems many people on the spectrum report. If you think you have any of them too, check the box.

Problems making friends:

☐ "I can't seem to meet people who have my interests."

☐ "I don't know where I should be looking for friends."

☐ "I can't figure out which acquaintances could be good friends."

☐ "I am intimidated by online social networking sites that many people use."

☐ "I can't seem to make 'small talk'—I can't keep a conversation going."

☐ "I have been told I am aloof and people think I am rejecting them."

☐ "I don't know how to join in when it looks like everyone knows each other."

☐ "I have been told I talk too much."

☐ "I am too shy—I would never start talking to someone I don't know."

Problems keeping friends once you have them:

☐ "I have been told I don't keep in touch with friends enough."

☐ "I can't seem to make time to do things with my friends."

☐ "I don't like to talk on the phone."

☐ "I like to be with a friend one on one, but I don't like group gatherings."

☐ "I don't know what to do when a friend is mad at me or vice versa."

☐ "I don't like being pressured to do something I don't want to do."

☐ "I am too afraid to say no when a friend asks a favor."

☐ "Sometimes I think my friends are using me."

☐ "I have been told I am too bossy or that I dominate the conversation."

☐ "I have been told I act arrogant or like a 'know-it-all.' "

☐ "I have been told that I don't think of other people's feelings."

If any of these thoughts have crossed your mind, you should read Chapter 11, which is full of exercises and strategies to help you reach your goals with regard to the quantity and quality of your friendships.

Social Life: Dating, Sex, and Marriage

Out of all the issues my patients are concerned about, this area of social life probably brings the most pain when it is not going well. Of course some people choose to stay single and/or celibate and are content with that. But you may want a romantic life that is more satisfying than the one you have. Maybe you have difficulty meeting people to date, knowing how to ask for a date, getting along with a partner, dealing with sexuality, or coping with the pressures of marriage or a committed relationship.

Remember *Noel*? He was struggling with dating. The story of Carla shows us how someone on the spectrum who is already married can still have some difficulty with romantic partners.

> *Carla, 34, works full time as a veterinary technician at an animal hospital. Her most difficult time of day is late night when it is time to go to bed. Her husband is very affectionate and likes to hold her and hug her, whether they have sex or not. Carla does enjoy sexual activity, but she finds it unpleasant to be held tight for long periods. Her husband gets annoyed with her when she rejects his hugs, and lately they have had more and more arguments about this. She finds herself wanting to avoid bedtime and sometimes stays up late, waiting for him to fall asleep before she goes to bed.*

Listed below are some other common problems reported by people on the spectrum. If any sound familiar to you, check them off.

Dating:

☐ "I don't know where to meet people to date."

☐ "I don't know when or how to approach someone I want to ask for a date."

☐ "I don't like to go to crowded places, like parties or bars."

☐ "I can't seem to make 'small talk'—I can't keep a conversation going."

☐ "I don't understand different gender roles or customs that apply on a date [e.g., how the woman should act, how the man should act, who should pick up the tab on a date]."

☐ "I want to meet someone to marry, but I have never had a girlfriend/boyfriend in my life—I don't know where to begin."

☐ "I have joined several online dating services over the past few years, and I never got a date."

☐ "I have had several relationships on the Internet, but they have all been with people who live far away, and we never seem to get to meet."

☐ "I have had several relationships on the Internet, but things always seem to fall apart after we meet in person."

Sex:

☐ "I feel very uncertain about how to handle sex."

☐ "I am embarrassed about being a virgin at my age."

☐ "I am very uncomfortable with my own sexuality."

☐ "I don't enjoy sexual activity."

☐ "I do not like to be touched."

☐ "I have had some unpleasant sexual experiences in the past, and I am afraid to be sexual again."

☐ "I doubt I can trust another person enough to become intimate."

☐ "I am afraid another person will not understand or accept what arouses me [e.g., specific types of touch or particular fantasies I might have]."

Committed relationships/marriage:

☐ "I don't know what to do when there is a disagreement with my partner."

☐ "My partner is unhappy with the amount of time I spend with him/her."

☐ "My behavior sometimes embarrasses my partner at parties."

☐ "I get so upset when my partner is upset, but I freeze and don't know what to do."

☐ "My partner tells me I am insensitive."

☐ "My partner embarrasses me when he/she corrects me in front of other people."

☐ "My partner gets annoyed at me for not doing more chores around the house."

☐ "My partner blames all of our problems on my ASD, and it makes me feel guilty."

If you are having any problems in the area of dating, sex, or committed partnership, be sure to read Chapter 12, where you will find positive strategies to improve the areas of your romantic life with which you are dissatisfied.

Health

Many of my patients have reported high levels of stress over their own healthcare—maintaining healthy self-care practices or trying to access treatment from professional healthcare providers.

Earlier you met **Meredith,** who was struggling with managing her diabetes. Dan feels overwhelmed by another health-related problem.

***Dan** lives by himself, is 51, and works for an information technology department in a hospital. The most stressful points of the day for him are mealtimes. Dan is very overweight and was recently told by his doctor that he needs to lose at least 60 pounds to become healthy. He has a girlfriend whom he has been with for about 3 years, and she also makes occasional comments about his need to lose weight. There is a history of heart disease in Dan's family, and he began worrying more about this vulnerability since he turned 50 last year. He knows he has poor eating habits but is overwhelmed by the idea of changing his routine. He is not even sure what his first step should be toward organizing a weight-loss plan. Meanwhile, he continues to eat the same things, feeling guilty throughout each meal.*

More comments from people on the spectrum regarding the stress caused by health concerns follow. Mark with a check those that seem familiar to you.

Personal care:

☐ "I have a chronic medical condition, and I feel overwhelmed by it."

☐ "I am afraid I will never be able to take care of my health on my own—I need help from my parents for everything."

☐ "I forget to take my medicine on some days."

☐ "I always forget to renew my prescriptions until it is too late."

☐ "My shower routine takes so long that I prefer to skip it."

☐ "I will wear dirty clothes because I can't get to the laundry."

☐ "I don't remember to brush my teeth every day."

☐ "I am overweight, and I can't seem to follow a diet."

☐ "I am a picky eater, and my diet is not balanced; I have been told I am underweight."

☐ "I hate to shave but don't like a beard either."

☐ "I sleep at odd hours, sleep too little, or sleep too much."

☐ "I get so focused on my diet or exercise routine that I have been told I am overdoing it or that I am 'obsessed' with it."

☐ "I find it hard to tolerate medication side effects, so I don't always comply with prescription instructions."

☐ "I can't find the time to exercise regularly."

Accessing healthcare services:

☐ "I don't trust doctors, so I hate going on appointments."

☐ "I can't keep track of all of my appointments."

☐ "Doctors talk too fast, and I can't follow what they say."

☐ "I constantly worry that something is wrong with me, but I am afraid to be examined by a doctor."

☐ "I am afraid to go to the dentist."

☐ "I get nervous when I have to talk to receptionists to schedule appointments."

☐ "I am afraid to ask questions when I don't understand what my doctor says."

☐ "I get confused when the pharmacy staff asks me about my insurance."

☐ "I become very angry if the office staff talks to me in a rude way."

☐ "I have difficulty describing my symptoms to a doctor during a visit."

☐ "I have been told I have a high pain threshold or I don't feel pain until a condition gets out of control [e.g., infected tooth], so I don't get help when I should."

☐ "I have been told I have a low pain threshold or I feel pain almost all the time, even when the doctors can't find anything wrong."

☐ "I never know whether to go to the doctor when I don't feel well because I have been told my pain is 'psychosomatic' or that I am a hypochondriac."

If you're having some difficulty with some aspect of caring for your health, read Chapter 13, which covers the strategies you can use to improve your self-care and/or work more effectively with professional healthcare providers.

■   ■   ■

In sum, you are probably under tremendous pressure to get along in a world that is populated and designed largely by people who do not operate the same way you do. This book will help you better understand the specific reasons you are struggling with certain activities and situations. Now that you've identified the areas where you have the most pressing problems, the next step is to focus on your strengths.

Human Strengths and the Autism Spectrum

When I started putting together my ideas for this book, it seemed only natural to base it on the psychology of human strengths. For years I have been listening to my patients tell me their stories of survival. Over and over again I have heard about incredibly creative strategies my patients have come up with, on their own, to help themselves endure extremely painful situations in their lives. One man, who was not diagnosed with Asperger syndrome until he was in his early 40s, had learned as a young man that he could comfort himself by listening to folk music. The lyrics of some songs, he found, validated his experience of loneliness and isolation and helped him feel more connected to other people, even though he had trouble relating to them in real-life situations. He eventually became a very knowledgeable fan of this music genre, and attending music festivals was a continual source of great enjoyment for him. After his diagnosis and entry into therapy with me, his capacity to use music for pleasure, self-soothing, and connection to others became an important foundation for our work. Through this experience and many others like it, I came to understand that "Nurturing what is strong must be part of therapy, not just healing what is weak." Those are the words of positive psychology scholars Martin Seligman and Christopher Peterson, and they encapsulate my approach to helping adults with AS and HFA improve their lives.

What Positive Psychology Tells Us about Happiness and Resilience

As I said in the Introduction, this whole book is based on the principles of *positive psychology*. But what is positive psychology? Once when I was introducing this concept to a patient of mine, he asked sarcastically, "What is that, only thinking about smiley faces, rainbows, and puppies?" Contrary to what you may think, this approach is not as simple as encouraging people to "think happy thoughts." Rather, it is a movement in the science of psychology away from the tradition of studying disease and distress and toward the study of human health and well-being. Instead of studying only things that go wrong with the way humans function, positive psychology looks at what goes right. Scholars are interested in what traits tend to be associated with happiness (or subjective sense of well-being) in humans, and that does not mean looking at people whose lives are free of adversity. It does involve looking at what characteristics help a person be *resilient* in the face of adversity. At its very core, positive psychology seeks to identify and understand human *strengths*.

The amount of material that has already been written on the topic is too much to cover here because this book is meant to be a practical guide, not a theoretical text. (See the Resources at the end of this book for a list of further readings on positive psychology.) But there are some key ideas that come from scholars in that field that guide the solutions I offer to you in the chapters ahead.

Human First

If you were to look in the index of a positive psychology textbook, you would find nothing about AS or autism. However, if you think about the phrase *the psychology of human strengths*, you can see that you really are included in this movement. After all, you are human. Also, you possess strengths, or you would not have survived up to this point. Granted, I have had people with AS and HFA tell me that they feel as though they function so differently from others that they might as well be considered a separate species. It is true that brains of people on the spectrum function in unique ways that often make them stand out from neurotypical people, and I will be giving you many examples of that in this book. But we in the autism community, professionals and affected people alike, can sometimes get so caught up in defining these differences that we lose sight of the fact that every person on the spectrum is bound to every neurotypical person by one thing, and that is a common membership in the same species. Your unique brain is still a human brain. For that reason, the science of positive psychology and human strengths has everything to do with you. After all, you are classified as a human first. Being a person on the spectrum comes after that, though it is just as important as the other factors that shape the individual human you are, such as your personality, gender, religion, and culture.

The scientific study of human strengths has shown that there are a number of characteristics that can buffer the effects of adversity and serve to prevent mental and physical health problems. Some of the key traits that have been named repeatedly by positive psychology scientists are:

- courage
- rationality
- insight
- optimism
- authenticity
- perseverance

- realism
- capacity for pleasure
- future-mindedness
- personal responsibility
- purpose
- interpersonal skill

In Chapters 2–5, I will cover this in more detail, but the features of AS and HFA can give a person the propensity to possess some of the characteristics on this list. Yet, when I work with my patients, I find that they may not see these strengths in themselves. By the time they reach my office, they have been repeatedly reminded that they are different, often cast in the role of a "patient" and defined as "suffering from a disorder." After years of being seen that way by others and themselves, it is not surprising that their perspective is more focused on differences as "defects" but not as strengths.

As an exercise, look at Worksheet 3. Take a moment to check off the characteristics on this list that you think you possess. Remember, nobody has all of them. As another exercise, give Worksheet 4 to someone who knows you well. Without revealing your answers, have that person check off the traits you have. Did any of the answers surprise you? Remember, no human being has all of these strengths. Even if you have just one trait on this list, it can be used as a foundation for your plan to improve your life satisfaction. Finding positive solutions to problems often involves tapping into a strength you already have, which may not have been obvious to you before.

Positive Solutions

In this book you will be shown how to approach your difficulties using the basic strategies of *problem solving* and *coping*. For each problem area you identify, you will be guided to:

1. define your goal
2. identify the obstacles or reasons you are being blocked from achieving your goal
3. choose positive solutions to address the obstacles and tailor them to your individual life

WORKSHEET 3

What Are Your Personal Strengths?

Look at this list of strengths that positive psychologists have found to be part of resiliency. Check off (✓) the ones you think you have. Don't think too hard about it. Go with your first impression.

☐ Courage   ☐ Realism

☐ Rationality   ☐ Capacity for pleasure

☐ Insight   ☐ Future-mindedness

☐ Optimism   ☐ Personal responsibility

☐ Authenticity   ☐ Purpose

☐ Perseverance   ☐ Interpersonal skill

From *Living Well on the Spectrum* by Valerie L. Gaus. Copyright 2011 by The Guilford Press.

WORKSHEET 4

Personal Strengths— Family and Friends Version

Your friend or loved one has asked you to fill out this sheet about him/her. Look at this list of strengths that positive psychologists have found to be part of resilience. Check off (✓) the ones you think your friend or loved one has. Don't think too hard about it. Go with your first impression.

☐ Courage   ☐ Realism

☐ Rationality   ☐ Capacity for pleasure

☐ Insight   ☐ Future-mindedness

☐ Optimism   ☐ Personal responsibility

☐ Authenticity   ☐ Purpose

☐ Perseverance   ☐ Interpersonal skill

From *Living Well on the Spectrum* by Valerie L. Gaus. Copyright 2011 by The Guilford Press.

The positive solutions offered by this book are coping strategies that have been shown to be effective in improving the quality of life for all kinds of people and can be tailored to meet your individual needs. *Coping strategies* are the "tricks" or "tools" that people use to adapt successfully to new situations or demands. Like most people, whether on the spectrum or not, you have a natural "bag of tricks" that you can draw from when faced with demands; those tricks come from your *strengths* and can make you more resilient in the face of change or adversity. As with any skill, people vary greatly in terms of the quantity and quality of strengths they have access to in any given situation. Chapters 2–5 will help you become more aware of how your AS/HFA has affected your bag of tricks for better and for worse, so you will finish Part I with a clear sense of which problem areas to focus on. The chapters in Part II will teach you the coping strategies you will need to address the specific problems you are having. These techniques will be explained in detail in Chapter 6. For now, here is a brief introduction.

Problem-Solving Techniques

Problem-solving techniques allow you to take a rational, step-by-step approach to a problem that might otherwise be overwhelming or upsetting. As you know, when you are very upset, it is hard to be objective and your judgment can be clouded. If you follow the basic formula of problem solving that will be presented in every chapter, you will be able to think more clearly and use your strengths to come up with solutions that make sense. The eight-step approach that will be used throughout this book is:

1. Identify and define your problem.
2. Define your goal.
3. Identify the obstacles in the way of your achieving the goal.
4. List several possible solutions to address the obstacle(s).
5. Consider the consequences of each solution.
6. Choose the best one(s) to try out first.
7. Implement the solution and track your progress.
8. Evaluate the solution to see if it met the goal you defined in Step 2.

This problem-solving model will be used to help you choose which of the following eight strategies are most appropriate for meeting your goal as you use problem solving in Part II.

Environmental Modifications

Sometimes a simple change in your personal space can go a long way toward solving a problem—moving furniture, removing an irritant, or changing a lighting source, for example.

Organizational Techniques

When a single environmental change is not enough, a whole system in your environment can be set up or redesigned to make it more user-friendly for you—organizing a backpack, desk top, kitchen drawer, or closet.

Scheduling Techniques

Most people rely on a schedule of some sort to guide them through the day, week, month, and year. If scheduling does not come naturally to you, there are many strategies and tools that you can use to make this part of your life run more smoothly.

Relaxation Techniques

Your body can become very tense and stay that way for prolonged periods due to extended emotional arousal, which is not good for your health. This book will encourage you to use relaxation tricks you already know and also introduce you to new ideas for how to relax the body and the mind.

Emotion Identification Techniques

Coping effectively with stressful situations often involves changing something to help yourself become more comfortable and functional and/or communicating your needs to another person. Knowing how you feel gives you a clue about what you need; for example, you might recognize that you need a break from your work only if you first recognize that you are feeling very nervous and pressured.

Thinking Techniques

Everyone has an "internal voice" that narrates everything that is happening, and sometimes that voice can say things that are negative and discouraging. Becoming more aware of negative "self-talk" allows you to challenge the irrational statements.

Understanding Other People

People on the spectrum often report that they can't understand other people or their behavior. That's because people on the spectrum have difficulty with *social cognition*, the ability to make good guesses about others' thoughts, feelings, intentions, and/or motives. Fortunately, you can learn techniques that will better enable you to make good guesses about other people, their intentions, and their needs.

Communication Techniques

Communication is a very complicated human behavior, but there are techniques for ensuring that you get your messages heard by others while also ensuring that you hear their messages.

■   ■   ■

I hope this chapter has gotten you to think about the areas of your life that are causing you the most stress. I also hope you have begun to think about your goals as well as your strengths. The next several chapters will describe how your brain may work differently because of AS or HFA. They will also illustrate how these differences can lead to both strengths and vulnerabilities.

2

A Unique Brain

How Thinking Differences Can Affect Your Daily Life

You now have a good idea of why your life feels stressful: being on the spectrum can cause difficulties that interfere with home life and school life, friendship and romance, work and play, even health. But *why* does being on the spectrum have such far-ranging effects?

To answer that question, this chapter and the next three will explain in depth the differences that come with an ASD. The fact that challenges seem to greet you everywhere can leave you feeling helpless. Ongoing stress naturally makes you focus on the negatives in your life. But if you are to shift to a problem-solving approach to improving your life satisfaction, you need to look at all sides of a problem. That is, you need to become *objective*. Acquiring knowledge of how your unique brain works is a major step toward objectivity. So we'll be looking at how the characteristics of ASDs can not only make you vulnerable but also bring *strengths* you can build on while implementing your problem-solving strategies.

Differences as Vulnerabilities, Differences as Strengths

The differences that come with ASDs are often responsible for the stress you feel. This is why it's so important to know exactly how these differences operate—so you can do whatever is possible to reduce the drain on your energy they can cause. It is, however, just as important not to overstate these differences. Focusing only on how you differ from neurotypical people is what leads to the feeling of being a member of another species expressed by some people on the spectrum, as mentioned in Chapter 1. Remember that you have many human characteristics in common with neurotypical people. For one thing, neurotypicals do not live completely without stress, and life for people on the spectrum is more than unremitting stress. I'll remind you where common ground exists between you and neurotypical people throughout the next few chapters. Also keep in mind that no two people are alike and no one person with an ASD has all of the characteristics that I will discuss in these chapters. Your goal should be to learn more about the differences that can interfere with happiness for people on the spectrum so that you can understand how these differences affect you specifically.

The four major categories of differences are:

- thinking differences
- social differences
- emotional differences
- sensory and movement differences

These differences can make you more vulnerable to the demands of daily life by hindering your "stress immune system." The two main reasons this happens are:

1. ASDs cause you to experience the world in unique ways and may lead you to encounter **stressful events more often** in your daily life than typical people.

2. ASDs can lead you to have **fewer coping strategies** available. You may feel uncertain about how to handle many types of problems and demands your life imposes on you. With fewer *buffers*, you may end up having longer-lasting distress than typical people. For example, it may not be obvious to you how to cope with an overbearing boss or a noisy home environment, leaving you in distress for prolonged periods without any opportunity to recuperate.

The remainder of this chapter will focus on thinking differences, while social, emotional, and sensory differences will be covered in the three chapters that follow this one. Each of these chapters will illustrate how these differences expose you to more troublesome events throughout the day *and* leave you with fewer coping strategies available when you need them.

Notes

✓ People with ASDs have unique brains that operate differently from those of neurotypical people.

✓ The ASD brain is associated with:

1. thinking differences
2. social differences
3. emotional differences
4. sensory and movement differences

✓ ASD differences are vulnerabilities and strengths at the same time.

Thinking Differences

What is really going on when you are "thinking"? Scientists refer to it as *cognitive activity*, which is a complex set of operations that your brain is performing continuously, even when you're asleep. Simply put, your brain is constantly processing information so that you can make sense of your world and respond in adaptive ways. Here, *adaptive* means you can get what you need from your world with minimal distress or discomfort. It means you are responding in a way that ends up productive. People on the spectrum think, or process information, in unique ways that make it harder for them to adapt comfortably to the things that happen in their lives as compared to neurotypical people. To understand this better, we'll start by considering how the human brain works in general. *Cognitive scientists* are the people who study human information processing, and the ideas outlined in this section are based on many years of their work.

Human Information Processing

Look at the diagram called "Human Information Processing" on the next page. It is a very simplified illustration of what each person's brain ought to be doing from moment to moment. When things are working smoothly, your brain should take the information that it receives from your senses and turn it into something meaningful to you. The box on the left side of the diagram, called "Input," represents what happens first. Your brain cannot possibly process every single thing that is going on in your environment at any given moment, so the brain's first task is to help you filter out, or ignore, the bits of information in the environment that are not important or relevant. This operation is part of what scientist call *perception*.

Once the brain lets in the information that it deems relevant, it starts to process it by carrying out several operations. These are illustrated in the second box on the diagram, called "Processing." The brain analyzes or interprets the information by comparing it to information that is already stored in memory from past events. Then the information is sorted and categorized to help the brain label it appropriately. Next the brain decides whether the information needs to be stored for future use and, if so, puts it away in the correct brain storage area. The brain then takes all of the information it analyzed and interpreted and tries to predict what might happen next in the environment. Based on those predictions, the brain decides what action would be best to carry out and then makes a plan. The plan is sent to the brain areas responsible for different types of behaviors, such as speech and movement. The real-life actions that are ultimately carried out are represented by the "Output" box on the diagram. For humans, the output generally takes the form of a verbal or physical behavior.

Let's look at a relatively simple piece of information to see what all the thinking steps look like.

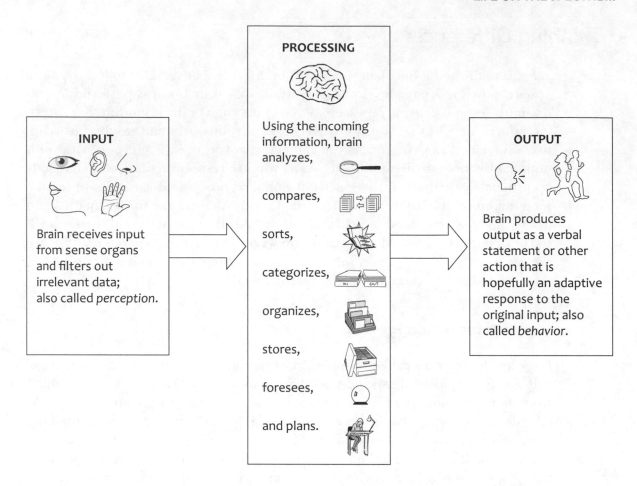

Human information processing.

Input

Picture yourself walking through your house or apartment on your way to the kitchen. On the floor in the middle of the hallway you see your keys. This visual information is input that comes through your eyes. Because the hall floor is usually clear, the novel sight of an object there makes the brain choose the keys as important information. Even though the wallpaper, moldings, floorboards, or carpet may be within your field of vision, your brain chooses not to focus on them, allowing only the visual input about the keys into the processing area of the brain.

Processing

As your brain begins to analyze the picture of the keys, it compares the picture to other pictures stored in memory. The brain concludes that the object belongs in the "key" category already on file, that it fits into a subcategory of "familiar keys," and even more specifically, that it looks identical to the picture on file called "my keys." Then the brain looks at the files in memory regarding where the keys are normally kept in the house and recognizes that the keys are not where they belong, which is on a hook by the door. The brain also tries to draw some conclusions about why the keys are on the floor instead, especially because there is no memory on file about putting the keys there. Hence the brain makes a guess that you dropped them by accident. Finally, the brain looks ahead in time and imagines a scenario in which you might want those keys. The brain might imagine your having to search for the keys and then feeling frustrated by the fact that they are not where the brain expected them to be. Because of this prediction, the brain makes a plan to pick the keys up and put them on the hook.

Output

You carry out the physical act of picking up the keys and putting them on the hook by the door.

This is such a simple action—putting your keys back on the hook where they belong after finding them on the floor—that it may be hard to imagine anything going wrong. *But what if your brain* ... did not filter out irrelevant information and you did not even notice the keys on the floor? ... did not identify the object on the floor as your set of keys? ... did not think ahead about the consequences of not having the keys by the door? ... did not make the plan to put the keys back by the door? ... did not keep your attention on the plan long enough to have you carry out the action of putting the keys back in their place?

Any person's brain could fail to carry out any of these operations at any given time for a variety of reasons. But research has shown that people on the spectrum are more prone to have difficulty with some of these operations than neurotypical people. Let's take a closer look at how these thinking problems interfere.

> ## Notes
>
> ✓ The human brain is processing information all the time—this is called <u>cognitive activity</u>.
>
> ✓ New information goes through three stages:
>
> > 1. Input   🗝
> > 2. Processing
> > 3. Output
>
> ✓ When all the stages run smoothly, the <u>output</u> is some action that helps a person adapt successfully to a situation—sometimes called <u>adaptive behavior</u>.

Thinking Differences as Vulnerabilities

The best way to understand the thinking differences involved in creating problems experienced by people on the spectrum is to break them down into two categories: (1) problems with the *management* of information and (2) problems with the *interpretation* of information.

Problems with Management of Information

In the story about the keys, I isolated one experience to illustrate how the brain processes information. However, throughout the course of your day, nothing really takes place in isolation. Your brain has to process many pieces of information at once, and in real life you don't have the luxury of having only one thing on your mind at a time. If you really did find your keys on the hall floor, your brain would be dealing with that new information in addition to all the other things that had happened to you that day, including whatever you were thinking about just before you found your keys on the floor. Managing all the information in a coordinated fashion is a very complex job that your brain has to do for you to function at your best. This coordinated management is often referred to as the *executive functioning* of the brain.

Imagine that your brain is an airport. The individual airplanes are the pieces of information flying all over your brain, but the air traffic control tower is the center that is responsible for keeping track of everything. The control center not only knows about every bit of information (each airplane), but also knows how each piece of information relates to or impacts every other piece, and decisions about what should go where when are made based on that coordinated "big picture." In your brain, this control center is responsible for all of the *executive functions*. For our purposes, it's not important to know which sections of the brain actually function as the control center, but you can read more about brain structure and executive functions if you like by using the Resources at the back of this book.

Notes

✓ When your brain works to manage and coordinate multiple pieces of information, it is carrying out operations that are called <u>executive functions</u>.

✓ People with ASDs are known to have problems with some of the executive functions of the brain.

✓ Executive function problems are <u>not</u> a sign of low intelligence; one can be highly intelligent but have executive function problems.

✓ Executive function problems can make the completion of certain types of tasks more difficult.

People with AS or HFA are usually bright, with a high level of intelligence and specific talents or abilities that are superior compared to the average neurotypical person. If you continue to imagine the brain as an airport, people on the spectrum have airports with incredibly sophisticated airplanes flying around them—aircraft with unique and advanced technology. However, their air traffic control centers are not equipped to manage the planes. The consequence, at best, is that these beautiful airplanes don't get to take off when they want to and don't get to land when they need to; at the very worst, it's that they endure crippling collisions and crashes.

Take a moment to fill out Worksheet 5 on the facing page. All the statements on the list are complaints of people on the spectrum who were having problems with information management or *executive functions*.

Thinking Differences
Information Management

Check off (✓) the statements that sound familiar to you or reflect experiences you frequently have in your day-to-day life.

☐ I can't seem to focus on more than one thing at a time.

☐ I get distracted easily.

☐ I have trouble completing tasks.

☐ I often enter a room without being able to remember why I went there.

☐ I can't get back on track after someone interrupts me.

☐ I have trouble keeping my belongings organized.

☐ I procrastinate.

☐ I lose things a lot.

☐ I can do only one thing at a time; I can't "multitask."

☐ I know what I want to do, but I never seem to get around to it.

☐ I get thrown off by unexpected changes in my routine.

☐ I have trouble setting goals.

☐ I have goals but I can't seem to get them done.

☐ I have trouble figuring out how to do new things.

☐ I hate change, because it takes me so long to learn new routines.

No one person has all of these problems, but if you checked off two or more, you may have some of the problems in executive function that will be described next. Scientists who study human information processing have found that people with AS and HFA have problems with these executive functions:

- Attention regulation
- Organization
- Goal setting and planning
- Working memory

In the next few sections you will find examples of these problems and see how they can affect your everyday life.

Attention Regulation

Being able to focus your attention on the right thing at the right time is a crucial thinking operation. The ability to *shift* attention in a flexible way is an important part of that skill. In the key scenario, being able to focus your attention on the keys, temporarily shift your attention away from other things, and sustain your attention on the keys long enough to place them by the door would all be necessary to adapt optimally to finding the keys unexpectedly on the floor. The difficulty that people on the spectrum tend to have with attention can show up in several different ways:

Blanca, the graduate student introduced in Chapter 1, cannot study at home because she gets distracted by all the family activity around her. When she tries to read in her room, for instance, she keeps thinking about the things her brother might be doing elsewhere in the house and ends up wandering out of her room. This is an example of a common *difficulty with staying focused on one thing long enough to address it appropriately–that is, being easily distracted.*

Jake, the young man who is afraid to drive, gets anxious behind the wheel partly because he always feels like he is concentrating on the wrong things. If he watches the other cars, he misses important signs and makes wrong turns; when he concentrates on signs, he fails to notice what other drivers are doing. This is an example of another common problem, which is *difficulty choosing the most relevant thing to focus on in a given situation.*

Henry, unemployed, feels particularly stressed out in the afternoon because he realizes another day has gone by without his getting much done. One reason he doesn't get much done is that he tends to "get lost" in activities for hours. When he goes onto his computer in the morning to check e-mails and job postings, he sometimes ends up visiting websites related to his hobby, always with the intention of looking up something quickly. But the next thing he knows, 90 minutes have passed without his awareness. This is an example of *difficulty with shifting attention from one thing to another thing where appropriate–that is, staying focused on one thing too intensely and/or for too long.*

Because problems with attention are so common among those on the spectrum, some of my patients have been misdiagnosed with attention deficit disorder at some point in life. The term *deficit* is a misnomer because people on the spectrum don't suffer from a lack of attention but from a disability in *controlling* or *regulating* attention. Think about how a gas stove works. Once a flame is ignited on a burner on most stoves, the intensity of the flame is controlled, or regulated, by a knob that turns like a dial. You can adjust the amount of heat that comes from the burner by turning the knob one way to raise it and the other way to lower it. You have a lot of flexibility in where you set the heat—from superhot to boil water, to very low to warm leftovers, to anywhere in between to cook different foods without burning them. You can also change the heat setting very quickly if you need to, for example, if a pot starts to boil over. Then you can instantly lower the heat without turning the burner all the way off. But what if all your stove had was an on/off switch? The burner would be either off or on full blast. You'd lose the flexibility to cook a variety of foods without burning everything except water that you were boiling for tea.

When it comes to attention, you might think of yourself as having only an on/off switch where neurotypical people have a dial. You have no problems paying attention—your "flame" goes on without a hitch—but your ability to regulate your attention effectively is impaired. As a result you can have problems adapting to whatever is going on in your surroundings.

Organization

Being able to sort information and recognize which category or location it belongs in is crucial for optimal functioning. This ability is involved in designing, setting up, and maintaining the spaces we all use from day to day. To deal effectively with finding keys on the floor, you would have to be able to recognize whom the keys belonged to (you) and that the keys were not in their proper place. Preceding that was your ability to have chosen a proper storage place for the keys (by the door). Being on the spectrum creates difficulty with these thinking operations. You may not be able to easily set up systems that work for you in various environments. Or you may be able to set up an organized-looking space but then have difficulty maintaining it over time. The types of spaces that we all need to organize range from very small, like a wallet or purse, to very large, like a basement, so this thinking difference can have far-ranging ramifications.

Blanca has difficulty getting herself organized in the morning, as mentioned in Chapter 1. One of the reasons for this is that she is unsure about how to set up her bedroom so that things are easy to find. She

---

Notes

✔ Some people with ASDs can have problems with "attention regulation."

✔ You may have difficulty shifting your focus from one thing to another in a smooth fashion.

✔ You may focus very intensely on one thing and not enough on something else.

✔ Where neurotypical brains are equipped with a dial knob to regulate attention, you may have been furnished with an on/off switch to regulate your attention.

Notes

✔ Some people with ASDs can have difficulty with organizing information, which involves sorting and categorizing.

✔ This can result in problems with setting up and/or maintaining organized spaces.

✔ Spaces that can be disorganized include wallets, purses, book bags, a car, a desk, or any room in the home.

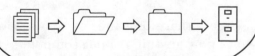

does not know what should be placed where, including which things should go in her book bag.

Goal Setting and Planning

To achieve success in life, people must be able to think about things that have not yet happened, which is often referred to as *foresight*. With this ability, people must be able to identify specific things they want to achieve at a future time (goals), then figure out a set of steps they have to carry out to accomplish the goals (plan). Back to those keys in the hallway: you would need to use foresight to imagine the next time you would want to have those keys. You would need to have a goal—to have your keys next to the door when you leave your house at a future time—and then design a plan for taking the steps necessary to achieve that goal. Despite the simplicity of this particular problem, some people on the spectrum may struggle with it and certainly will have difficulty with more complex life issues. This is because ASDs make people prone to difficulty with foresight, which affects their ability to set goals and/or to design plans that will get them to their goals.

> ## Notes
>
> ✔ **People with ASDs may have difficulty with planning.**
>
> ✔ **This may be due to one or more of the following processing problems:**
>
> 1. **Problems imagining what has not yet happened (foresight)**
> 2. **Problems choosing or clearly defining a goal**
> 3. **Problems formulating and sequencing the smaller steps necessary to achieve the goal**

Dan is the man you met in Chapter 1 who is concerned about being overweight. He does have the foresight to imagine that he could develop heart disease or other health problems in the future. He also believes he should lose weight, which represents the beginning of a goal. He is stuck, however, because he does not know how to turn that belief into a concrete goal and certainly does not know how to go about mapping out a set of steps that he could carry out toward that goal. Even neurotypical people not struggling with lack of foresight will tell you how hard it is to start a diet. Dan's thinking difference makes the task even more challenging than it might be for a neurotypical person.

Working Memory

Every person's brain has a "temporary" memory that stores information just long enough for a task to be carried out. If you know anything about computers, the RAM of a computer operates the same way as the working memory of a human brain. Information stored there is not usually put into permanent storage but has to stay there as long as needed. Using the key example again, you would have to be able to keep those keys in your "online" memory long enough to bring the situation to closure. If you forgot about the keys before you even picked them up or forgot where you were going after you picked them up, the keys never would have been put back. Of course once you do put the keys back on the hook by the door, you may very well forget about the whole event by the end of the day with no adverse consequences.

People on the spectrum seem to have less storage space for temporary information than typical people. Interestingly, many people with ASDs seem to have superior ability to remember large quantities of information across long periods of time. Using the computer analogy again, it is as if you have a huge amount of hard drive space but a very small amount of RAM. The way this plays out in everyday life is that you may appear to be able to keep only one piece of information at a time in temporary storage, whereas typical people may be able to store multiple pieces of information in their working memory.

Do you usually prefer to tackle only one task at a time? This is a function of working-memory differences. Working on more than one task at a time requires you to hold and manipulate several pieces of information simultaneously, so many people on the spectrum have a lot of trouble multitasking. In a simple example, if you were talking on the phone while cooking, you would have to keep information "online" about the topic you were discussing while also keeping track of a recipe, ingredients, equipment, and oven temperature. If you have problems with working memory, you could lose track of the conversation if you focused on the food or lose track of your cooking if you focused on the phone conversation.

Meredith, the woman with diabetes and a law degree, has always struggled because she can manage only one task at a time, and the steps of self-care she must carry out daily for her diabetes are incompatible with the busy life she would surely have if she pursued a career in law.

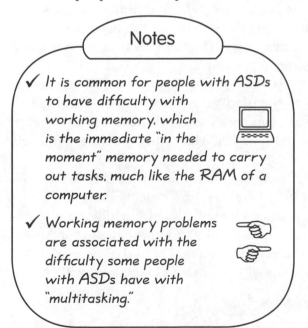

Notes

✔ It is common for people with ASDs to have difficulty with working memory, which is the immediate "in the moment" memory needed to carry out tasks, much like the RAM of a computer.

✔ Working memory problems are associated with the difficulty some people with ASDs have with "multitasking."

Problems with Interpretation of Information

If information management operations are complex, then information interpretation functions are doubly complicated—and less understood by cognitive scientists. One of the things that separates us humans from other species is that we can take bits of information and attach *meaning* to them. Coming up with a theory that your keys ended up on the floor because you must have dropped them by accident is an example of interpreting the information received in the here and now.

Cognitive scientists have found that human beings normally try to understand events in their world. When something new occurs, the human brain tries to figure out what it *means*. The brain tends to ask *why* it happened and then tries to answer by explaining what *caused* it to happen; another word for this process is *attribution*. The brain will also draw some type of *conclusion* from it that involves an expectation about what might happen next. If you refer back to the "Human Information Processing" diagram (page 42), the term *analyzes* in the middle box includes all the operations mentioned here. When things are working smoothly, a good analysis or interpretation of an event is going to lead a person to adaptive output. Remember, that means the person either says or does something that is productive.

To operate efficiently, the brain uses a lot of *shortcuts* while interpreting new information. The brain may go ahead and draw a conclusion about something without examining every single piece of information available. For example, if you encounter a small two-legged creature that has feathers and wings, your brain will quickly conclude that it is a bird even if the bird is a color and shape you never saw before. The brain took just a few pieces of information (number of legs, presence of wings and feathers), skipped past unfamiliar information (color and shape), and labeled the creature; via this shortcut you could recognize what it was without inspecting it closely or looking it up in a book. If you came to the conclusion "I must have dropped my keys by accident," you did so without having actual proof—you did not need to see yourself on camera dropping the keys on the floor to be comfortable believing they ended up there that way.

Shortcuts are necessary to function successfully because we don't have enough time to examine every detail of every situation we encounter. The downside to using shortcuts, however, is that it can sometimes lead to errors. Have you ever made an assumption that turned out to be wrong? Have you ever caught yourself jumping to a conclusion too quickly?

Human beings show individual differences in how they use shortcuts. Patterns of preference or tendencies to use (or fail to use) certain shortcuts are called *biases*. The biases that people have are determined by many things, including personality, past experiences, family background, and culture. You have biases formed in these ways like anyone else. But cognitive scientists have found that people on the spectrum are also prone to certain kinds of biases that come along with AS or HFA, such as:

- a tendency to look at details more than the whole
- a tendency to see things in an all-or-nothing fashion; things are black or white, all good or all bad, and there is very little attention to dimensions or "shades of gray"

These tendencies are a great example of differences that are strengths as well as vulnerabilities, and those strengths will be covered later in the chapter. As to the vulnerabilities:

Orientation to Detail

Research has shown that people on the spectrum can sometimes spend too much time examining the minute details of a situation and miss the gist or central theme of a collection of information. Researchers call this bias *weak central coherence*, and it can cause difficulties with catching the "big picture" of situations in your life. You may have heard the phrase "You can't see the forest for the trees." A person on the spectrum who looks at a collection of 100 trees of varying sizes and species growing close together is likely to see each individual tree and all the details about each individual tree. He or she may even try to identify the species of each tree. A neurotypical person is more likely to group the trees together into a unit and label it as a "forest" or "woods." As another example, take a look at the illustration below. What do you see?

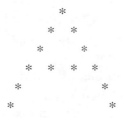

If your answer is "I see the letter *A*," then your mind used a shortcut and demonstrated central coherence. Even though 13 separate images are displayed above, your mind put them together and saw them as a unit. But if your answer was anything like "I see 13 stars," then you saw 13 separate images rather than a unit, which means you did not demonstrate central coherence. Interestingly, if you saw 13 stars, you were actually giving the more accurate description of what is displayed in the diagram. Yet, in everyday life, the more detail-perfect accurate description of something may not be the most efficient, practical, or functional interpretation.

Remember **Jake,** the young man who recently dropped out of college, partly because of his discomfort with driving? One of the reasons he has difficulty with highways and busier roads is that

Notes

✓ People with ASDs tend to pay attention to details but not to the whole or the "big picture" of a situation.

✓ This means you may be more prone to see individual parts of a picture but miss what the parts make up.

✓ For example, you may look at each of the 12 trees pictured below and notice them individually but miss the idea that there is a picture of a forest.

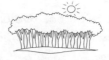

he focuses too much on one thing in his field of vision at a time. He has difficulty scanning his surroundings to assess the status of the road as a whole because he will focus intently on one car, missing what other cars are doing. He has had several close encounters because he failed to notice a changing traffic pattern until he got dangerously close to another car.

Dichotomous Thinking

People on the spectrum tend toward inflexibility. They also tend to interpret things literally. Both of these inclinations are related to a tendency to see things in an all-or-nothing, black-or-white fashion. When combined with the fact that you are more likely to experience stressful and negative life events if you have AS or HFA, this difference makes you more prone to engage in unproductive *negative self-talk*.

What do I mean by "self-talk"? The information-processing operations that I have been describing in this chapter are usually aided by an internal voice of some type. You may not always be aware of it, but you do have a "commentator" in your head who is continuously narrating what is going on in your surroundings. This voice is really your voice, and it helps you analyze information, draw conclusions, and direct you to carry out tasks. In the example of the dropped keys, it was your internal voice that said, "I must have dropped them by accident." All of the things that the voice says are referred to as *self-talk*. Don't worry; you are not crazy for hearing a voice in your head. Self-talk is actually a useful tool that all healthy people rely on.

Self-talk can become negative and unproductive, however, if your brain is using too many shortcuts, leading to interpretation errors. Psychologists call these errors *cognitive distortions*. Even for neurotypical people, cognitive distortions can lead to problems with anxiety and depression. Negative self-talk could be seen in the dropped key story if we added one more line. Let's imagine that, when explaining to yourself how the keys got on the hall floor, you said, "I must have dropped the keys by accident. *I am such an idiot.*" That last line really changes the tone of the story, doesn't it? How do you think you might feel if you were called an idiot, even if it was by your own voice? You might feel ashamed, angry, or sad.

Negative self-talk is playing a role in **Henry's** story. Remember him, the unemployed man who lives with his father and who gets anxious in the afternoon? His anxiety is fueled by the statements his internal voice is making to him, such as "I can't

Notes

✓ Self-talk refers to the internal voice that all people have that narrates what is going on from moment to moment.

✓ Self-talk refers to the thoughts people have that help them make sense of things and direct themselves.

✓ Self-talk can be positive or negative; either way it influences how we feel and behave.

believe another day went by and I haven't gotten any job leads. I am never getting a job. I am doomed to live with my father for the rest of my life."

You can also see how negative self-talk is affecting **Charles**, the married teacher who has difficulty interacting with his son in the afternoon. He feels guilty because he is not enjoying his son's company at that time of day, and he is beginning to get depressed as he tells himself, "I should be able to enjoy my son all the time. He's not doing anything wrong. I'm sure other fathers want to be with their kids all of the time. I am such a bad father."

Listed below are some of the cognitive distortions that people on the spectrum are prone to, along with examples of the self-talk associated with each. Interestingly, these distortions are also common in neurotypical people who are suffering from depression or anxiety disorders.

All-or-nothing thinking: There are only two categories for everything. You see things in terms of "black or white," "good or bad," "smart or stupid," "beautiful or ugly," and so forth. It's hard for you to see things on a continuum or in "shades of gray."

Catastrophizing: You exaggerate the possible negative outcomes of an incident. A minor problem is assumed to have catastrophic implications. For example, "I lost my car keys, so that means I am developing Alzheimer's" or "My boss reminded me of an upcoming deadline, which means he is getting ready to fire me."

"Should" statements: You have a set of strict rules about how you or other people are supposed to act or handle things and exaggerate the consequences if a rule is violated. For example, "I should be able to keep my room organized at all times or clse I am irresponsible" or "Bank tellers should always be polite or else they should be fired."

Personalization: You overestimate your role in the actions of other people, including strangers. You assume you are the reason for others' behavior without considering alternative explanations. For example, "My professor did not call on me when I had my hand up because she thinks I am an idiot" or "A store clerk gave me the wrong change because he knows I am a sucker."

Labeling: You engage in negative name-calling by assigning unfavorable labels to yourself or other people without having evidence for your conclusion. "I am a *loser* because I couldn't get a date" or "He is a *selfish bastard* because he would not help me with my project."

Mental filter/disqualifying the positive: You have a filter in your mind that allows only negative information in; you will pay attention only to the negative details about yourself or others and "filter out," ignore, or disqualify positive information. For example, you focus on one mistake you made at work as a sign of failure, but you ignore the positive feedback you recently got from your boss.

Mind reading: You assume you know what other people are thinking or what their intentions are, even if you have no evidence for it. For example, "She mentioned her vacation because she knows I don't have enough money to take a trip and she wanted to hurt my feelings."

Emotional reasoning: You let your feelings guide your reasoning. You use the logic "If I feel it, it is true." For example, "I am afraid to fly, so it must be dangerous."

Overgeneralization: You base global statements and conclusions on isolated events. For example, "I could not get the lawnmower started today—I am terrible with mechanical things" or "My daughter did not do her chores this week. She is never going to be a responsible person."

Did you recognize yourself in any of these examples? Take a moment now to fill out Worksheet 6. There you can check off any distortions that you might be prone to.

Thinking Differences as Strengths

This chapter has focused up to this point on the ASD thinking differences that can set you up to experience more stress in your life. However, the very same differences that can make you vulnerable to pressure have also given you strengths. Remember the list of strengths presented in Chapter 1 on Worksheet 3? Those are the attributes that scientists in the field of positive psychology have linked with resilience and human happiness. The next few sections will describe how some of the thinking differences found in ASDs can lead a person to possess some of these positive characteristics.

Attention and Focus

If you are like many people with ASDs, you may have the ability to focus intensely on one task or subject over a long period of time. When this type of attention is applied to an activity that is adaptive or constructive, we often use the term *perseverance*. We may also refer to a sense of *purpose* when we observe someone dedicating a lot of time and effort toward one goal.

Margaret, the 61-year-old endocrinologist mentioned in Chapter 1, spent large amounts of time during adolescence reading and doing science experiments. Her dedication and ability to focus intensely on tasks allowed her to persevere through her medical training. Even though she has had many interpersonal struggles, she has had a meaningful career because she has a strong sense of purpose and can persevere despite obstacles.

Orientation and Memory for Details

A tendency to focus on the details instead of the "big picture" can be a very useful skill in many situations. As a very simple example, I was once talking with the

Thinking Differences
Interpretation

COGNITIVE DISTORTIONS

Check off (✓) the cognitive distortions that you may be prone to in your day-to-day life.

☐ *All-or-nothing thinking:* There are only two categories for everything. You see things in terms of "black or white," "good or bad," "smart or stupid," "beautiful or ugly," etc. It is hard for you to see things on a continuum or in shades of gray.

☐ *Catastrophizing:* You exaggerate the possible negative outcomes of an incident. A minor problem is assumed to have catastrophic implications.

☐ *"Should" statements:* You have a set of strict rules about how you or other people are supposed to act or handle things and exaggerate the consequences if a rule is violated.

☐ *Personalization:* You overestimate your role in the actions of other people, including strangers. You assume you are the reason for others' behavior without considering alternative explanations.

☐ *Labeling:* You engage in negative name-calling by assigning unfavorable labels to yourself or other people without having evidence for your conclusion.

☐ *Mental filter/disqualifying the positive:* You have a filter in your mind that allows only negative information in; you will pay attention only to the negative details about yourself or others and "filter out," ignore, or disqualify positive information.

☐ *Mind reading:* You assume you know what other people are thinking or what their intentions are, even if you have no evidence for it.

☐ *Emotional reasoning:* You let your feelings guide your reasoning. You use the logic "If I feel it, it is true."

☐ *Overgeneralization:* You base global statements and conclusions on isolated events.

mother of a young man with AS, and she told me that her son's "eagle eyes" came in handy whenever she dropped something small on the floor, such as an earring or a screw. Ever since her son was a toddler, he had been able to find the dropped item in an instant; without his help it would take her and her husband a long time to find it, if they ever did. The ability to notice details that others might not see at all can be developed into countless job or career skills. In addition, despite the problems with working memory mentioned earlier, people with ASDs often have a superior ability to *remember* details over a very long period of time.

Together the ASD tendencies to focus on and commit details to long-term memory allow a person to be more realistic than neurotypical people in some situations. In my own therapy practice, I have observed that *realism*—one of the positive psychology strengths—is indeed a common characteristic of my patients with ASDs, and those who possess it benefit greatly from their keen observation skills, applying it to their homework between sessions. These individuals are often able to be more objective than my neurotypical patients when tackling problems in their lives.

Richard, the unemployed 25-year-old you met in Chapter 1, was feeling more hopeful about finding a job because testing done by his vocational counselor had revealed that Richard had a strong aptitude for detail-oriented work. Combined with his English degree, this talent could lead him to some work as a copyeditor. His extreme shyness had been a major obstacle to working up to this point, but the copyediting job could be done at home with minimal interaction with other people. Though he did not want to work at home for the rest of his life, at least he could make some money while he continued to work on addressing his shyness, all due to the talent he had for noticing details.

Dichotomous Thinking

The tendency to see things in an all-or-nothing fashion can, at times, be an asset. One of my patients explained to me that his brain works according to "binary code," the system by which computer programs give instructions to computers. Traditionally, all computer commands are written in a language based on numerical, rather than alphabetical, units. Only two numbers are used, 0 and 1. At its very fundamental level, binary code is used to convey complex information by stringing together unique sequences of "off" or "on" statements. Because there are only *two* possible symbols to be found at any single point of a sequence, 0 or 1, the term *binary* captures the all-or-nothing nature of the system.

My patient used the term to describe his thinking style because he was well aware of his tendency to see things in an all-or-nothing, black-or-white fashion. How this can contribute to stress has already been discussed, but it can also be an advantage, because, like a computer, a "binary" mind is also a logical mind. Logical reasoning involves coming to a valid conclusion by walking yourself through a series of "if, then" statements (e.g., "If _____ is true, then _____ must be true"). Philosophers, lawyers, and computer programmers all must be good at this, and I would guess that people drawn to those professions have minds that can operate easily in the binary mode, without being sidetracked by irrelevant information or emotional reactions. *Rationality* appears as an important resilience factor on the list of strengths highlighted in the field of positive psychology. The ASD brain, as discussed above, is one that is well equipped to demonstrate rationality.

For my patient, this type of thinking was sometimes a protective factor. While he was suffering from an anxiety disorder caused by various factors, he seemed to be immune to the type of collective anxiety that can be brought on by media hype about impending disasters for which there is no hard evidence. For example, when many people were bracing themselves for the Y2K disaster that was sure to happen at midnight on January 1, 2000, he had worked out a logical thinking sequence and had drawn a conclusion that there was not going to be a disaster. Similarly, in the wake of 9/11, a series of terrorism scares were triggered by anthrax attacks and warnings about mass assaults with lethal gas. At one point, there was a widespread recommendation that people reinforce the seals of their windows with duct tape. My patient, who did indeed suffer from severe anxiety about certain things in his life, had used his logic to arrive at the conclusion that the gas attack was unlikely; he disregarded the duct tape recommendation, stating "The most danger I could possibly be in right now would be in the Home Depot parking lot, where I am likely to be run over by someone rushing in to buy duct tape." In this instance, his logical mind served as a buffer in the face of mass anxiety, and in therapy with me he often tapped this strength to address the anxiety that pervaded other areas of his life.

Thinking Differences as Strengths

ASD Thinking Difference	Associated Strengths
Ability to focus intensely on one subject or task	👍 Perseverance Purpose
Orientation and memory for details	👍 Realism
Dichotomous or "binary" thinking	👍 Rationality

All of the thinking differences outlined in this chapter—as both strengths and vulnerabilities—are related to the social differences discussed in the next chapter. If any of the concepts are unclear to you, they will be covered several times again in Part II. There the chapters about problems in daily life will give you more examples of how thinking differences can affect you and also how these issues can be addressed through problem-solving techniques.

3

How Social Differences Can Be Vulnerabilities and Strengths

It's impossible to talk about ASDs without discussing problems with social functioning. Remember *Noel*, the 37-year-old single man who was frustrated by the fact that he never seemed to get second dates with the women he went out with? You met him in Chapter 1. You also met *Arnold*, the college student who was having difficulty joining in with his college roommates and their friends. Then there was *Margaret*, the 61-year-old doctor who was so uncomfortable during her lunch hour because she didn't know how to make small talk with the staff at her office. Scientists and clinicians describe these difficulties as "impairment in social interaction," but that phrase doesn't seem to do justice to the struggle and pain involved in so many of your encounters with others.

When you think about your own typical day, as I asked you to do in Chapter 1 when you filled out the worksheet with the clock on it, do you think your most stressful times of day involve social situations? Remember, when we focus on social functioning, we are including *any situation in which you must interact with at least one other person*. People often think that "social life" is about friendship, parties, and dating. While those areas are certainly important parts of social functioning, just as crucial are the brief and simple encounters you have with a store clerk, a bank teller, a mail carrier, or anyone else you interact with even briefly during your day. The story of *Richard* is a good example. He's the 25-year-old unemployed man who

Notes

✓ People with ASDs have unique brains that operate differently from those of neurotypical people.

✓ The ASD brain is associated with:

1. thinking differences
2. social differences
3. emotional differences
4. sensory and movement differences

✓ ASD differences are vulnerabilities and strengths at the same time.

lives with his mother and is almost completely housebound because of his fear of having an encounter with any person outside of his home. His lack of skill and confidence around even simple interactions with strangers is keeping him from using important resources in his own community.

Human Social Cognition

As with the cognitive differences discussed in Chapter 2, ASDs involve social differences that can affect you in many ways, in all of the arenas of your life. To understand the social ramifications of having an ASD, it will help to know how neurotypical people operate successfully in social situations. How do neurotypical people understand other people? How do they seem to know what to say and do, even in brand-new situations? If you're on the spectrum, you may very well have pondered these questions as you observed your neurotypical family members and friends navigating the social world with apparent ease. But these questions have also been asked for decades in an area of scientific psychology called *social cognition*. Researchers in that field study how people process and use information in social situations. The definition from a classic textbook called *Social Cognition* by Susan Fiske and Shelley Taylor says it is "the study of how people make sense of other people and themselves."

While your neurotypical counterparts may make social interaction look easy, it really involves a very complex set of operations. Those operations parallel the ones you learned about for human information processing in Chapter 2. In fact, social cognition is about information processing, but with a focus on how people process information specifically *about other people*. Remember the diagram in Chapter 2, which illustrated the steps of human information processing? There is a similar one for social cognition at the top of the next page.

The diagram illustrates the input, processing, and output steps that must be carried out by your brain for you to behave appropriately during social interactions. But what is "appropriate"? For the purposes of this discussion, appropriate responses are those that are *expected* by the other person(s) you are interacting with, based on the *circumstances* at hand as well as the *norms* of the culture in which you are operating. *Norms* are social rules regarding people's *expectations* about behavior within a particular group or society. This is not to say that people do exactly what others want them to do, like puppets or robots. Rather it means that people make *informed decisions* about their responses, based on a good *understanding* of the social scene and the norms involved.

The process by which people make these informed decisions about what to do or how to act when they enter a social situation (any encounter with one or more other human beings) involves several cognitive steps. Scientists have called this process *social inference*. The decision is an *inference* because the person must "guess" what is going on to some extent. Most situations a person encounters are

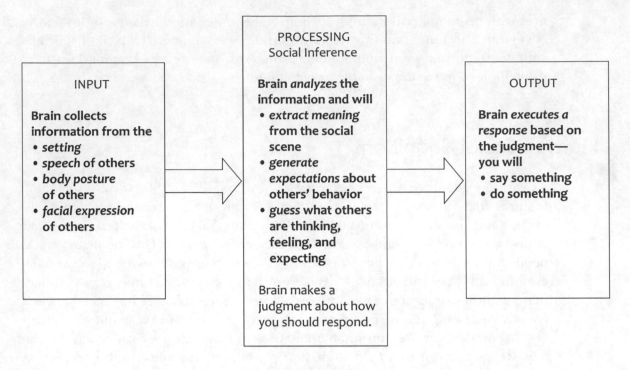

Social cognition.

not *identical* to any previous one in every regard, and in most situations a person is not provided any explicitly stated instructions for what to think and do. Neurotypical people guess correctly most of the time (though not always) because they are using *educated* guesses. Their decisions are based on information they gather and analyze very quickly, while referring to their preexisting fund of knowledge about social rules or norms. The study of social cognition over several decades tells us that people must make fairly accurate guesses to be successful in social situations.

Let's look at an example that shows how involved the social brain must be, even when we are doing things that do not seem that social on the surface. The man in this example does not have a goal to socialize. He simply wants to get himself something to eat.

Mr. Jones is on a business trip in an American city that he has

> **Notes**
>
> ✔ To understand the ASD social brain and its differences, we have to understand a little about the neurotypical social brain.
>
> ✔ When human beings process information about other people it is called <u>social cognition</u>.
>
> ✔ Scientists who study social cognition can lend us a hand in understanding how the neurotypical social brain works and also how the ASD social brain works.

never visited before. It's lunchtime, but he does not have very much time between meetings, so he decides to quickly purchase a sandwich. He enters a crowded deli, where he'll have to go through all the steps of social information processing shown in the social cognition diagram—input, processing, and output—to get himself some lunch. In each of the steps described below, you'll see in *italic type* what Mr. Jones might say to himself as he accomplishes the steps. Upon entering the store:

1. Mr. Jones must **collect the most relevant information properly**. This is the **input step**. First he must decide what information to gather. *I must find out where the line starts.* He will base his decisions on his fund of knowledge and past experiences with similar situations (because he has never been in this exact situation before). This allows him to know where to look. *I will look at the layout of the deli and also the other customers and see where they are standing and which way they are facing.* Scientists tell us that at the beginning of a successful social encounter, people pay attention to details about the setting (the physical environment and the purpose of the gathering, or goal shared by all the people present), as well as the speech, body posture, and facial expressions of the other people in the setting. For Mr. Jones, this means collecting information like (but not necessarily limited to) the following:

- *Setting:* Where is the deli counter, cash register, entry and exit doors? Where are the other people situated in the physical setting?
- *Speech:* Who is talking, who is not talking, and where are the talking people versus the quiet people?
- *Body posture:* How are people standing? Is there a group of people standing one behind the other, all facing the same way?
- *Facial expression:* Though all the people are strangers, which people have neutral expressions, happy expressions, annoyed expressions, and so forth?

2. He must **analyze the information and make a judgment**. This is the **processing step,** in which a person has to make sense of the information gathered so as to decide what to do in that setting. Mr. Jones has to assume several things based on the information he has gathered *and* based on his knowledge about and experience with similar situations in his past. As with all social situations, he has to understand the purpose of the gathering, which is the shared goal of everyone in the room; in this case there is an unspoken assumption that everyone has gathered in this place either to sell food or to buy food at lunchtime. Processing information involves these smaller steps:

- *Extracting meaning:* Mr. Jones must know about how typical delis work within this culture, even if he has never been in this exact one, and use that knowledge to make meaning of the things he observes in this deli. He must have the capacity to recognize which people are customers, differentiate them from employees, and see them as a group.

■ *Generating expectations:* He must be able to predict how others will act. If he sees several customers standing one behind the other, all facing the same way, he must be able to recognize and label that group, saying to himself *Oh, there is the line.* He *expects* that the people in that line are going to behave in a particular way; they will all keep moving forward as each person takes a turn, in the order of the line, buying lunch.

■ *Guessing other people's thoughts and feelings:* He has to be able to guess what the other people in the deli are thinking, feeling, and, more important, expecting him to do in the setting. Based on all of this knowledge and analysis, he assumes what is expected of him. He says, *Since I am a customer, I am expected to do what the other customers are doing.*

■ Now Mr. Jones is ready to *make a judgment* about what he should *do* based on how he interpreted the information: *I think I should go stand behind the last person in the line.* This judgment is based on the information at hand as well as his prior knowledge of and experience with the social norms of his culture (in this case, typical expectations in typical delis).

3. Finally he must **execute a response** that is based on the judgment he made from his analysis of the situation. This is the **output step.** In this case, he must actually walk over to the place in the deli that he has identified as the end of the line. He must also withhold any impulses he may have to ignore the line and go straight up to the counter, especially if he is in a hurry; he must exercise patience.

If all goes well in this example, Mr. Jones will end up getting his lunch, which is what he set out to accomplish. That sounds pretty mundane, doesn't it? So why did I just make it sound like so much work? And if a simple task seems hard, imagine what must be involved if you want to mingle at a party, ask your boss for a raise, ask someone out on a date, or assert yourself with someone who is mistreating you! For most neurotypical people, the steps of social cognition are all executed in a fraction of a second and without much conscious thought; some would describe their behavior as based on *intuition.* For them it is usually not so much work because their brains are wired to do many of these tasks automatically. But, as you well know, these operations are not so automatic for people on the spectrum. The next section will describe the aspects of social cognition that are difficult for people with ASD.

Notes

✓ Social cognition scientists have mapped out the steps involved for successful social behavior.

✓ A person is successful who is able to do the following with relative accuracy:
  1. <u>Collect</u> the most relevant information
  2. <u>Analyze</u> the information
  3. <u>Make a judgment</u> about what to say or do
  4. <u>Execute</u> the response

Social Differences as Vulnerabilities

Autism research has provided evidence that people with ASDs are prone to problems with performing some or all of the steps of social cognition outlined above: difficulty *collecting* relevant social information, *analyzing* that information, *making judgments* about what to do, and then *executing* responses appropriate for a given social situation. Most of the social operations that are crucial to success are information-processing or *thinking* activities. That is, the *thinking differences* described in Chapter 2 may frequently lead to "social mistakes" in the behavior (or *output*) that comes at the end of the social cognition process.

Many adults on the spectrum have told me they know they are making social mistakes by the unfavorable responses they get from others and the fact that their personal social goals elude them. Maybe you too have received some clues like these:

- Being ignored
- Being given vague, indirect feedback (e.g., "You are insensitive" or "That was inappropriate") without specific details
- Getting frequent angry or hostile responses from others
- Lacking the friendships you desire
- Lacking the dating experiences you wish to have

While these hints are useful signals that you've made social mistakes, they don't provide the information needed to improve social success. Many of my adult patients say they don't know precisely what's going wrong, and so they can't correct their errors. This is frustrating in the short term, but when it happens repeatedly over the course of many years, it can lead to chronic stress, anxiety, self-blame, and depression. *Noel* is continually frustrated by never getting a second date and also never getting any feedback about why. *Arnold* is mostly ignored by his college roommates and their friends but cannot figure out what he should be doing differently. And *Margaret* has been told by her office manager that she is not well liked by the staff in her medical practice but not what she should do to change how they feel about her.

Noel, Arnold, and Margaret are getting either no specific feedback about their behavior or feedback that is mostly vague or indirect. In this sense, most of the social mistakes they make are innocent—they are oversights or slips made with no intent to cause harm or conflict. This is little consolation, however, when you are meeting with indifference, annoyance, or rejection by other people. Also, just knowing you're making mistakes *without* an explanation does nothing more than create more pain. The rest of this section is therefore designed to explain what goes wrong socially for many people on the spectrum. This knowledge should help you begin to understand the types of social mistakes you might be making—*not* to give you reason to *blame* yourself but to lay the groundwork for the solutions in Part II of the book.

Take a couple of minutes to fill out Worksheet 7 below, remembering as you check off hints about your social mistakes that these problems are not the result of character flaws or a true lack of consideration for others. Rather, you have a unique brain that may lead you to make social mistakes, but those errors can be addressed without shame or guilt, with the help of this book.

So you can see how social cognition problems can contribute to social mistakes, let's pretend Mr. Jones has AS and look at the "social mistake" that he might make at the deli. We'll start at the end of the social cognition process because this is the only part of the process that is observable by other people and the part that they respond to directly.

Imagine that Mr. Jones walks directly to the deli counter, disregarding a long line of customers ahead of him, and tells the employee behind the counter what he wants. She ignores him because she is serving another customer. Having noticed

---

Social Differences
My Hints

Check off (✓) the statements that reflect experiences you have had which may be hints people have given you about your social differences.

☐ It seems like I get ignored when I am in a group—people act like I am not even there.

☐ I have been told I am too quiet or that I should talk more.

☐ I have been told I talk too much.

☐ I have been told I am too opinionated.

☐ People seem to get frustrated with me and I do not know why.

☐ I have been told I am pushy.

☐ I have been told I have no feelings.

☐ I have trouble getting along with people—I get into a lot of arguments.

☐ I have often been told I am acting inappropriately.

☐ More than once I have been told that I give people the creeps.

☐ It seems like I say the wrong thing at the wrong time.

☐ I have been told I should pay more attention to other people.

☐ I don't have the number or quality of friendships I would like to have.

☐ I don't have a romantic partner even though I would like one.

only that he was ignored by the employee, Mr. Jones repeats his request in a louder voice. Because this behavior would be labeled as "cutting into line" within the norms of his culture, most people in the deli are likely to consider it rude. The other people in the deli see only the *response executed* by Mr. Jones and not the faulty social cognition that has led to his behavior, and so they react with unpleasant and hostile comments. There are numerous points at which Mr. Jones could have made an information-processing error, each coinciding with the steps outlined in the social cognition diagram on page 60:

1. He may have failed to *collect* the most important information about the deli scene. He may have made the wrong decision about what to look for in the setting; he might have decided to look only for the location of the deli counter and not at the other customers. Or he may have known what information to gather but not how to collect the right information. He may have looked for other customers but not have known to look at their body language (standing position).

2. Mr. Jones may have gotten the first step right, but then did not *analyze* the information correctly. He may have seen the way the customers were standing, but did not cluster them together as a group and/or did not recognize them as a "line." Perhaps he did not generate the right expectations about the way people would be moving in a line or make the right guess about what others would expect from him.

He may have looked for, collected, and analyzed the information correctly, but made a poor *judgment* about what he should *do*. That is, he may have located the customer line and identified it as such, but he may not know the social rule about waiting at the back of a line, or, more realistically, may not understand its importance; he may know the rule but thinks it does not apply to him if he is in a hurry, for instance.

3. He may have done all of the above without error, but couldn't inhibit his impulse to bypass the line and therefore made a mistake when it was time to *execute* the appropriate response.

Although this example is somewhat simplistic—and possibly not a mistake you would make—it does illustrate how difficult it is for someone on the spectrum to carry out a social interaction that most neurotypical people would find easy. Even if you would not have any difficulty navigating a deli, you may be able to think of other scenarios that you do find difficult to figure out. The worksheets you filled out in Chapter 1

Notes

✓ People with ASDs are prone to have difficulties <u>collecting</u> and <u>analyzing</u> social information.

✓ This is related to problems making <u>judgments</u> about what to say or do.

✓ When an unsuccessful response is the result, it is considered a "social mistake."

may have included some of those. The chapters in Part II will help you assess these types of situations and will provide you with some strategies to make them easier. Because of the thinking differences of the ASD brain, social processing is extra challenging due to the multifaceted, ever-changing, and fast-paced nature of social interactions.

There are two major categories of problems that autism researchers have identified in the social processing operations of the ASD brain. They are *social perceptual* problems and *social communication* problems.

Social Perception Problems

Autism researchers have shown us that people on the spectrum have several types of problems "reading" other people. Each of these parts of social perception has been studied by social scientists:

- Noticing and interpreting social cues
- Mind reading
- Empathizing

Social Cues

Social cues are part of the *input* of social cognition. When you *collect* information from a social scene, attention to the *setting*, as well as the *speech*, *body posture*, and *facial expressions* of other people is crucial at the outset of an interaction. Without this information, you cannot make good inferences and judgments about how to behave. Researchers have shown that people on the spectrum miss a lot of cues that come from these sources. There are two ways this can happen:

- Some people with ASDs tend to overlook a certain kind of cue; they simply do not see it, as if they are blind to it (e.g., some people miss the fact that a person has an annoyed facial expression).
- Other people with ASDs may see the cue but not deem it relevant to the interaction (e.g., they notice the annoyed facial expression but don't realize it's relevant to what is going on at the moment between the people in the scenario).

You may recall reading in Chapter 2 that people on the spectrum tend to focus on details and not on the big picture or whole scenario (even with nonsocial information). This tendency may contribute to failing to see the relevance of social cues. Also, it's important to pay attention not just to the words spoken but also to *how* the speaker is *using his or her voice*. People on the spectrum often have very strong verbal skills and therefore rely heavily on spoken or written words, but less ability to process the nonverbal parts of human communication. Nonverbal social cues come in the form of the tone, volume, inflection (ups and downs of tone), and prosody (rhythm and pace) of what is being said.

Arnold's difficulty relating to his roommates and their friends is affected by problems he is having reading social cues. He is never certain about when to join in with them because it seems like they are constantly talking and laughing and there is no opportunity for a newcomer to start talking. Yet he has noticed that some of the friends come in at different times after a gathering has begun. He has tried watching what they do as they ease into the conversation but has not been able to figure out what they are doing and how they are doing it.

Mind Reading

A large part of *analyzing* the information taken in from a social scene involves guessing (inferring) what another person is thinking, feeling, expecting, and planning to do next. To do this, you first have to assume that another person may have thoughts, feelings, or expectations that are *different from yours*. Social cognition researchers who study autism refer to this ability to think about other people's internal states as *theory of mind*. Trying to sort out what another person is thinking or feeling is called *mind reading* or *perspective taking*. It does not refer to clairvoyance or ESP but is the process by which a person forms a theory, hypothesis, or guess about what another person is thinking or experiencing.

As a very simple example, imagine you and another person are sitting at opposite sides of a table, facing each other. Say there is a picture of a mountain landscape on the table between you, and it is oriented so that you see it right side up. Does the other person see the image exactly as you do, or will that person see the image in a different way? Obviously, the mountain landscape will appear upside down to that person. If you realize that, you are practicing the simplest form of *perspective taking*; you know that another person may not be experiencing something the same way you are. There is a very large body of research that tells us people on the spectrum have great difficulty with this. The degree of the difficulty varies with the severity of the autism symptoms as well as the presence of intellectual impairment. For instance, a person with mild symptoms of autism and a high level of intelligence may perform some theory of mind tasks very well (e.g., would automatically assume the mountain landscape in the example is not seen the same way by the other person), but will show impairment when the tasks are very complex (navigating a business meeting or cocktail party). If you are not aware of another person's perspective, you are at risk of saying things out loud that might offend that person. People on the spectrum are often described by people who know them as "brutally honest" because they will say what they think without considering the impact it may have on another person. This is not because they are callous or uncaring, but usually because they were simply unaware of the other person's perspective.

Margaret's discomfort with her coworkers is partly due to her problems with mind reading. One reason she doesn't understand "small talk" is that she hasn't figured out that the people working at her office have a wide range of different life experiences. She has never thought much about the fact that others have diverse backgrounds and interests that influence their social behavior. Also, she has never attempted to learn about other people's experiences because she never knew it was important to her own social life.

Empathy

Empathy is the ability to understand another person's feelings even when those feelings are different from yours. In a simple example, if you attend the funeral of someone you do not know (because you do know a surviving relative), and you see the loved ones of the deceased crying, you may understand that those people are sad about their loss even if you did not personally experience the loss (you do not know the deceased). You are experiencing empathy because you can guess how the other people are feeling and perhaps feel a little sad yourself, even though you are not going through the same experience. For your empathy to have social value, you must also be able to express it to the people around you. The diagram called "Empathy" below illustrates how the most complete empathy experience would go: *Think* about another person's experience, *identify* the emotion he or she is having and why, *feel* some of the emotion yourself, and *express* it by letting the other person know you can imagine their experience.

Empathy is very closely related to mind reading, in that you must be able to

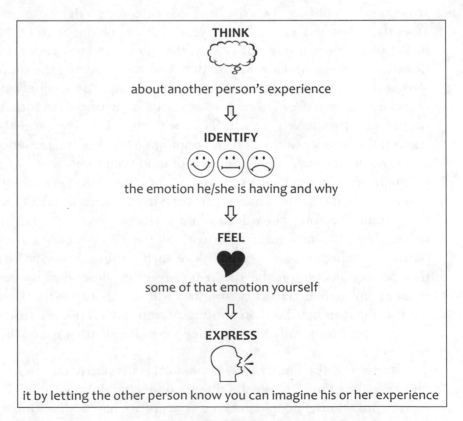

THINK

about another person's experience

IDENTIFY

the emotion he/she is having and why

FEEL

some of that emotion yourself

EXPRESS

it by letting the other person know you can imagine his or her experience

Empathy.

engage in theory of mind processes before you can experience or express empathy. You wouldn't be able to guess that the loved ones of the deceased at a funeral are sad without the ability to imagine what they might be thinking about (that they lost someone they love). However, people who can mind-read are not necessarily empathic. At a funeral you might be able to guess that the people are thinking about the deceased person but fail to guess that they are sad. And even if you guess correctly that the mourners are thinking about their loved one *and* feeling sad, you won't be seen as empathic unless you can express your empathy.

Unfortunately, because people on the spectrum experience and express empathy differently than neurotypical people, they have traditionally been viewed as *lacking* empathy and feelings for others. Recent research has not supported this idea, however. Researchers have divided empathy into *cognitive empathy* and *emotional empathy*. Cognitive empathy happens when you think about another person's feelings without necessarily *feeling* anything yourself. In the funeral example, this would be the point at which you say to yourself, "The relatives of the deceased are sad," but you don't necessarily feel sad yourself. Through a purely intellectual exercise you have arrived at a correct answer. Emotional empathy happens when you not only correctly identify the other person's feeling but also *feel* some of the same emotion yourself. In the funeral example, you would be experiencing emotional empathy if you said to yourself, "I *feel* sad when I think about how sad these people are." Your sadness is coming not from the fact that you lost someone (you did not even know the deceased) but from your empathy for the people who did lose someone.

Interestingly, some recent research has revealed that on tests of cognitive empathy people with ASDs tend to score lower (show less cognitive empathy) than neurotypicals. However, on tests of emotional empathy, people with ASDs scored *higher*, indicating that people on the spectrum actually *feel more* intense emotion in the face of the troubles or distress of another person(s). Some people on the spectrum report, in fact, that they get very anxious when someone else is in distress because they believe it is their responsibility to alleviate the other person's pain by fixing the problem. The pressure they put on themselves can get overwhelming if they don't know what to do to help. So why do people with ASDs have a reputation for lacking empathy? Let's look again at the components of a complete empathy experience as numbered steps:

1. *Think* about another person's experience.
2. *Identify* the emotion he/she is having and why.
3. *Feel* some of that emotion yourself.
4. *Express* it by letting the other person know you can imagine his or her experience.

People with ASDs tend to miss the social cues in a situation that would give them the information necessary for Steps 1 and 2—to *think* about and *identify* the experience of the other person. You need to notice cues you are getting from the setting, speech, body posture, and facial expressions of another person to get these steps right. And if you miss the first two steps, you cannot possibly do the second two steps. In addition, people on the spectrum may not *express* empathy clearly, even when experiencing it. Due to differences in information-processing speed, you may sometimes need extra time to realize that another person needs help or support. By the time you realize it, the opportunity to express empathy to the other person could be lost (e.g., realizing a friend is troubled many hours after an occurrence).

Noel's problems with dating are related to his unique experience and expression of empathy. Noel gets very nervous on dates and becomes very preoccupied with the impression he is making on his date. It has never occurred to him that most people, including the women he has gone out with, are a little nervous on a first date. Because he has not thought about the possibility that his dates might be nervous, he has never done anything to try to help the other person feel more comfortable on the date. People who know him well would describe him as very kind and caring. However, his focus on his own anxiety on dates has caused him to ignore the needs of his dating partners, which has probably made him appear aloof or disconnected from those women.

Take a moment to fill out Worksheet 8 on the facing page, which is a checklist of some typical experiences of adults on the spectrum. This is by no means a clinical diagnostic tool like the ones you may be given if you were to be evaluated by a licensed or certified mental health professional. Rather, it is an exercise meant to start the self-evaluation process that will continue throughout the chapters in Part II, intended to increase your self-awareness and understanding of why you have struggled in these areas.

Notes

✓ Problems with <u>collecting</u> and <u>analyzing</u> social information are also called problems with <u>social perception</u>.

✓ The most common social perception problems for people with ASDs are difficulties with:

1. using social cues
2. mind reading
3. empathizing

Social Communication Problems

Another major area of social difficulty for people on the spectrum is communication. Interestingly, it is common for people with AS and HFA to have excellent vocabularies and strong language skills in the academic sense. However, they have difficulty with the *social use* of language, an area that professional speech–language pathologists call *pragmatics*. That is, a person on the spectrum may struggle to understand the many ways people use language in social situations. They are also prone to difficulties using language in a flexible way, which is crucial to social success.

Autism researchers have identified several key problem areas in the language

Social Differences
My Social Perception

Check off (✓) the statements that sound familiar to you. These may be clues to social perception problems.

NOTICING SOCIAL CUES

☐ I can't sort out what is going on when I try to join a group of people who are already engaged in a conversation.

☐ It seems like people are picking up on things that I am missing.

☐ Sometimes people around me will start laughing about something that is happening, but I can't figure out what it is.

☐ I don't always notice right away when someone is trying to get my attention.

☐ I have been told that people give each other messages with their eyes, but I don't know what that really means or how to do it.

MIND READING

☐ Sometimes people get annoyed at me and I don't know why.

☐ I get confused when people don't just say what they mean.

☐ I hate it when people expect me to guess what they are thinking.

☐ I find it hard to believe that other people don't think the way I do.

☐ I sometimes don't understand what people want from me.

EMPATHIZING

☐ I have been told I am insensitive or uncaring.

☐ I get really upset when someone else is upset.

☐ I am slow at realizing someone is in need of my help or support; sometimes I think of it when it is too late.

☐ When I am worried about someone I care about who is having a problem, I want to help but don't know what to do.

☐ I don't know how to tell someone when I feel sorry about something bad that happened to him or her.

☐ When someone I like is upset, I will avoid that person because I feel so overwhelmed.

use and communication of people on the spectrum. In simple terms, people on the spectrum are most prone to have:

- unique ways of processing the language they hear
- unique styles of speech and expression
- difficulty with conversation skills

Unique Ways of Processing Language

People on the spectrum sometimes have problems with slow processing speed when it comes to hearing language. If another person is speaking too fast, or more than one person is talking at once, a person on the spectrum may miss a lot of the content. This is not a hearing problem; it is happening at the brain level.

Another common problem is the tendency to interpret information in a very literal way. You may take everything you see or hear "at face value." The hidden or unspoken meanings of things might be hard for you to figure out. With enough life experience, you may already have figured out what the most common *idioms* or *figures of speech*—words that don't mean exactly what they say—mean. You may know that expressions like "Hit the road" and "Pull yourself together" are not meant literally. But you may find yourself surprised and confused by unfamiliar phrases. **Arnold** has difficulty joining in when his roommates are talking with friends because he doesn't understand some of the slang words and phrases they use. He keeps getting confused when people use grammatically incorrect phrases or terms that have no meaning to him, such as "My bad" or "That's sick."

Also, because of the tendency to take things at face value, people on the spectrum may have difficulty learning about the unspoken or unwritten rules of behavior in certain settings. Every group has its own subculture with rules of its own, which can be very difficult for even the most intelligent person on the spectrum. For example, if the manager of an office has her door closed, it may be known in the office "culture" that this means she does not want to be disturbed. In another office with a different "culture" the door may always be closed but the manager expects people to come and knock when they need to talk to her. A neurotypical person may be quick to figure out a rule like that when changing jobs, but a person on the spectrum may have great difficulty with this.

Unique Styles of Speech and Expression

People on the spectrum also have some unique ways of expressing themselves. These issues cause them to stand out, draw unwanted attention, and/or be seen as odd. One common feature seen in people on the spectrum is *pedantic speech*. This means you may be prone to use very formal language (even in informal settings), may be very detailed with your descriptions, and might attempt to correct the errors made by other people. None of these behaviors are problematic, per se, as there is a time and place for each. However, it is the inflexible nature of this formal and exact style that can cause social problems. For example, it may be appropriate to use formal language when addressing the person interviewing you for a job, but the exact same style may seem odd at a family barbecue with people you have known all your life.

The other feature of speech that you may be prone to is unique *prosody*. This term is the one speech–language pathologists use to refer to the rhythm, pace, and tone of speech. Neurotypical people may use ups and downs in their voice, vary the volume of their voice, use pauses, and elongate some words while saying others quickly, all to convey different meanings and feelings. People on the spectrum are less likely to exhibit those speech habits. You may not vary your voice as much as neurotypicals. You may speak in a consistently monotone voice, consistently too loud, low, fast, or slow. The key word here is *consistently*. All people speak in these ways at different times, but they vary it according to the social situation. People on the spectrum are more prone to speak just one of these ways and then keep it that way all the time.

Noel may have been affected by this issue, as he was told by one date that he was talking like a computer. He was not exactly sure what she meant, but she may have been referring to his loud, monotone voice.

Difficulty with Conversation Skills

Most people on the spectrum have some problem with conversations. The exact nature of their problem varies from person to person, however. One major area of difficulty making people on the spectrum prone to conversation skill deficits is *verbal fluency*. Despite the fact that people on the spectrum can have strong language skills and vast vocabularies, they cannot always access the words they need in a spur-of-the-moment fashion. If you have ever heard the phrase "I am at a loss for words," it means there was a temporary interruption in verbal fluency. In certain circumstances, you may find that you simply cannot think of what to say. These word-finding difficulties are a common complaint of people on the spectrum; they can stop you from initiating a conversation and make it difficult to maintain one that has started.

The other area of difficulty in conversation for people on the spectrum is *turn taking*. A conversation is a temporary partnership with another person in which you agree that there will be an *exchange*

Notes

✔ People on the spectrum are prone to <u>social communication</u> problems, even if they have strong verbal skills.

✔ The problems with the social use of language most common to ASDs are:

1. processing what they hear
2. styles of speech and expression
3. conversation skills

of ideas and information. Because of problems with flexibility and social perception, people on the spectrum have great difficulty participating in this type of give-and-take activity. You have to be able to constantly pay attention to and read the other person to know when to talk and when to listen, and these cues from the other person are often nonverbal and hard for you to read. Some people on the spectrum deal with this difficulty by saying nothing; others deal with it by talking incessantly. Neither approach is good for conversation.

Margaret's trouble at lunchtime comes largely from her problems with conversation skills. She has problems thinking of what to say and also has difficulty knowing when to start talking even when she has something to say.

Now go to Worksheet 9 on the facing page, a checklist of some typical social communication issues for adults on the spectrum. Again, this is not a diagnostic test, and I cannot repeat enough that you should use the tool for *self-awareness but not for self-blame.*

Social Differences as Strengths

Just like thinking differences (Chapter 2), social differences that are part of ASDs can be strengths—and used to enhance your relationships—as well as vulnerabilities. Look back at the list of strengths presented in Chapter 1 on Worksheet 3 (page 35). These are the characteristics found in the field of positive psychology to be associated with happiness. Two of these positive characteristics, *authenticity* and *personal responsibility*, can be enhanced by some of the social processing differences found in ASDs.

When I meet with the family members of my patients on the spectrum, I often hear tremendously positive descriptions of their character. So often the loved ones of my patients report a genuine enjoyment of being in relationships with these people because of their unique qualities. The most common terms I hear in their descriptions are:

- honest
- patient
- sensitive
- funny
- helpful

Lack of Attention to Social Cues and Unwritten Rules

Because people on the spectrum may not pick up on social cues and may not understand the unwritten rules of conduct, they will speak without thinking about the impact of what they say. For this reason, it is not uncommon for a person with an ASD to be "the voice of reason" in a group. You may find yourself being the one person in a group to speak with clarity and honesty at the right time and for the benefit of the whole group.

Social Differences
My Communication

Check off (✓) the statements that sound familiar to you or reflect experiences you frequently have in your day-to-day life. These may be clues to communication problems.

PROCESSING LANGUAGE I HEAR (OR DON'T HEAR)

☐ I don't understand the expressions people use sometimes.

☐ People speak too fast for me—I miss a lot the first time someone says something.

☐ I don't understand how everyone around me seems to know the rules of the place even though they are not written anywhere.

☐ I can't seem to keep up with the latest slang terms—I feel so out of touch.

☐ I know I take things too literally, but I don't figure it out until it is too late.

MY SPEECH AND EXPRESSION

☐ I have been told I speak too loudly.

☐ I have been told I speak too quietly.

☐ I have been told I speak too fast.

☐ I have been told I speak too slowly.

☐ I have been told my voice is weird or strange.

CONVERSATION SKILLS

☐ Sometimes I want to say something but don't know what to say.

☐ I don't know how to ask another person to do something for me.

☐ I don't know how to join in a conversation that is already in progress.

☐ I often "go blank" in a conversation and can't think of the words I want to say.

☐ I can't tell when it is my turn to talk in a conversation—I never know when to pause and when to speak.

☐ I have been told I talk too much and should let others say something—have been told I go on and on.

☐ I don't know what to say if I get bad service or a store clerk makes a mistake.

Margaret, for example, is usually the one to ask questions and make comments to keep the discussions at the weekly staff meeting, run by an office manager who tends to go off on tangents, focused on the agenda. Most people at the meeting, who are neurotypical, are afraid to prompt the office manager because the unwritten rules of the office tell them that the boss should not be challenged. However, these neurotypical people are usually sitting at the meeting secretly wishing that the office manager would not go off on tangents. Margaret is not tuned in to that rule and is therefore not too inhibited to move things along. In that regard, Margaret is appreciated by everyone at the office. Her honesty is an asset in this setting.

Perhaps you can think of examples from your own life where you spoke honestly and the people around you expressed appreciation. This tendency is linked to the positive psychology trait called *authenticity* and is one important characteristic that has been observed in people who are resilient and successful.

Strong Desire to Solve Problems

As mentioned earlier, people on the spectrum can be determined to express an idea, sometimes at the expense of a conversation partner, and are committed to ensuring things are "right." Their pedantic speech often involves correcting people and ensuring that at least the written rules of conduct are followed. Because the pursuit of what is right is very important to many people with ASDs, they often have a strong sense of *personal responsibility* and will work very hard to solve a problem once committed to it. Related to this is the phenomenon I described earlier when discussing empathy. People on the spectrum will often get very upset when someone else is upset because they believe they must alleviate the person's distress. If this has happened to you, you may feel overwhelmed by a sense of pressure to solve the problem, and this can be a source of great anxiety for you. But it is also associated with a sensitivity to another person's problem and, again, a sense of *personal responsibility*.

Authenticity and a sense of personal responsibility can strengthen relationships and make you an important member of a group. Part II of this book will show you how you can take advantage of your social differences in specific settings of your daily life. The table below summarizes the social differences that can also be strengths.

Social Differences as Strengths

ASD Social Difference	Associated Strengths
A tendency to speak honestly without filtering	👍 Authenticity
A strong desire to solve problems and alleviate the distress of others	👍 Personal responsibility

4

The Role of Your Emotional Differences

As you read in Chapter 3, you have a unique way of perceiving the emotions of other people that may be causing you social problems. But there are also differences between how people on the spectrum and neurotypical people perceive and respond to their *own* emotions. *Jake*, the 20-year-old man you met in Chapter 1 who had dropped out of community college, was having difficulty managing the *anxiety* he felt while driving. *Meredith*, the 46-year-old woman with a law degree who was struggling with diabetes, felt overwhelmed by *anxiety* as she tried to manage her diabetes and also *sadness* over her lost opportunities to practice law because of her difficulties. Thirty-one-year-old *Fred* was running the risk of losing an old friend because he could not control his *anger* during their get-togethers at the sports bar.

Notes

✓ *People with ASDs have unique brains that operate differently from those of neurotypical people.*

✓ *The ASD brain is associated with:*

1. *thinking differences*
2. *social differences*
3. *emotional differences*
4. *sensory and movement differences*

✓ *ASD differences are vulnerabilities and strengths at the same time.*

Look again at the clock worksheet you filled out in Chapter 1 (page 16). Does your least favorite time of day involve some difficulty in managing your emotions? Don't be surprised (or worried) if your initial answer to that question is "I'm not sure." As you will see in this chapter, the experience of emotion is very subjective and therefore more difficult to describe than some other scientific concepts discussed in this book so far. And not just for people on the spectrum. Scientists have been studying emotion for decades and are still debating the best ways to define and measure it.

Just as your unique brain creates thinking and social differences for you (as well as sensory/movement differences, discussed in the next chapter), it creates differences in how you experience, manage, and express emotions. These differences, too, can be both vulnerabilities and strengths, as you'll see in the following pages. To understand how the ASD emotional brain is different, however, you need to know how emotions work for everyone. As you try to understand the behavior of neurotypical friends and loved ones, as well as your own unexpected reactions to various situations in your daily life, you may feel like Mr. Spock from the original *Star Trek* TV series. Some of my patients have said they feel like Mr. Spock when trying to decipher emotions because, from their perspective, emotions just don't make sense.

Emotions: Why Humans Have Them

Although scientists disagree about the exact nature of emotion and acknowledge that we have a lot to learn about the phenomenon, a few fundamental ideas have emerged from that field of study that can help you implement some of the problem-solving strategies in Part II:

- *Emotions* are distinguishable from *thoughts*.
- There are basic human emotions that can be categorized by a list of four words. They are *joy, sadness, anger,* and *fear.*
- Each of the basic emotions serves an important survival purpose for everyone, those with ASDs as well as neurotypical people.

> ### Notes
>
> ✓ Scientists who study human emotion have a long way to go before giving us all the facts. The following three assumptions came from some of their findings:
>
> ✓ <u>Emotions</u> and <u>thoughts</u> are different from one another.
>
> ✓ There are basic human emotions that can be described by these four words:
>
>   1. joy
>   2. sadness
>   3. anger
>   4. fear
>
> ✓ Each basic emotion serves an important function to help us survive.

Emotions versus Thoughts

Thoughts and emotions have some things in common: Both are *internal states*, meaning they happen inside of a person and are not completely observable by others. In that sense they are both considered *subjective* experiences. You read in

Chapter 3 about how important it is in social situations to know about the internal states of other people (through mind reading and empathizing) and how challenging it can be when you have to rely on guessing (inferring).

Even though thoughts and emotions are both internal, they are distinct processes involving different parts of the brain and body. *Thoughts* are ideas, beliefs, images, memories, or utterances we make to ourselves during self-talk, as described in Chapter 2. *Emotions* are feelings, or changes in physical arousal, that can be either pleasant or unpleasant to the individual. Thoughts involve what scientists call "higher-order" reasoning and appear to involve the parts of the human brain that are more evolved and complex than in other species, primarily the area scientists call the *neocortex*. This is the wrinkly outer tissue of the human brain that is visible in the information-processing diagram you saw in Chapter 2. Thoughts can be images (pictures in our minds), memories, or comments we make with our internal voices. Thoughts are also often tied to language, which is another higher-order ability controlled by the neocortex (e.g., self-talk is completely language based). Emotions, on the other hand, can be experienced without thought or language and seem to involve parts of the brain that are less evolved—parts that we share with many animal species, including nonmammals, that are much more primitive than humans. These parts are located deep inside the brain and are components of something scientists call the *limbic system*. They are covered by the wrinkly neocortex and are not visible in the picture that is part of the diagram in Chapter 2. When we experience emotions, our entire body is involved; we go through changes in heart rate, respiration rate, blood flow in muscles, digestive activity, skin temperature, and sweat-gland activity. Putting it simply, thoughts occur in our heads, while emotions occur across the whole body. There may really be scientific support for that old-fashioned notion that decisions based on *thoughts* and reasoning are made when you "follow your head" and those based on *emotion* are made when you "follow your heart" or "follow your gut."

The chart on the next page, called "Differences between Thoughts and Emotions," may help you remember how these processes are different. As you look through the points on the chart, remember that the science of emotions is far from settled on a lot of these issues. None of the statements about thoughts or emotions can be made with absolute certainty for all humans in every situation. That is why I used words like *more* or *less*—to reflect the fact that these statements represent some *trends* of scientific findings. They have been simplified here for the sake of explanation, but you can read more about the science of cognition and emotion in some of the resources listed at the back of the book.

It's important to know the difference between thoughts and emotions for reasons that will become clearer as you read on, but it's also important to know that thoughts and emotions often occur together and actually influence each other. For instance, a thought you have can lead you to feel an emotion, which in turn shapes further thoughts about the situation, which in turn influence the emotion you are feeling, and so on, much like this:

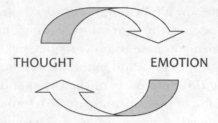

THOUGHT   EMOTION

To grasp this interconnection, imagine that you love to eat lobster. If you know you are going to your favorite lobster restaurant tonight, you may have *thoughts* about it in the form of self-talk ("I am really looking forward to that lobster!") or images (e.g., visualizing what the lobster looks like based on your memories of past lobster meals). It is very likely that you will also *feel* happy in connection with this scenario. So the thoughts about the lobster and the emotion of happiness are occurring together. If the happy feeling then triggers further thoughts about the dinner, which in turn prolongs the happy feeling, you're experiencing the interaction of these two processes.

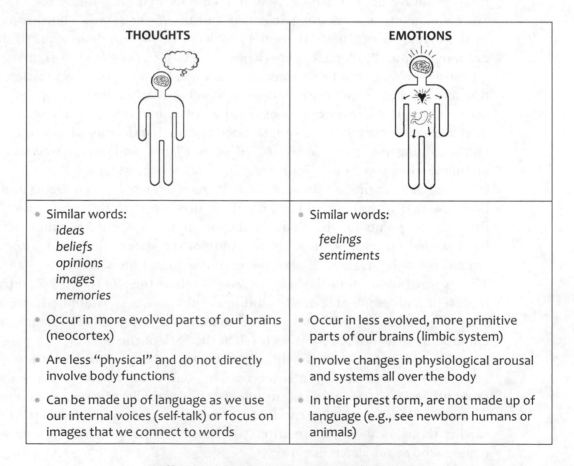

THOUGHTS	EMOTIONS

• Similar words:
    ideas
    beliefs
    opinions
    images
    memories
	• Similar words:
	
	    feelings
	    sentiments

• Occur in more evolved parts of our brains (neocortex)	• Occur in less evolved, more primitive parts of our brains (limbic system)
• Are less "physical" and do not directly involve body functions	• Involve changes in physiological arousal and systems all over the body
• Can be made up of language as we use our internal voices (self-talk) or focus on images that we connect to words	• In their purest form, are not made up of language (e.g., see newborn humans or animals)

Differences between thoughts and emotions.

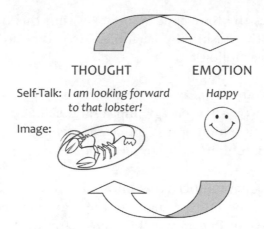

THOUGHT   EMOTION

Self-Talk: *I am looking forward to that lobster!*   Happy

Image:

The Basic Human Emotions

Human emotion is complicated, and a person's emotional responses at any given moment can be tough to sort out, even for neurotypical people. So you may be surprised to learn that many scientists and practitioners believe there are only four basic emotions (each with an image of its typical corresponding facial expression):

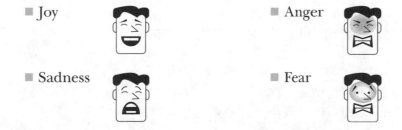

- Joy
- Anger
- Sadness
- Fear

These emotions are basic in the sense that apparently we don't need to learn them. Studies of newborn babies, for example, have suggested that humans are born with an innate ability to experience and express these four feelings. They are part of our "primitive" selves and can also be observed in less evolved species. If you own a pet, for example, you can probably remember enough situations where you were sure the animal was experiencing joy, sadness, anger, or fear.

Each of these emotions is either pleasant (joy) or unpleasant (sadness, anger, and fear). Different levels of physiological arousal accompany the experience of each of these emotions. Some emotional experiences involve high arousal, during which the body is in a charged-up, high-energy mode (joy, anger, and fear). Other ones involve low arousal, during which the body is in a slowed-down, low-energy mode (sadness). Defining emotions along the unpleasant ⟷ pleasant dimension and the high arousal ⟷ low arousal dimension can be another useful way to understand what they mean. The chart called "Defining Emotions on Dimensions" below places the four basic emotions within this framework. Find each emotion and notice the position of each one. According to this approach, we can define these terms as follows:

- ■ *Joy* is a high-energy pleasant feeling.
- ■ *Sadness* is a low-energy unpleasant feeling.
- ■ *Anger* is a high-energy unpleasant feeling.
- ■ *Fear* is a high-energy unpleasant feeling.

You may have noticed that only one of the four emotions is pleasant. You may have also wondered why anger and fear are defined identically with this dimensional approach. The answers become clearer when you know something about the purpose of emotion.

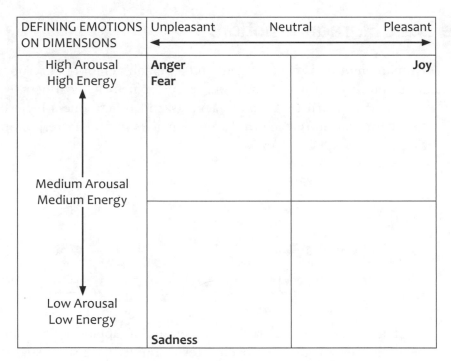

DEFINING EMOTIONS ON DIMENSIONS	Unpleasant	Neutral	Pleasant
High Arousal High Energy	**Anger** **Fear**		**Joy**
Medium Arousal Medium Energy			
Low Arousal Low Energy	**Sadness**		

The Purpose of Emotions

If you shared Mr. Spock's view that emotions are senseless before you began this chapter, you may believe that even more strongly at this point. After all, if three out of four of our basic emotions are unpleasant, aren't emotions primarily bad? If we are hardwired to feel emotions that are three-quarters unpleasant, aren't we doomed to suffer 75% of the time? Actually, the answer to both of those questions is no. All of our basic emotions, though not all pleasant, are good because they lead us to act in ways that are self-preserving and can literally keep us alive in the face of threats and danger. So, unpleasant does not equal bad. And we are not doomed to suffer perpetually, because emotions are experiences that are meant to be temporary; they are designed to kick in and stay in process only long enough to allow us to address the situation that triggered the emotion in the first place.

To understand the function of emotion from a scientific point of view, we have to consider the process of evolution. You may remember studying in school the Darwinian concept of "survival of the fittest." Because there is no room here to describe the science of evolution, I will borrow the crude synopsis I always use when teaching Introduction to Psychology to college freshmen. I ask you to imagine that at one time, very early in the history of human beings, we lived in caves. We had to hunt and gather our food and had close-knit bonds with the other members of the groups in which we lived. It was not outside the ordinary to be attacked by large cats, bears, wolves, snakes, spiders, and rival groups of primitive humans. It might also have been common for people to fall off cliffs or get stuck in crevasses. The people who did not have the ability to avoid or fight off these threats died young and did not pass on their genes. And the people who did have the ability to deal with these situations lived long enough to reproduce and pass down their genes. The traits most useful for survival surely involved physical strengths and abilities but also included emotional and behavioral characteristics. Some of these useful traits might be tendencies to avoid large cats, bears, wolves, snakes, spiders, rival groups of humans, cliff edges, and tight spaces. Also important were urges to fight with any of the animals or humans who may try to attack group members, invade the group's territory, or steal food from the group when resources were scarce. That's the end of the evolution lesson. (If anyone reading this book is a real anthropologist, please forgive me for the injustice I am doing to your field of study throughout this section!)

It's very likely that our ancestors who lived in caves passed down the hardwiring we continue to possess for experiencing basic emotions. Emotions did several important things for them that they continue to do for us. Emotions:

1. *signal* to us that something needs immediate attention
2. *trigger physiological changes* that prime the body to *perform* the behavior that is needed at the moment
3. *motivate* us to act in some way that will address the situation about which we received the signal
4. *dissipate* after the immediate situation is over

So how were the four basic emotions valuable when we humans lived in caves? Here's a plausible theory:

■ *Joy* is the signal to play. It is associated with increases in arousal and physical readiness to become active in a pleasant way—to have fun. Play serves two purposes: (1) to practice in a relatively safe way the skills needed for survival and (2) to bond with other humans to increase the strength of the group. When we lived in caves, games that involved hiding, chasing, and wrestling sharpened the skills that would be needed for evading predators, hunting food, or fighting intruders. Playing with other people in our groups strengthened our bonds, motivating us to stay together and defend each other, which was crucial during a time when a single person could not possibly survive alone. Joy and play were also crucial to the process of mating and reproduction. Even solitary play served a purpose—for example, stacking or arranging objects (stones, branches) might have sharpened the skills needed for building shelters, designing tools, or making weapons.

■ *Sadness* is a signal to lie low and withdraw. It is associated with decreases in arousal that put the body in a slow-moving or inactive state. It is normally triggered by some kind of loss. When we lived in caves, it served a function to withdraw and become inactive after a loss. If one or more of our group members died or disappeared, for example, our group could suddenly be more vulnerable to predators and invaders. Until we figured out what our new group hierarchy and plans were going to be, it was best to become less active so we would not attract the attention of unwanted visitors. A period of sadness is really an opportunity to go into hiding until we "regroup."

■ *Anger* is a signal to fight. It is associated with increases in arousal that put the body in a very charged-up, active state. It is normally triggered by some kind of threat. When we lived in caves, getting charged up when a predator or invader was trying to hurt us or steal our food enabled us to effectively chase and fight the intruder, furthering the survival of the individual and the group.

■ *Fear* is a signal to run away. Like anger, it is associated with increases in arousal that put the body in a very charged-up, high-energy state. It is also triggered by threat. When we lived in caves, it served the purpose of getting us to take drastic action to avoid contact with predators, invaders, or dangerous situations. This usually meant running away but could also involve "freezing" so as not to be detected or simply avoiding a place where a known threat was located (e.g., bears, snakes, cliff edges, crevasses). It could also

Notes

✓ Basic emotions help us, as they did our early ancestors, to survive.

✓ Unpleasant emotions are not bad; they are just as important to us as the pleasant ones.

✓ Basic emotions:

1. <u>signal</u> to us that something needs attention
2. <u>trigger physical changes</u> that prepare our bodies to perform needed actions
3. <u>motivate</u> us to either approach or avoid a situation for the sake of survival
4. <u>dissipate</u> after the situation is passed

mean fighting as a last resort, at which point this emotion would be serving a very similar function to anger.

The early humans who did *not* experience these emotions very likely died off because their own emotional systems were failing to prompt them to engage in adaptive survival behaviors, as outlined above. Those who did have these emotions are our ancestors, and the genes that program each of us to experience these emotions today were passed down to us from them. In this sense, even Dr. Spock would agree that emotions have a purpose. But do they have any value in the world we live in today? Most of us don't live among groups in caves and don't face the daily threat of being attacked by a wild animal. While some people live in dangerous environments and may be relying on their basic emotions in a more primitive way, our world has become much more complicated, and so have our emotional lives.

Why Is Human Emotion So Complicated?

Wouldn't life be simpler if we needed to know about and understand only the four basic emotions of joy, sadness, anger, and fear? That's not possible because we have more sophisticated brains than our early ancestors did. In fact we have elaborate information-processing systems (see Chapter 2), and thanks to the neocortex, we can recognize "false alarms" and adapt accordingly. We might realize, for example, that a scary-looking animal coming toward us is actually just a big friendly dog and we don't need to be as fearful as we felt upon first sight. We're equipped to recognize when we are becoming overaroused and take steps to calm ourselves down. Adapting like this is called *regulating* our emotions. It involves the capacity to put all kinds of twists on the basic emotions, which helps humans do what they need to in all kinds of situations. But it also makes it so much harder to understand ourselves and each other because human responses go so far beyond those four basic emotions.

There are two major ways that our advanced information-processing skills—or, as one of my patients put it, "our big fat brains"—make emotions complicated for us:

Notes

✓ Modern humans have complicated emotions; we experience the basic four, plus a whole lot more.

✓ Our brains can put twists on the basic four to create countless types of emotional experiences.

✓ Our information-processing centers let us do more with emotions than our early ancestors or other species:

1. mix <u>thoughts</u> and emotions together
2. use <u>language</u> in our emotional experiences
3. use thoughts and language to <u>regulate</u> emotion

1. Our cognitive or thinking ability gives us countless ways to experience and remember emotions; we can mix thoughts and emotions together.

2. Our language gives us a vast vocabulary of words that are meant to describe the wide range of experiences humans can have.

Mixing Thoughts and Emotions: Varied Emotional Experience

When our cave-dwelling ancestors felt an emotion, it was likely to have been simple and fleeting, even if intense. Likewise, when an animal with less sophisticated thinking ability, such as a dog or a cat, experiences an emotion, it is normally short-lived and disappears once the situation that triggered it has passed. Scientists believe that many less evolved mammals can think in terms of images and sensory-based memories and make up strategies to solve simple problems, such as getting at some food that is not easily accessible. Anyone who has tried to keep squirrels away from the bird feeders, or who has owned an escape-artist dog or cat can tell you that. But animals have less ability to influence their emotions with their thinking. We modern humans, on the other hand, have very sophisticated language, which allows us to tangle our thoughts and emotions together in a much more elaborate way than any other creature on earth. Mainly, there are two ways our thinking makes us experience so much more than the basic emotions:

1. Thoughts and emotions that occur together can become blended into an experience that is like a *thought/emotion cocktail*.

2. Thinking *about* a particular emotion can trigger the onset of an additional emotion, which called a *secondary emotion*.

Thought/Emotion Cocktails

Because our thoughts and emotions tend to occur together, we often blend the two ingredients together to create something that seems like a single experience. A good example of a cocktail is being "overwhelmed." This can happen when you find yourself with more tasks to do than you have time to complete. Perhaps you are behind on a project that has a deadline, you have too many assignments at work or school for the time in your schedule, or an unexpected event arises in your life that suddenly demands all of your time (e.g., an illness or accident in your family). These are common experiences for all adults (neurotypical and on the spectrum), and for the duration of these periods in our lives, we may describe our experience as "overwhelming." If I say I am feeling overwhelmed, it may appear as if I am reporting on an emotion. But that term does not really describe a single emotion, nor does it reflect a single thought. The experience I am having is really a thought/emotion cocktail with two ingredients. The *thought* is about there being more tasks to do than there is time, and my thoughts may be in the form of self-talk like "I don't have enough time to complete my tasks" and/or images of stacks of paper, a clock, or a calendar. The *emotion* is anxiety (a form of the basic emotion of fear). See the recipe card for this cocktail below.

Cocktail Recipe

Name of Cocktail: **"Overwhelmed"**

1. Gather all thought ingredients:

   a. One shot of self-talk—for example, *"I do not have enough time to finish!"*

   or

   b. One shot of images—for example,

2. Add emotion ingredients:

   a. One shot of anxiety (fear)

3. Mix well and serve immediately.

Secondary Emotions

Another way our thoughts make our emotional experiences so varied is by allowing us to think about our emotions. Sometimes the mere experience of an emotion becomes an event to react to. For example, let's say a man named Mr. Smith has a *fear* of public speaking that he has been working hard to overcome. He has been taking on extra speaking opportunities at his job just so he can get used to it because it's very important to him to improve in this area. After several months he begins to feel more comfortable, and he carries out several successful presentations at work. Then, one day, as he prepares for another presentation, he is struck by the sudden onset of *fear* that is more intense than any he has felt in a long time. He immediately becomes *angry* about the fact that he is afraid because he believes he should be over this by now. In this case Mr. Smith's *anger* is a secondary emotion because it's the result of his thinking about his initial emotion of *fear*. In generic terms he is upset because he is upset. Only humans can do this to themselves!

Language and Our Emotion Vocabularies

Human languages are rich with large numbers of words that can be used to describe emotions. This can be great for people who enjoy reading or writing fiction because there is always a new way to describe age-old human experiences. But it can also make things very confusing when we are trying to understand our own emotions in everyday life. You and Mr. Spock may still say, "Why can't we just stick to the basic four emotion words—aren't joy, sadness, anger, and fear plenty to go on?" As discussed in the previous section, modern humans experience emotions in such a variety of ways that we need a lot of words to capture all of those possibilities. We rarely experience joy, sadness, anger, and fear only in their pure forms. There are two types of vocabulary words that help us describe the variations. (1) *Synonym*s for the four basic emotions can help us capture variations in the intensity of these emotions. (2) *Hybrid* words help us capture internal states that are actually cocktails like the ones just described.

Synonyms

If you have ever used a thesaurus, you know there are always several words in the English language to express the same idea; they are synonyms. For emotion words, like the synonyms for joy, sadness, anger, and fear, the meanings may differ from the basic word only in terms of intensity. For example, *rage* is a synonym for *anger* but suggests a more intense version of that emotion. In scientific terms, the intensity differences that we can see in our own emotions have to do with the level of physiological arousal that our bodies may go through while experiencing each of the different feelings. I cannot possibly give you a complete list of emotion synonyms, but the chart below gives some examples.

Basic Emotion Words	Joy	Sadness	Anger	Fear
Synonyms	Happy Ecstatic Content Serene	Depressed Miserable Devastated Down	Enraged Annoyed Frustrated Irritated	Terrified Anxious Tense Nervous

To illustrate how these words reflect variations in the intensity of each emotion, I have placed the synonyms on the dimensional chart that appeared earlier. Each emotion synonym is placed along the two dimensions in relation to the basic emotions words, which appear in **bold** print (see the chart at the top of the facing page).

Hybrids

As mentioned, a single moment of internal experience may really be made up of a thought and emotion mix (thought/emotion cocktail) or may be a mix of two emotions. We have many vocabulary words that describe those mixes. The word *overwhelmed* is one such word, which was defined earlier. In the boxes in the middle of the facing page are some other examples of thought/emotion hybrid words and emotion/emotion hybrid words. Each is listed next to the suggested components or "ingredients."

DEFINING EMOTIONS ON DIMENSIONS	Unpleasant Neutral Pleasant	
High Arousal **High Energy** ↑	Terrified Enraged **Anger** **Fear** Anxious Nervous Irritated Tense Frustrated Annoyed	Ecstatic **Joy** Happy
Medium Arousal **Medium Energy** ↓		Content Serene
Low Arousal **Low Energy**	Down Depressed **Sadness** Miserable Devastated	

THOUGHT/EMOTION HYBRID WORDS		
WORD	THOUGHT	EMOTION
Satisfaction =	Belief that something went well	+ Happiness
Worry =	Belief that something will go wrong	+ Anxiety

EMOTION/EMOTION HYBRID WORDS		
WORD	EMOTION	EMOTION
Disappointment =	Frustration	+ Sadness
Jealousy =	Fear	+ Anger
Impatience =	Frustration	+ Anxiety

Emotional Differences as Vulnerabilities

It was once thought that people with ASDs were *lacking* emotion, but now there is no doubt that people on the spectrum experience all the basic emotions as well as some of the complex ones. The major area of difference for people with ASDs is in their *emotion regulation* ability. You may learn as you read the next section that you have difficulties regulating your emotional experiences, which can lead to a whole host of problems in everyday life.

Emotions work best for us when they *signal* a need, *trigger physical changes* to ready the body to perform a key behavior, *motivate* us to either approach or avoid something, and then *dissipate* when no longer needed. For them to work this way, however, your brain has to be able to perform a number of functions that don't come easily to people on the spectrum. When you have trouble with any of these functions, you'll have trouble with one or both of the two types of emotion regulation: (1) *self-regulation* involves being able to monitor and alter your own emotional reactions so you can adapt to the situation you're in; (2) *mutual regulation* involves understanding and interpreting the internal states of other people, expressing your feelings to them, and using their help.

Problems with Self-Regulation

> ### Notes
>
> ✓ People on the spectrum experience all of the basic emotions plus some complex ones.
>
> ✓ People on the spectrum differ from neurotypicals in that they have difficulty with the <u>regulation</u> of emotion.
>
> ✓ The use of strategies to manage emotional arousal is difficult for people with ASD in terms of:
>
>   1. <u>self-regulation</u>, or using strategies to manage emotions alone
>   2. <u>mutual regulation</u>, or using other people as helpers to manage emotions

One of the reasons you and other people on the spectrum have problems monitoring and altering your emotions is that in the same way that you may have an on/off switch to regulate your attention (see Chapter 2), you may have an on/off switch for emotional arousal. Neurotypical people have a dial knob for both. Just as you tend to pay either all or none of your attention to something, you are either highly aroused, and you become that way very quickly, or underaroused in a situation that warrants arousal. As one patient described it, his anger goes from "0 to 60 in a millisecond" once his engine is started, but that is only after a long delay in responding to the "gentlemen, start your engines" cue. Another difference that exists in the ASD brain is that the more sophisticated higher-order brain (i.e., neocortex) is not communicating very well with the more primitive emotional brain (i.e., limbic system). Where the thinking brain of neurotypical people has the power to influence the emotional brain, such as when thoughts and emotions blend together and interact with each other, there seems to be a poor connection between these two brain areas in people on the spectrum. ASDs seem to hamper the ability to use the thinking brain to influence feelings and arousal. If your system operates this way, it will be difficult for you to:

1. recognize your own physiological/emotional state
2. identify the need signaled by that emotion
3. attend to the things in the environment that may be important to address the need

4. use your behavior to regulate (adjust the intensity of) the emotion
5. use cognitive strategies to cope with very intense experiences

Remember *Jake*, the young man who has been avoiding driving? Let's see how he experiences each of these stages of self-regulation difficulty.

Recognizing Emotions

When you experience emotion, your body goes through changes in arousal states. You may have difficulty recognizing when that is happening and/or being able to label the experience appropriately. For example, when *Jake* drives a car, his heart races, he sweats profusely, and he has difficulty concentrating. He is usually not aware of what is going on inside his mind and body when he is in the middle of it. When he is out of the situation (e.g., at home and not in a car), all he knows is that he wants to avoid driving because he has a vague sense that it is a highly unpleasant experience for him. He is having difficulty *recognizing* and *labeling* his experience as "fear" or "anxiety" in the moment.

Identifying the Need

Even if you can recognize and label your emotion, as mentioned above, it is not useful information until you can identify what the emotion is *signaling* to you—what is the need that warrants your attention? If you can't pinpoint it, then you can't begin to resolve it. In *Jake's* case, his anxiety is signaling to him that he needs to look for strategies that will allow him to feel safer behind the wheel. If he cannot identify that need, he will not know where to begin to solve his problem, which is crucial for regulating his anxiety.

Attending to the Situation in the Environment

Let's say you recognize and label your emotion, and identify the need that is being signaled, but you don't know where to look for tools or help. Once again, you are not going to be able to regulate the emotion that is activated. You must be able to scan your environment and look for useful objects or opportunities that can help you solve your problem and regulate your emotion. *Jake* may need to shift his attention while driving to different things in the environment (e.g., learn to focus on merging cars using his peripheral vision while paying more attention to the road ahead). If he cannot change the direction of his focus, he will have difficulty regulating his anxiety.

Using Behavior to Adjust the Intensity of the Emotion

Even if you carry out all three previous steps of regulation perfectly, it will do you very little good if you can't use adaptive behavior to address the need. What is adaptive behavior? It is any action (or inhibition of an action) that leads to an outcome that is helpful for you and does no harm. People on the spectrum may be prone to use maladaptive behaviors to adjust the intensity of their emotions because their arousal is so extreme when activated. As you well know, being extremely aroused can be so unpleasant that you're desperate to feel relief. You will do anything to make the unpleasant feeling go away. You may have learned that certain behaviors provide you with relief but are not adaptive or helpful in the long run. For example, hitting yourself, banging your head, or screaming can immediately release tension but may cause injury or be hurtful to other people. Running away and escaping the situation that triggers the unpleasant feeling can also provide immediate relief but is maladaptive in many cases. This is what is going on for *Jake*. He has learned that he can escape his unpleasant feeling by simply avoiding his car. But this has meant he had to quit school. A more adaptive behavior may be to look for more active ways to increase his confidence in his driving skills by, let's say, taking driving lessons and practicing more so he can feel safer behind the wheel. If he can't identify that option, he won't be able to regulate his anxiety effectively to adapt to this situation.

Using Cognitive Strategies to Cope

Finally, even if you carry out all of the steps above successfully, it will be hard for you to practice adaptive behavior if you can't use your thinking brain to plan and reinforce the behavior. In the introduction to this section, I mentioned that in people on the spectrum the part of the brain that produces thoughts and language and the part of the brain that produces emotions do not communicate with each other as well as they do in the brain of a neurotypical person. That makes it hard for thoughts and language to influence emotions in a positive way. In *Jake's* situation, he may benefit from using self-talk to direct himself through some of the anxiety-producing situations he has encountered while driving. However, because his brain does not do that naturally and automatically for him, he has missed out on the benefit of those cognitive strategies and therefore has not been able to successfully regulate his anxiety.

Now look at Worksheet 10 on the facing page, which may begin to help you pinpoint some self-regulation problems that are affecting you in your everyday life.

```
╭─────────────────╮
│      Notes      │
╰─────────────────╯
```

✓ *Self-regulation is difficult for people on the spectrum because:*

1. *emotion arousal systems work with an on/off switch* *instead of a dial/knob*

2. *the thinking brain does not communicate with the emotional brain; it is difficult to use thoughts and language to influence emotion*

Problems with Mutual Regulation

Effectively regulating your emotions often means involving other people in the process. This is called *mutual regulation* because two or more people are participating in an

Emotional Differences
My Self-Regulation

Check off (✓) the statements that sound familiar to you. These may be clues to self-regulation problems.

☐ I sometimes get extremely upset, and it seems like there is no reason.

☐ When I am nervous or angry, my stomach gets so upset I almost throw up. Sometimes I can't eat for the rest of the day.

☐ When I am nervous or angry, I get a headache that I can't get rid of—I usually have to lie down for the rest of the day.

☐ It can take hours for me to calm down after something upsets me.

☐ Sometimes I have fits that seem to come out of nowhere. I am fine one minute and the next I feel like screaming.

☐ When something really upsets me, I get paralyzed. I just don't know what to do to make it better.

☐ I can sometimes come up with good solutions to solve my problems, but not when I am in the middle of being upset—I think of the answer hours later, when it is too late.

☐ When I am really upset about something, I don't notice things that could help me—it is almost like I am blinded by my feelings.

☐ When I get angry, I often kick or punch walls, slam doors, or break things.

☐ When I get angry, I hit myself or bang my head on something hard.

☐ I get embarrassed because I overreact to minor problems.

☐ By now I know exactly what makes me overreact, but I still can't prevent it no matter how hard I try.

☐ I cannot think clearly when upset.

From *Living Well on the Spectrum* by Valerie L. Gaus. Copyright 2011 by The Guilford Press.

exchange of information that can help all parties regulate the arousal level of an individual or a group. The skills necessary to participate in mutual regulation are many of the same abilities discussed in Chapter 3 on social functioning. Because of the difficulties people on the spectrum have with social cognition, several aspects of mutual regulation are difficult for them. Also, the poor connection that exists between the thinking/language brain and the emotional brain that was mentioned in the previous section can affect mutual regulation. If you are subject to these differences, you are going to have some difficulty with the following steps of mutual regulation:

1. understand and interpret the internal states of others; identify potential helper(s)
2. express emotions and needs to another person(s)
3. ask for and accept help from others

When you met *Fred* earlier in the book, he was having difficulty with anger outbursts while out with his friend at a sports bar. Let's see how he has difficulty at each of these steps of mutual regulation.

Understanding and Interpreting the Emotional States of Other(s)

Neurotypical people often rely on cues from other people to help them appraise a situation and manage their own emotional reaction. But if you have the social cognition problems that are part of ASDs, you'll have trouble doing this. *Fred* is getting overaroused and angry every week during his get-togethers with an old friend. Disagreements about sports topics usually trigger his arousal. He is unfortunately missing the nonverbal cues his friend is giving him that he is uncomfortable with Fred's increasingly loud voice volume and concerned that Fred may draw unwanted attention and possible ridicule from others (e.g., friend will look around to see if others in the bar are noticing the loud voice, will use hand gestures to signal Fred to lower his voice). Fred's friend is trying to help him, but Fred is missing the signs of that. His anger only escalates.

Expressing Emotions and Needs to Another

Even if you can identify others' emotions and ability to help you, doing so can be beneficial only if you can find the words to tell the other person how you are feeling *and* what you need. Some people on the spectrum have difficulty accessing the words in their vocabulary to describe their feelings, especially in the "heat of the moment" when they are experiencing strong feelings. They are also prone to have difficulty identifying something they may need that would be helpful. *Fred* tends to get angriest when arguments occur in public (as opposed to on the phone with his friend or in more quiet settings) because he is also embarrassed when his friend disagrees with him. He has the misconception that his friend is putting him down in front of others when they disagree in the bar. He has not been able to pinpoint that feeling and thought, nor has he been able to express it to his friend. He would benefit from watching Friday night games in a more quiet setting such as his home or his friend's. He cannot express that need because he is not fully aware of it himself.

Asking for Help and Accepting Help

Let's say you can pick up cues from others when you're upset, you can identify a potential helper, and you can express your feeling and your need, but you don't know how to ask someone to do something specific for you that would be helpful, or you don't accept help when it's offered. You'll still miss out on the chance to involve another person in the regulation of your emotion. If *Fred* can't ask his friend to make a change in their Friday night routine (e.g., ask him to meet at one of their homes instead of the bar), he won't be able to adapt and regulate this anger effectively.

Now fill out Worksheet 11 (page 96), which might help you identify some ways that mutual regulation problems are causing you difficulties in your daily life.

> ## Notes
>
> ✓ Mutual regulation is difficult for people on the spectrum because:
>
> 1. social cognition problems make it hard to read and utilize other people
> 2. problems using language to describe emotions make it hard to ask for help

Emotional Differences as Strengths

Looking back again to Worksheet 3 in Chapter 1 (page 35), you can see there are three helpful characteristics that can be enhanced by the emotional differences found in ASDs. They are *capacity for pleasure*, *courage*, and *optimism*.

As mentioned above, your emotions tend to occur in an "all or nothing" fashion, and your thinking brain does not communicate very easily with your emotional brain. Therefore, you may not be able to use your thoughts and language to "put the brakes on" when something triggers your arousal. This can make life very intense, but there are several ways this can make life interesting and fun, specifically when the pleasant emotions are activated:

All-or-Nothing Emotions

When you engage in an activity you enjoy, you probably have more fun than a neurotypical person would doing the same activity. Because all of your emotions are experienced in an intense way, you get the benefit of extreme joy! This will make your *capacity for pleasure* one of your strengths. You have probably already learned to use that strength to help yourself throughout your life. In Part II, where I will provide you with positive strategies to enhance your life, I will be calling on you to use it some more. For many people on the spectrum, this characteristic contributes to their development of their passions and interests, which often lead them to make connections with others or can enhance their work life.

In the case of *Fred*, his extreme enjoyment of sports contributed to the positive aspects of his relationship with his friend, because they both shared a passion for activities related to it. *Meredith* is disappointed that she is not working as a lawyer,

WORKSHEET 11

Emotional Differences
My Mutual Regulation

Check off (✓) the statements that sound familiar to you. These may be clues to mutual regulation problems.

☐ I don't seem to react to things the way others want me to. People tell me I am cold or insensitive.

☐ My reactions to some situations seem to upset other people, but I don't know what to do about it.

☐ When I get upset, it seems like no one around me understands.

☐ Sometimes when I have an upsetting problem, I feel helpless but don't know whom to ask for help.

☐ I wish I could get some help sometimes, but I don't know what to say to people to get them to help.

☐ I am too embarrassed to ask for help when I need it. I am afraid it is a sign of weakness or immaturity.

☐ When I am upset, I become speechless.

☐ I don't like it when people try to help me if I am in the middle of trying to solve a problem. I would prefer to solve it on my own.

but the pleasure she takes in horticulture and plants enabled her to get her garden center job, which she does enjoy and succeed at. This is something that would not be present in her life if she did not so passionately enjoy being around plants.

Less Communication between the Thinking and Emotional Brains

When you feel your emotions so intensely, as described above, you are less apt than a neurotypical person to use self-talk to regulate the level of arousal. Because you may not always think about your own reactions to events, your passion may at times cause you to persist in your pursuit of something despite "rational" reasons to stop. This tendency is probably behind the incredible *courage* and *optimism* I see in so many of my patients.

Richard is the 25-year-old college graduate in English literature who lives at home with his mother. He is so motivated to be independent that he is willing to try things that are associated with the unknown. The strong positive emotions he associates with an independent life are not marred by negative thoughts while he is experiencing them. This is not to say he has no negative thoughts; indeed he does, which is why he has some of the problems he has. But his persistence toward his goal is driven by a strong positive feeling, and because his brain is not so prone to use thoughts to halt emotions, he can experience the pleasant feeling to its fullest. This gives him the *courage* to try new things that can in many ways be scary to him.

Noel is the 37-year-old single man who is trying to meet a woman to date. Although he is frustrated by his lack of success, his strong desire to experience the positive feelings that he associates with family life motivates him to keep trying. His pleasant emotions around this subject are not being mediated by thoughts regarding failure. He strongly believes that if he can get help with the mistakes he is making, he'll be successful. This type of *optimism* is associated with positive outcomes for the patients with whom I work.

Emotional Differences as Strengths

ASD Emotional Difference	Associated Strengths
All-or-nothing emotions	👍 Capacity for pleasure
Less communication between the thinking and emotional brains	👍 Courage
	👍 Optimism

5

How Sensory and Movement Differences Can Affect Your Interactions with Your Environment

Autism spectrum disorders can have profound effects on the way the brain processes and responds to information that comes in from the physical senses and then how it sends movement messages back out to the body. As a person on the spectrum, you're likely to experience your physical environment and your own bodily sensations differently from neurotypical people. These differences can cause problems like the ones you saw in the lives of some people introduced in Chapter 1. *Charles*, the high school teacher who has difficulty interacting with his son when they both get home in the afternoon, feels so tense partly because he is very sensitive to noise. By the end of his workday, he has expended a lot of energy just trying to tolerate the constant loudness at school. *Richard*, the unemployed college graduate who lives with his mother, is aware that he's afraid to go out on errands by himself because of his fear of talking to strangers. But something else that is affecting him is sensitivity to bright indoor lighting, especially fluorescent bulbs. The harsh lighting in many public buildings makes him even more uncomfortable around people he doesn't know than he might be if the lighting were soft or dim. *Carla* is the married woman whose relationship with her husband is being affected by her sensitivity to certain types of touch because it makes her reluctant to give or receive hugs.

These three people are struggling with sensitivities to *sound*, *light*, and *touch*. Other people have differences in the way they experience *taste* and *smell*. Especially during childhood, people on the spectrum commonly have sensory systems that are either overresponsive or underresponsive to environmental events, and this is closely tied to the way they move their bodies. While these issues are not as well studied in adults with ASDs, there is some evidence that these characteristics are most extreme early in life and taper off or become less significant in adulthood.

Notes

✓ *People with ASDs have unique brains that operate differently from those of neurotypical people.*

✓ *The ASD brain is associated with:*

    1. thinking differences
    2. social differences
    3. emotional differences
    4. sensory and movement differences

✓ *ASD differences are vulnerabilities and strengths at the same time.*

Some of my adult patients with ASDs are not affected by these issues, but many report at least some degree of difficulty related to their sensory experiences.

Consider again the clock worksheet you filled out in Chapter 1. Is it possible that your least favorite time of day is being affected by your unique senses? As with your emotions (discussed in Chapter 4), you might not be sure. People with sensory problems are not always immediately aware of how significant a role they are playing in day-to-day stress. I hope reading this chapter will help you evaluate whether they are affecting your daily struggles. As with the cognitive, social, and emotional differences that come with ASDs, your sensory/movement differences can be vulnerabilities but also strengths.

How the Human Brain Manages Sensation and Movement

By now you're probably pretty familiar with the idea that the brain is an information-processing device. In addition to social and emotional information, your brain processes sensory movement information, going through the stages of input, processing, and output.

How Many Senses Do We Really Have?

When you were in grade school, you were probably taught that we have five senses; sight, hearing, smell, taste, and touch. While we do indeed have all of those senses, the fifth one, touch, is really part of a trio of senses that are sometimes called the *body senses*. They include touch, balance, and motion and are called body senses because they involve information being communicated about and between the brain and areas below the neck. These are distinguished from sight, hearing, smell, and taste because for them all communication occurs in the head and about the head region. This means that we really have seven senses. Each of these has an "input device" (sense organ), which is a specialized part of the body with built-in sensors (receptor cells) to pick up a particular type of physical information. If you compare a computer to a brain, the computer must have input devices to be a useful tool; even a computer with a very powerful processor is going to be idle if the processor cannot receive new information from the environment. A personal computer, for example, relies on a keyboard, mouse, or touch screen to interface with the environment (which includes a human operator), and the brain relies on the sense organs in much the same fashion. The sensors in those organs translate physical information into a nerve impulse that is sent via specialized pathways to the brain, where it can be processed. The way this happens for each of the seven senses is described below and is also summarized in the table called "Our Seven Senses," which appears below.

Sight

Sight involves the translation of *light* into nerve impulses by the specialized cells in the *eye* that can be found in the retina. This is called *visual* information, and it gets sent from the eye to the brain through a specific nerve path.

SENSE	Common Term	Technical Term	Organ or Sensor
	Sight	Visual	Eye
	Hearing	Auditory	Ear
	Smell	Olfactory	Nose
	Taste	Gustatory	Tongue plus nose
	Touch	Tactile	Skin
	Balance	Vestibular	Inner ear
	Motion	Kinesthetic	Joints and muscles

Our seven senses.

Hearing

Hearing involves the translation of *vibrations* in the environment into nerve impulses by the specialized cells in the *ear*. This is called *auditory* information, and it gets sent from the ear to the brain through its own special nerve path.

Smell

Smell involves the translation of *gases* into nerve impulses by the specialized cells in the lining of the nose. This is called *olfactory* information, and it gets sent from the nose to the brain through a special nerve path.

Notes

✓ *Humans have seven senses:*

1. *sight*
2. *hearing*
3. *smell*
4. *taste*
5. *touch*
6. *balance*
7. *motion*

✓ *Each sense has a specialized organ and set of sensors that send signals to the brain for processing—this is a type of* input*.*

Taste

Taste involves the translation of *chemicals* into nerve impulses by the specialized cells on the *tongue*, which can be found in the taste buds. This is called *gustatory* information, and it is complex in that it incorporates some information about the smell (olfactory) of the food that is collected from the nose while it is being sent to the brain through its own special pathway.

Touch

Touch involves the translation of *pressure* and *temperature* into nerve impulses by the specialized cells in the *skin*. This is called *tactile* information, and it is sent to the brain through a complex network of neural pathways channeled through the spinal cord.

Balance

Balance involves combining information about body orientation in relation to the ground, and it relies on the physical presence of *gravity*. The specialized sensors that detect this are found in a liquid-filled chamber of the *inner ear*, which acts much like a carpenter's level. The liquid is always level in relation to the ground, no matter how much your body may tip—so your inner ear can measure the difference between the orientation of the liquid (which is constantly level) and the orientation of your body (which may or may not be level). This is called *vestibular* information, and it is sent to the brain via its own special nerve path.

Motion

Motion translates information about the *physical position* of the body and each separate part (e.g., arms, legs) that is translated by special cells in our joints and muscles. Movement is detected whenever the position changes. This is called *kinesthetic* information, and it is sent to the brain via a complex network of neural pathways channeled through the spinal cord.

How the Brain Processes Sensory Information

What does your brain do with all of the sensory information sent its way? Look at the diagram called "Human Sensory/Movement Processing." The layout should look familiar, as it has the same components as the information-processing diagrams in Chapters 2 and 3. Once a signal has been delivered by a sense organ, the brain must go through four processing steps before the information can be useful to the person with that brain:

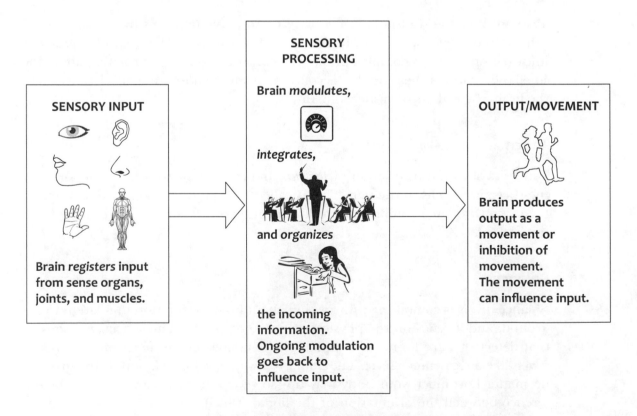

Human sensory/movement processing.

1. Registration
2. Modulation
3. Integration
4. Organization

Registration

Just because a signal is *sent* to the brain does not mean the brain agrees to accept it. The process of accepting a signal is called *registration*. This happens when the brain responds to the signal by beginning to process the information. Signals that are not registered, while they have been physically sent by the sense organ and connecting nerves, just die out on the spot, and the brain does nothing with them. Sometimes, for example, you might not notice a particular background noise, like the humming sound of an air conditioner. The noise is there, and your ears pick it up and send it to the brain, but the brain does not register it, so you're not conscious of the sound.

Modulation

One reason the brain might not register a sound like the hum of an air conditioner is that through a process called *modulation* the brain decides what's most important and then amplifies some input signals and tunes out others. No one's brain could possibly handle all the physical information that hits the sense organs at any given moment. Even if you're just sitting still and alone in a room, there is light reflecting off objects on all sides, sounds coming from inside (the hum from a computer or air conditioner) and outside the room (car engine, lawnmower, birds, dogs barking), and numerous things touching the body (clothing, furniture), as well as odors (cleaning product residue, indoor plants, residual odors in the upholstery and rugs). The human brain cannot efficiently process all the information at once or make any good use of it, so it has to pick and choose. It does so by regulating the amount and type of sensory input it is dealing with at any given time, using a "dial knob" to adjust the amount in gradients—similar to the *attention regulation* process described in Chapter 2 and the *emotion regulation* process discussed in Chapter 4. Two processes are involved in modulation.

Habituation is the process by which the brain initially registers a signal, but then "gets used to" it if it is continuous or repetitive and deemed insignificant by the brain. When you enter a room where an air conditioner is on, you probably hear the hum at first but then gradually become less aware of it. Your ear is still physically picking it up, but the brain is tuning it out because it has decided it's not worth spending the energy to process it.

Sensitization is the process by which the brain initially registers a signal but then amplifies it because it is novel (new) or unexpected and deemed by the brain to be significant or essential to process. The air conditioner sound just mentioned might fade into the background the longer you're in the room, but if it started to fizz, sputter, or hum more loudly, your brain would switch gears and start paying attention. The human brain has evolved to do this because unexpected events or changes in the environment can signal a possible threat and must be attended to. Sensitization to important signals allows us to assess a situation more effectively in case defensive action is necessary. Once the brain has ruled out a threat, it doesn't need to amplify the sensory signal, and it may then fade back via habituation.

A typical human brain can balance sensory habituation and sensitization in a fluid and flexible fashion. It can smoothly change the focus of its processing operation in response to what is going on in the environment. It can also backtrack and affect the actual sensory input. For example, you could turn your head a certain way so that some things to which you've become habituated are no longer in your field of vision and so are not even being picked up by the sense organ.

Integration

Sensory information that has been registered and modulated must then be integrated into sets of information that are already being processed. For example, when you listen to a band or an orchestra, you are literally hearing each instrument, but your brain is integrating each separate piece of auditory information in a way that allows you to experience it as a single and rich event. If your brain could not do that, you would hear a collection of separate sounds that would be experienced as chaotic and/or unpleasant. The same thing happens when you eat something that has several ingredients. Your taste buds are literally taking in the separate chemicals that make up the ingredients and sending all of the signals to the brain, but your brain is integrating it to give you a single flavor experience. Even more interesting is the brain's ability to integrate information coming from different senses. If you walk through a well-designed garden, for example, your enjoyment of this singular experience may really be the result of your brain integrating visual (colors and shapes of the plants and flowers) with olfactory information (fragrances from the flowers).

Organization

Finally, your brain has to organize the sensory information that it has registered, modulated, and integrated. It has to be sorted into categories and then stored for future reference, or discarded if deemed no longer useful or relevant. One simple illustration of this would be sorting sensory experiences into the categories of "pleasant" or "unpleasant." This sorting and storing influences your actions in the future. If you eat a lamb chop and you find the flavor experience unpleasant, your brain will store that piece of information away for future reference, and this will stop you from eating that again. Likewise, if you hear a new song on the radio that you find pleasing, you are likely to seek it out again. Avoiding situations that produce unpleasant sensory experiences (e.g., bad taste could be a signal that something is toxic) and approaching situations that produce pleasant sensory experiences has survival value.

How Sensation and Movement Are Interrelated

Sensation and movement are often studied separately by scientists, but it's very difficult to discuss them separately in a book about your everyday life, because they are so intricately intertwined. Movements are dependent on sensation, and sensation is dependent on movement.

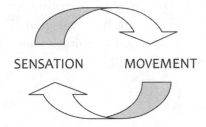

Movement represents the *output* that comes after a bit of sensory information has been processed. For example, you may move to catch a ball, which is *output* after you've processed the *visual* (sensory) information that allowed you to know the ball was coming toward you. Or you may move to uncover a pot on the stove (movement output) after processing the *olfactory* (sensory) information involved in detecting some delicious-smelling food cooking. Or you may move your whole body forward (movement output) after you process the *vestibular* (sensory) information that told you your chair was tipping backward.

Not only is movement part of the output of sensory processing, but it is also very involved in the *input*. As we move around our environments, the changes in our orientation to what is around us produce new sensory input. If you move from one part of a room to another, you may smell something that you did not smell before you moved. The body senses are almost always triggered by movement; moving your hand across a soft blanket triggers a touch sensation, moving through an exercise routine will produce various *vestibular* (balance) and *kinesthetic* (motion) sensations.

Furthermore, movement is very involved in how sense information is *processed*. Its most important role is in the *modulation* of sensory information. If you turn your head to include or exclude something in your field of vision, that motion is going to affect the modulation of certain visual information. Or when you move your hand to shield your eyes from bright sunlight, that motion helps you modulate and regulate the intensity of the visual information.

Our brains perform certain key functions involved in physical movement: *coordination, planning*, and *inhibition* of movement. Specialized movement areas in the brain carry out these operations by communicating with other key parts of the brain.

Coordinating Movements

Most of the tasks of daily living require you to perform a collection of simultaneous movements that are smoothly coordinated. For example, something as simple as walking across a room involves several muscle groups. Your brain has to be able to signal each set of muscles to do certain things at certain times in concert with all the others. Functions that involve the whole body in big movements, like climbing steps, riding a bike, or dancing, are called *gross* motor tasks. Movements that involve our hands in more intricate or small motions, like writing, sewing, or doing a jigsaw puzzle, are called *fine* motor tasks. When you engage in any motor task, gross or fine, your brain is working hard to coordinate the muscle movements so that you can accomplish your goal. The movement called *facial expression* that is so important to social cognition (see Chapter 3) requires coordination of the muscles of the face, just like any other movement.

Planning Movements

Movements of your body require planning by your brain. If you want to take the lid off a pot on the stove to see what's cooking, your brain maps out the movement before you make it. You may not always be aware when this is happening because it is often so rapid, but your brain imagines the motions necessary to uncover the pot even before your arm moves toward doing it.

> **Notes**
>
> ✔ *The brain uses sensory information to help guide the body's movements in several ways:*
>
> 1. *coordination of movements*
> 2. *planning movements*
> 3. *inhibition of movement*

Inhibiting Movements

There are many times a day when your best move is *not* to move, so inhibition of movement can be a very important brain function. Sensory processing often leads the brain to the conclusion that an action should not be carried out. If you smelled something delicious cooking on the stove, you would want to see what it was, you would move toward the stove, and your brain would plan to have you uncover the pot. But when your hand came into contact with the pot lid, your sense of touch might tell your brain that the lid was very hot. Not only would you then move your hand away, but your brain would have to inhibit the initial impulse you had to take the lid off.

Sensory and Movement Differences as Vulnerabilities

The sensory experiences and movements of people on the spectrum are different from those of typical people in a number of ways. These differences can set you up for some extra stress, as they can make common everyday events very difficult to manage.

Sensory Problems

Your senses are the tools that allow you to interface with the environment. You rely on them to bring accurate information to your brain without overloading your nervous system. But the sensory systems of people on the spectrum may *overrespond* to sensory stimulation (hypersensitivity) or *underrespond* (hyposensitivity), meaning your brain may not get the information it needs to help you reach your goals, or your nervous system may be overwhelmed, also blocking you from your goals. Some people with ASDs are overresponsive at some times and underresponsive at others, which can cause a problem with the *modulation* of the incoming sensory information.

Overresponsiveness

If any one or more of your senses is overresponsive, or hypersensitive, you may experience certain sensory experiences as more intense than a neurotypical person might. For some people with ASDs, only one sense is affected, while others may have more than one area of hypersensitivity. This may be happening for you if you find yourself getting overwhelmed or dramatically turned off by certain kinds of light, sound, odors, or foods. You may also find certain kinds of touch or fabric textures very unpleasant, or find yourself easily feeling off balance or unsettled by certain kinds of motion. All of the people presented at the beginning of the chapter were having problems with overresponsiveness. *Charles* is very sensitive to the noise in his work environment and has not found a way to modulate it. *Richard* is hypersensitive to some kinds of light and has not yet found a way to address it. *Carla* is sensitive to the mix of light touch and deep pressure touch that comes with hugs and has learned to deal with it by simply avoiding hugs. See the chart called "Sensory Processing Differences in ASDs" on page 108 for specific examples from each of the seven senses. Scientists have tried to figure out whether overresponsiveness is coming from the sense organs themselves, the nerves that communicate between the organ and the brain, or the brain's use of *sensitization* at the wrong time or in the wrong place. Sensitization is a normal process that occurs in typical brains all the time, but it may just be overused by the ASD brain.

Underresponsiveness

If any of your senses are underresponsive, or hyposensitive, you may be oblivious or numb to sensory experiences that neurotypical people respond to. This may be happening to you if others have told you that you're failing to notice important things, seem indifferent to sights or sounds, seem unaffected by pain or extreme

SENSE	Process	Overresponsive	Underresponsive
	Sight	Low tolerance for certain lights or patterns	Difficulty detecting depth, tracking a moving target, indifference to some visual cues
	Hearing	Low tolerance for certain sounds, exaggerated startle responses to loud or sudden noises, difficulty filtering out background noise	Lack of response or indifference to certain sounds
	Smell	Strong aversions to some smells	Failure to notice some strong smells
	Taste	Strong food aversions	Lack of interest in some foods
	Touch	Sensitivity to light touch, deep pressure, fabric textures, clothing labels, clothing fasteners, or temperature changes, or low pain tolerance	Indifference to temperature extremes, high pain tolerance
	Balance	Easily feeling off balance	Failing to sense when the body is dangerously off balance
	Motion	Low tolerance for movement, inaccurate perception of the position of body parts	Failure to notice movement, resulting in involuntary movement

Sensory processing differences in ASDs.

temperatures, or have a slow response time. Look again at the chart to see specific examples for each of the seven senses. Once again, it's unclear where this problem is based in the sensory processing experience—input or processing (modulation). One possibility is that *habituation*, a normal process, is simply being overused by the brain of a person with ASD.

Modulation Difficulties

Because of the mixed problems of underresponsiveness and overresponsiveness observed in people with ASDs, scientists have recently been studying the *modulation* or regulation processes in people on the spectrum. One way modulation may be problematic in the ASD brain is that, as mentioned above, the brain is failing to discriminate between the best times to use *sensitization* and the best times to use *habituation*. The brain is using both, but the timing or the context is off. For modulation to be most adaptive for a person, the brain has to be able to switch back and forth between sensitization and habituation frequently and for different sensory modalities. For people on the spectrum it may get stuck one way and not switch back and forth in a flexible way. Also, remember from previous discussions about attention (Chapter 2) and emotion (Chapter 4), ASD brains tend to be equipped with on/off switches to control different functions, while neurotypical brains have dial knobs that allow for a more gradated approach to changing the intensity level of experiences. The same applies to sensory modulation—the ASD brain tends to be all on or all off in terms of processing a particular sensory signal.

Now take a look at Worksheet 12 on the next page and check off the statements that sound familiar to you. This will help you see if you are experiencing sensory problems and, if so, pinpoint the specific ways you are being affected.

> ## Notes
>
> ✓ People with ASDs have sensory differences that can be related to three major problems:
>
> 1. overresponsiveness
> 2. underresponsiveness
> 3. problems with modulation of sensory information

Movement Problems

The sensory problems just described have obvious implications for movement. In fact, the senses of balance and motion are going to be discussed again here because, out of all the seven senses, they are the two that are most interconnected with the movement differences experienced by people with ASDs. Those on the spectrum can have movement-related problems with:

- movement coordination
- motor planning
- regulating activity level
- repetitive or involuntary movements

Movement Coordination Problems

Almost all physical tasks and activities involve several muscles, each playing a separate role. Whether it is a gross motor task or a fine motor task, your brain must make sure those muscles are synchronized for the movement to be smooth and efficient. People on the spectrum may have problems with gross motor tasks, fine motor tasks, or both. Examples of gross motor coordination problems might include an unusual gait while walking or running, difficulty with some sports, or awkwardness while dancing. Examples of fine motor coordination problems are difficulty with handwriting, sewing, using utensils, or using hand tools. *Meredith*, who has a law degree and is trying to manage her diabetes while working at a nursery, is affected by fine motor coordination problems. One of the reasons her self-care tasks are so difficult for her is that she often drops important items on the floor (e.g., glucose meter, syringes). This makes the tasks all the more stressful for her.

Sensory Differences

Check off (✓) the statements that sound familiar to you. These may be clues to sensory problems.

☐ I often feel the lights are too bright in some places.

☐ I get a headache from squinting all day at work because the fluorescent lights bother me.

☐ I cannot listen to someone talking to me if there is any background noise at all (TV, radio). I can't tune out the background.

☐ I avoid situations that involve certain sounds (e.g., bells, whistles, buzzers, high-pitched sounds, crowds of talking people).

☐ I don't even notice sounds that seem to bother other people (e.g., sirens, fire alarms).

☐ I can't stand to be around certain smells (e.g., perfumes, cleaning products).

☐ I don't notice odors that seem to bother others (e.g., something rotting in the fridge will be missed by me but not the person I live with).

☐ I have a really limited diet because there are certain foods I love, and the rest I absolutely hate.

☐ I avoid some foods because I can't stand the texture, even if the taste is OK.

☐ I couldn't care less about eating. I do it because I know I need nourishment to survive, but most foods taste bland to me—eating brings me no particular pleasure.

☐ People are surprised by the things I wear in the winter—I don't feel the cold the way others do, and I sometimes go out with no coat or wearing shorts.

☐ I don't seem to notice when it is hot outside—I have to be told by someone else when to stop wearing my winter coat in the spring.

☐ I often feel unsteady on my feet—as if I am going to tip over.

☐ I avoid certain kinds of motions (e.g., won't sit on a swing, can't ride backward on the train).

Motor Planning Problems

For every physical action you carry out, your brain knows about your goal ahead of time, plans for the necessary movements, and helps you initiate them. For example, you may know you have to do the dishes, and may have every intention of doing them, but your brain may not map out the actual physical movements that are needed and/or does not connect a plan to the initiation of a movement. If you have this problem, you are very likely to let the whole evening pass without doing the dishes. Any person you live with has likely labeled you a procrastinator, even though the problem may be neurological. Professionals call brain dysfunction involving motor planning *dyspraxia*.

Regulation of Activity Level

People on the spectrum may have problems regulating their level of activity, which means they may be overactive (hyperactive) or underactive (hypoactive). The hyperactivity has to do with a problem inhibiting movements, which means people with ASDs may not always be able to stop themselves when they have a strong urge or impulse to do something. For this reason, hyperactivity can be a feature of ASDs; many adult patients of mine have been diagnosed with attention-deficit/hyperactivity disorder (ADHD) in the past. This is also related to a tendency to repeat an error, even after the person is well aware that it is an error. For example, if you were using a watering can to water a plant and you spilled the water because you tipped it too fast, you could be unable to stop the error from happening on the next plant because you cannot inhibit the motion of tipping the watering can, so you spill the water again.

The other regulation problem has to do with the initiation of movement. As mentioned in the motor planning section, some people with ASDs are very slow to initiate tasks because that process does not occur naturally for them. Some people on the spectrum report a problem with both initiation and inhibition in that they have difficulty getting started on a task but then find it difficult to stop the task once they get going. Related to the physics concept of inertia, whatever is in motion stays in motion. This can result in problems with time management, scheduling, and getting tasks done on time. *Dan*, the 51-year-old man who is struggling to start a weight-loss program, is being affected by this. While there are many factors that are complicating his efforts, many of which affect neurotypical people as well, Dan's tendency to just keep doing what he is doing, despite knowledge that it is not good for him, is being driven by this "inertia" issue.

Repetitive or Involuntary Movements

The final movement difference is related to the unusual mannerisms many people with ASDs display. Like the sensory issues, these problems are often more pronounced in children and then become less frequent and intense in adulthood, particularly for people with high cognitive ability. However, they are still present, though not constant, in many adults on the spectrum. Examples include finger flicking, hand flapping, body rocking, tics, or facial grimaces. These behaviors can serve a lot of different functions for people on the spectrum, including anxiety reduction or escape from unpleasant tasks. One possible factor, the one most relevant to this discussion, is the need to use repetitive behaviors to regulate sensory experiences. There is some evidence that some of these repetitive movements are a person's way of compensating for the fact that the brain is not properly regulating sensory experiences. So, for example, if your brain is not properly modulating your sense of balance and you have an unpleasant, unsettled feeling, repetitive rocking may actually even things out for you so that you no longer feel off balance. While these movements may be helping the person with an ASD adapt to a difficult challenge, they can have negative consequences if they are too intense (e.g., hitting oneself to regulate an experience can cause injury) or can look odd enough to make others shy away from or ridicule the person. The chart below summarizes how overresponsive or underresponsive senses can be affecting these movement problems.

Now take a look at Worksheet 13 on the facing page and check off the statements that sound familiar to you. This will help you assess whether your life is being affected by movement issues.

Notes

✓ *People with ASDs have movement differences that can be related to four major problems:*

1. *movement coordination*
2. *motor planning*
3. *regulating activity level*
4. *repetitive or involuntary movements*

SENSE	Process	Overresponsive	Underresponsive
	Balance	Difficulty changing speed and direction, contributing to coordination problems	Difficulty staying still, sensation seeking (rocking, crashing into things)
	Motion	Due to inaccurate perception of the position of body parts, lack of coordination	Difficulty inhibiting movement, odd gestures, ticlike mannerisms

Senses most affecting movement differences in ASDs.

Sensory and Movement Differences as Strengths

Two characteristics on Worksheet 3 in Chapter 1 can be more likely to be found in a person with an ASD because of the associated sensory and movement differences. They are *capacity for pleasure* and *perseverance*.

Movement Differences

Check off (✓) the statements that sound familiar to you. These may be clues to movement-related problems.

☐ I often feel clumsy because I drop things and trip over things a lot.

☐ I have never been good at sports involving a ball because I cannot move quickly enough.

☐ I can't seem to sit still, and my hyperactivity sometimes causes problems for me.

☐ I have trouble getting tasks started.

☐ I have never been good with my hands—I can't use tools to fix things.

☐ People tell me I am rocking when I sit for a long time, but I am not even aware that I am doing that.

☐ I can't carry two things at once without dropping something.

☐ My handwriting is so hard for others to read that I try to avoid it altogether.

☐ I sometimes catch myself flapping my hand or flicking my fingers, especially when I am feeling tense or overloaded. It is a habit that I can't seem to break.

The reasons you may have these strengths are both sensory and movement related. Your sensory experiences can be very intense. Your *all-or-nothing* sensation can be overwhelming at times, but when the sensation is pleasant, you will likely experience things in a much richer way than neurotypical people. In terms of movement issues, there may be some physical tasks that you can perform better than others. Despite the coordination problems mentioned earlier, when people on the spectrum do learn and practice a set of movements, they may be better than the average person in that particular area. This might be seen when a person on the spectrum is a gifted musician (fine motor superiority involved in playing an instrument) or athlete (gross motor superiority involved in sports). Also, in another movement area, you may have a tendency to *keep moving once you are moving*. You may have difficulty stopping yourself once you are involved in a task (lack of inhibition), and that can have consequences that are not favorable at times, but it is an asset when you are working on an important task.

All-or-Nothing Sensation

If you have a sense or senses that seem to be more intense in you than in the people around you, your *capacity for pleasure* may be heightened. Depending on what sense is most affected by this, your enjoyment of a sunset, a piece of music, a walk in the woods, a tasty meal, or a ride on a sailboat is going to be so much greater than that of a person without your sensitivity. Likewise, having a talent or gift for either fine motor performance (playing a musical instrument, painting or drawing) or gross motor performance (tennis, baseball, swimming, or dancing) can add to your pleasurable experiences. Your special interest or hobby is likely enhanced by your sensory and motor experiences. I mentioned in an earlier chapter a patient of mine who had become a folk-music enthusiast because it had helped to calm him down when he was anxious. The music was so powerful for him not just because of the lyrics, but also because of the melodies and sounds produced by the instruments.

Charles, the high school teacher who is bothered by his noisy work environment, also has a great appreciation for music of all genres. He enjoys listening to both classical music and opera when he is working on chores by himself on the weekends. In addition, he enjoys classic rock and roll as well as contemporary rock, and this is one arena in which he connects with his son, who is also a music lover, and himself a talented guitar player. *Richard*, who is anxious about going into the community by himself and is affected by fluorescent lighting, also loves hiking in the foothills near his town, even though he rarely gets to go because he will go only if his mom comes along. He finds the views very pleasing, and his sensitivity to visual information is probably enhancing his experience. He also notices that he feels very relaxed and happy after those walks.

Once Moving, Keep Moving

People who have "inertia" issues, who have difficulty getting moving, but also difficulty stopping movement once it starts, are going to be good at task persistence or *perseverance*. If you are working to complete a task that has an outcome that is desirable to you and/or the people around you, you are not likely to quit until it is done. This can lead you to success in many areas, and you may have already noticed that about yourself by this point in your life.

Margaret, the doctor we discussed earlier, got through medical school and her postdoctoral training because of this trait. She encountered many obstacles and difficulties along the way (particularly in the social domain), but she persisted because, once in motion, she stayed in motion. In various workplaces along the way, some people who disliked her personality appreciated her dedication and willingness to stick with a task until it was finished. The same applies to *Meredith*, who managed to complete college and law school with very good grades, despite a lot of obstacles along the way. *Henry*, the 29-year-old man who is unemployed and lives with his father, is also capable of great perseverance. At the moment, this plays out when he is doing Internet job searches. He stays with the task for a long period of time each day. His lack of awareness that this particular technique is not paying off is a problem for him, but once he figures out that he may need to use other strategies, his persistence has the potential to help him in his occupational life.

Sensory and Movement Differences as Strengths

ASD Sensory/Movement Difference		Associated Strengths
All-or-nothing sensory experiences	👍	Capacity for pleasure
Tendency to keep moving once a task is under way	👍	Perseverance

Part II

Positive Solutions for a Quality Life

6

Positive Solutions
Your Bag of Tricks

Part I of this book was designed to show you how your brain may work differently from the brains of neurotypical people and various ways those differences could be contributing to both your struggles and your strengths. Part II will help you use that understanding to define and assess the key sources of stress in your life and then design a solution plan. Starting with Chapter 7, each chapter will offer solutions you can use in a specific area of life that people on the spectrum commonly find stressful. This chapter will orient you to the problem-solving process by introducing you to all the positive solutions that will be referred to throughout the rest of book. As mentioned in the Introduction, these strategies are designed to help you:

- remedy problematic differences that can be improved
- accept and compensate for problematic differences that cannot be changed
- strengthen the positive differences that can enhance your quality of life and promote happiness

As you can see from this list, *problem solving* does not always mean *eliminating* your problem. In this book, *solutions* are strategies meant to alleviate suffering and increase peace of mind. Sometimes that means changing something in your environment. At other times it involves changing something about your behavior. And at still other times it might mean changing only the way you view the problem, coming to *accept* something for what it is. Since acceptance implies a lack of action, it might not on the surface seem like much of a strategy. But if we look again at the definition of intelligence offered in the Introduction, we can see that acceptance is really an active process that is quite compatible with problem solving. To use concepts from the field of positive psychology, you will be most successful if you can:

■ define success in your own terms, which may or may not correspond to societal or conventional definitions of success
■ adapt to, shape, and select the environments you are in
■ do all of the above by capitalizing on your strengths and correcting or compensating for your weaknesses

This concept of success was meant to refer to human beings in general, but of course it is particularly meaningful for you. Your differences from neurotypical people require you to define success in ways that *may not correspond to conventional definitions* and to be an *active* participant in shaping the places in which you live, work, and play. To do that, you must be able to actively *accept* how your mind works, for better and for worse—for better to capitalize on strengths and for worse to compensate and not struggle against a problematic difference.

Problem Solving

Problem solving is an evidence-based therapeutic approach that comes from the field of cognitive-behavioral therapy and has been used to help people with all types of difficulties over the last 40 years. I find it useful with my patients who have ASDs because it is not a single technique as much as it is a *way of thinking* about difficulties. If you can train your brain to think this way, you can approach any problem, no matter where or with whom it is happening, in a more objective way.

Problem solving involves eight steps that were introduced in Chapter 1:

1. **Identify and define your problem.**
2. **Define your goal.**
3. **Identify the obstacles in the way of your achieving the goal.**
4. **List several possible solutions to address the obstacle(s).**
5. **Consider the consequences of each solution.**
6. **Choose the best one(s) to try out first.**
7. **Implement the solution and track your progress.**
8. **Evaluate the solution to see if it met the goal you defined in Step 2.**

These are the steps that you'll follow when you apply all the strategies in Part II. I will walk you through the steps using general instructions in the next few pages, but I don't expect you to master the approach on this first read-through. You will be given more instructions and worksheets as well as specific examples of the steps in every chapter, starting in Chapter 7, when **Blanca** uses the tools to solve one of her home-based problems. Once you get used to the structured steps, you will probably be able to think more clearly about any situation that now feels overwhelming to you, just as Blanca did.

To complete each step, you'll be asking yourself a certain question, shown in

1. **What is bothering me in this situation?**

PROBLEM

2. **How do I wish it could be different?**

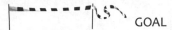

GOAL

3. **What is getting in my way?**

OBSTACLE

4. **What are the possible solutions for the obstacle(s)?**

POSSIBILITY LIST

5. **What are the pros and cons of each solution?**

CONSIDER EACH POSSIBILITY

6. **Which solutions should I try first?**

CHOOSE

7. **Now I will try the solution(s) and track my progress.**

IMPLEMENT AND TRACK

8. **Did the solution meet my goal, or do I need to try a
different solution?**

EVALUATE, CELEBRATE, OR

ADJUST PLAN

Problem-solving steps.

the "Problem-Solving Steps" diagram on page 121. In each chapter in Part II, you will find boxes in which to insert your answers, applied to the specific area of daily living covered in that chapter (e.g., home issues in Chapter 7). Also, a problem-solving worksheet that brings all the steps together is provided at the back of the book, and you can photocopy that as many times as needed to address any problems you have now and in the future.

Problem-Solving Instructions

Step 1: Identify and Define Your Problem

What is bothering me in this area? To start the process of choosing a problem to work on, look back at Worksheet 2, the second clock worksheet you filled out in Chapter 1. What do you wish was different at that time of day? Your answer gives you your first clue as to what kind of problem you would like to address and which chapters you will read. For example, if you are most stressed in the early morning at home, you may end up identifying a home-based problem, which means you will read Chapter 7. Finding that you are most stressed on weekend evenings because you have so few opportunities to socialize might suggest that you are having problems with friendship and should read Chapter 11 and/or dating and should read Chapter 12. If you identified more than one area of your life that you are concerned about, you may read several of the chapters, each one providing you with blank problem-solving question boxes.

Which one should you tackle first? Usually it's best to start with the one that is causing the most distress for you and/or the people around you. There are two ways you can figure that out:

■ *Rank the problems in order of most to least concern on your own.* Look back at Chapter 1 and the checklists you filled out for each of the seven areas of life covered by this book. In which areas did you check off the most concerns? Use Worksheet 14 on the next page if you're having difficulty deciding which problem to work on first. The example from Richard on page 124 shows how he decided to read Chapter 10 first and Chapter 7 second.

■ *Talk this over with someone you trust.* If there's a person in your life who has been helpful to you—listening to you, providing support, or offering guidance—that person may be willing to help you sort out the problems you should be working on by using this book.

Step 2: Define Your Goal

What would you like to see change to minimize the problem you identified? What would have to be different for you to feel less bothered by the problem you identified? The goal you lay out is simply the opposite of the problem you listed.

WORKSHEET 14

Prioritizing Your Problem List

Check off (✓) the areas of your life that are being affected most by problems identified when you filled out the worksheets and checklists in Chapter 1. In which of these areas is your worst time of day? In which of these areas did you check off the most problems? You may pick any number of the following areas. If you choose more than one, rank them in *order* of importance. Think about how much distress the problem causes you and/or the people around you. Put a number 1 next to the highest source of distress, a 2 next to the second highest, and continue until all of your chosen areas have a rank.

PROBLEM AREA	RANKING		CHAPTER
☐ Home	_____	⇨	Chapter 7
☐ Work	_____	⇨	Chapter 8
☐ School	_____	⇨	Chapter 9
☐ Your Community	_____	⇨	Chapter 10
☐ Building Friendships	_____	⇨	Chapter 11
☐ Dating, Sex, and Marriage	_____	⇨	Chapter 12
☐ Health	_____	⇨	Chapter 13

From *Living Well on the Spectrum* by Valerie L. Gaus. Copyright 2011 by The Guilford Press.

Step 3: Identify the Obstacles in the Way of Your Achieving the Goal

What is getting in the way of your goal? Here it is particularly important to consider your ASD characteristics as hidden players in your problem. As you go through this step, you may rely on the information about your ASD differences that you were given in Part I. One of the reasons I gave you so much information about the ASD brain and how it works is so you could put those ideas to use here.

Thinking Differences

"How might my *executive functioning* issues be contributing to my identified problem? For example, do I have difficulty planning, which causes me to procrastinate? Do I find it hard to concentrate on more than one task at time, causing me to get very few things done each day? How might my *negative self-talk* be contributing to my problem? What am I saying to myself that is putting more pres-

Example for Richard
WORKSHEET 14

Prioritizing Your Problem List

Richard is the man introduced in Chapter 1 who is anxious about running errands on his own, but is also frustrated with his restricted life at home. He filled out this sheet as follows:

PROBLEM AREA	RANKING		CHAPTER
☑ Home	_2_	⇨	Chapter 7
☐ Work	_____	⇨	Chapter 8
☐ School	_____	⇨	Chapter 9
☑ Your Community	_1_	⇨	Chapter 10
☐ Building Friendships	_____	⇨	Chapter 11
☐ Dating, Sex, and Marriage	_____	⇨	Chapter 12
☐ Health	_____	⇨	Chapter 13

sure on me? Could I be engaging in perfectionistic thinking, all-or-nothing thinking, or catastrophic thinking? For example, do I set up unrealistic expectations for myself, like 'I must clean out the entire basement in one day or else I am a failure?'"

Social Differences

"How might my *social perception* be contributing to my identified problem? Am I sometimes misunderstanding what another person is trying to tell me? Is it possible that this person is not communicating clearly enough about what he/she expects from me? How might my *social/communication skills* be contributing to my problem? Is my problem caused partly by my not knowing what to say or do when dealing with a key person?"

Emotional Differences

"How might my emotional reactions to things be affecting my identified problem? Do I have difficulty *regulating* my emotions? Do I have difficulty *identifying* my feelings or *asking for help* when I am upset? Do I take too long to calm down after an upsetting incident? Am I over- or underreacting to things that happen in this setting?"

Sensory and Movement Differences

"How might my sensory issues be contributing to my identified problem? Am I *oversensitive* or *undersensitive* to certain types of light, sound, smell, taste, or touch? How could my *movement* and *coordination* issues be contributing to my problem?"

Step 4: List Several Possible Solutions to Address the Obstacle(s)

What are the possible solutions for the obstacles? To answer this question, try to list as many ideas as possible. Sometimes people refer to this process as "brainstorming." Of course, you are probably a literal thinker, and that term could trigger a whole host of bizarre images! But when neurotypical people refer to this process, they don't mean you should have a storm in your brain. What they mean is that you should generate as many possibilities in your mind as you can, in an uninhibited fashion. In other words, don't judge or evaluate any solution that comes to mind—just write it down no matter how weird or silly it seems. You want your brain to be able to produce a blast of ideas without caution, the way a storm produces wind and precipitation. Psychology research has shown that people produce the most useful ideas when they "pull out all the stops" and consider anything and everything. What is the worst thing that can happen if you write down a silly idea? In Step 5 you will weed through them and discard any that are not useful, so no harm can be done.

Of course I don't expect you to know all the strategies that research has found effective in addressing ASD differences. So this chapter includes a section called "Positive Solutions" that lists and explains a lot of them. And at the end of the chapter you'll find a "Cheat Sheet" that shows which types of strategies usually work best for each type of ASD difference. This handy reference will be helpful during all of your brainstorming exercises in the chapters ahead. Finally, try to consider your *strengths* as you complete this step because they also play an important role in your solutions. Refer back to Worksheets 3 and 4 in Chapter 1 for ideas.

Step 5: Consider the Consequences of Each Solution

What are the pros and cons of each solution? Now you will rate each item on your list and put it to the test of how feasible or helpful it will be toward the goal you wrote down in Step 2. You'll use the following scoring system, included on the full problem-solving worksheet, to evaluate each option.

How likely is it to get me closer to my goal?				
Very Unlikely	Pretty Unlikely	Hard to Tell	Somewhat Likely	Very Likely
0	1	2	3	4 ⇨

How much effort, cost, or damage would this strategy involve?				
None	Almost None	Some	A Lot	Extreme
0	1	2	3	4

Step 6: Choose the Best One(s) to Try Out First

Which solutions should I try first? Now that you have scored all of your options, choosing the one or two strategies to start with should be easy. Which of your options had the highest total score? That score demonstrates that, according to your own rating, the highest score has the most benefit compared to the cost, effort, or damage it could involve. If you have two solutions with high scores, you may choose to combine them into one plan that you will implement in the next step.

Step 7: Implement the Solution and Track Your Progress

Now I will try the solution and track my progress. Once you have chosen your strategy, it's time to put it into motion. On the worksheet you will find questions to guide you in making your new plan. With the solution you picked:

- *Where will you do it?* Write down the location(s) in which you will practice the solution.
- *When will you do it?* Write down the times and days you will practice the solution.
- *What do you need to do it?* Write down any materials you may need to practice the solution.
- *How will you do it?* Write down what you will be doing in the location and time mentioned above.
- *Who can help you, if needed?* You don't have to do this alone. Write down the name of any person you think may be helpful to you in the process.
- *How will you keep track of your success?* Look back at your goal. Turn that statement into something that could be measured. Then pick a way to keep track of it. Choose from the following list or design your own measuring technique.
  - *Keep a running count.* If your goal is to increase or decrease the frequency of something (e.g., I want to leave the house on time *more often* in the next month), find some way to keep track of occurrences. You can choose whatever approach is going to be easiest for you, such as:
    - keep a log of relevant instances on a simple piece of lined paper
    - keep a log of relevant instances in your PDA, cell phone, smart phone, or computer

◆ make a checkmark (✓) or tally mark (/) on your calendar for every relevant instance

◆ throw a penny, marble, or chip into a jar each time you observe a relevant instance

● *Use a rating scale.* If your goal is to change your subjective feeling about something (e.g., "I want to *feel less nervous* when I go to the bank; or I want to *feel more confident* when I go out on a date"), do a daily rating of that feeling. Here is a simple rating scale you can use for any feeling. Just fill in the blank with the feeling you are trying to change and write down your rating every day or every time you are in the relevant situation.

Today I felt _____ to the following degree:										
0	1	2	3	4	5	6	7	8	9	10
None		A Little			Moderate			A Lot		Extreme

Step 8: Evaluate the Solution to See If It Met Your Goal

Did the solution meet my goal, or do I need to use a different solution? At this point, you have tried out your new solution. To see if it helped you meet your goal, tally up the data you collected and look at the trend. Then answer the following question as a method of evaluating your progress.

How would you rate your success, on a scale of 0–100% success for meeting your goal?										
0	10	20	30	40	50	60	70	80	90	100
None		A Little			Moderate			A Lot		Total

Positive Solutions

The problem-solving steps just described will lead you to effective solutions to whatever problem you're addressing. In this section I'll give you a collection of solutions from which you can choose—eight sets of strategies that have proven helpful to people dealing with the differences common among people on the spectrum:

■ Environmental modifications
■ Organizational techniques

- Scheduling techniques
- Relaxation techniques
- Emotion regulation techniques
- Thinking techniques
- Techniques to understand other people
- Communication techniques

I did not design any of the strategies I'm about to describe. They are drawn from the scientific and clinical literature on what has been shown to help adults with the problems associated with ASDs, and my patients have found them useful in solving their own unique problems. Which ones work best for you will depend on your personal circumstances. Think of the problem-solving model as a train that I have invited all readers to ride. The individual solutions represent different stops along the route, and each reader will decide which "stations" are most important to him or her.

One way you'll decide is by completing Step 3 and knowing which ASD differences are obstacles to reaching your goal. Each set of strategies (or "station") is most useful with certain ASD differences. Across the top of the "Cheat Sheet" chart on page 164 are the four major ASD differences, and down the far left column are the solutions described in this chapter. If you know from Step 3 that *thinking differences* are at play in a problem, for example, you'll see dots in the boxes for environmental modifications, organizational techniques, scheduling techniques, and thinking techniques. This means these sets of strategies are the ones to try *first*, because they have been shown in the scientific and clinical literature to be most effective for that problem.

If you try a number of the strategies you've identified using the Cheat Sheet and feel you're making little progress, you may need the help of a licensed practitioner, such as a mental health professional, speech–language pathologist, or occupational therapist. Chapter 14 presents a set of guidelines you should follow to figure out if you need professional help.

On the other hand, you might find that you get even more benefit than you expected from your problem solving. Because ASD differences overlap in real life, one strategy could actually help reduce the problems created by more than one ASD difference. You could, for example, make an environmental modification to cut down on the background noise that is making you tense in your office and find that the strategy helps not only with your sensory differences but also with your thinking differences, improving your ability to concentrate on your work.

And if you find that a particular strategy works so well for you that you'd like to learn more about it (or find other, similar solutions), you may decide to do some further reading about it. The list of resources at the end of this book includes many relevant books, CDs/DVDs, and websites related to these topics.

Environmental Modifications

These approaches—changing something about your physical surroundings to help yourself—should be considered first when you're struggling with *thinking* differences, particularly executive function problems, or with *sensory/movement* differences. Some examples:

- Changing a light bulb or fixture to change brightness or color
- Moving furniture to make a room or office easier to use in some way
- Adding a white noise generator (sleep sound machine) to a room to screen out some other type of noise
- Making wardrobe changes to appear neater while also accommodating a touch sensitivity
- Installing or changing a window treatment to modify light coming into a room or office
- Changing the type of bag and/or wallet used to carry personal items throughout the day
- Changing the type of clock used in a room or adding a certain type of clock to a room
- Changing where something is stored to make it more accessible

The environmental checklist (Worksheet 14) on the next page is useful for assessing the environmental factors that you may be able to change to help you function better in a specific space.

Organizational Techniques

When you're struggling with *thinking* differences, particularly executive function problems, organizational techniques are another set of strategies to try first. These approaches branch off from the preceding environmental modifications but involve several more steps. You are indeed modifying the environment when you organize, but you're doing more than just adding or moving one thing. Here you're designing a system to make an environment really work for you. The main objectives of any organization system are:

1. to keep the things you need from day to day accessible and easy to find
2. to prevent things from getting lost
3. to reduce or eliminate clutter

Some examples of organizational systems are:

- a filing system at home that keeps your important papers and bills in order and easy to find
- a filing system at your office to help keep your assignments in order and easy to find

Environmental Checklist

Use this when considering changes to the environment to help with thinking and sensory/ movement differences. Bring this checklist and walk through the environment in which you are having some difficulty. Answer the questions one by one. Don't be surprised if you notice something important that you never did before.

☐ *Lighting:* Look at the lighting source and focus on it. Is it natural light (window/skylight), fluorescent, or incandescent? Is it a possible irritant for you? If so, can it be changed? If not, can you accommodate to it somehow (e.g., hat with visor, dark glasses)?

☐ *Noise:* Close your eyes and listen for a minute. What do you hear? A lot of people talking to each other? Mechanical sounds coming from machines or electronic devices (e.g., buzzing, humming, banging)? Is there noise coming from outside the room? Is it too quiet for your comfort? Could any of these noise factors be irritants? If so, can anything be changed? If not, can you accommodate to it (e.g., with earplugs, iPod, white noise/soothing sound machine)?

☐ *Air quality/smell:* Close your eyes and take a deep breath. Are there any unpleasant odors? Does the air seem stuffy? Could there be irritants in the air? If so, can anything be changed? If not, can you accommodate to it (e.g., frequent breaks involving a walk outside)?

☐ *Food:* If your problem centers around a mealtime, are food choices that meet your needs and tastes available to you? Can you change the menu? If not, can you prepare your own food, do your own shopping, or make some other accommodation?

☐ *Temperature:* Is it too hot or too cold? If so, and if that's an irritant for you, can it be changed? If not, can you accommodate to it (e.g., different clothing choices)?

☐ *Clothing:* Is there a dress code or uniform in this setting? Do your clothes irritate your skin, feel scratchy or painful? If so, can that be changed, or can you accommodate to it?

☐ *Furniture:* Look at the furniture in the setting. Is it arranged in a way that makes you uncomfortable or makes it hard to get around? Is your chair, bed, or desk uncomfortable? Is it possible the furniture is irritating you in some way? If so, can it be changed? If not, can you accommodate to it?

☐ *Crowding:* Are you in close physical proximity to a lot of other people? Is there a lot of movement around you, others too close, bumping into you, touching your arms or shoulders, shaking hands, or hugging more than you are comfortable with? If so, could this be changed by simply moving where you sit or changing which rooms you use?

- an incoming–outgoing station by your main door so you don't need to search for the most important things on your way out
- a system for storing tools at home or work so that they are easy to identify and access
- a routine for discarding unnecessary items
- a well-designed system for your purse, wallet, briefcase, or backpack to have only the things you need every day and to make them easy to reach quickly
- a system in your car glove compartment or console to ensure you have necessary items on hand and easy to access

If you've already tried a lot of simple organizing systems but ended up frustrated because they've fallen apart, it will help to know why this happens so commonly and what you can do to make such ideas work.

Why Organization Systems Fail

It's not setting up organization systems that's so hard; it's maintaining them. Here's why they crumble so easily:

1. *The system is too complicated or ambitious.* Enthusiasm when starting out can lead you to make the system too elaborate and therefore hard to use. For example, using 15 different colors in a color-coded filing system can make it hard to remember from day to day which colors represent which category. Losing track kills enthusiasm quickly.

2. *The tools are hard to use.* Tools that create a struggle for you every day are hard to stick with. One patient of mine bought a big multicompartment pill organizer to help him keep track of his many medications, but the compartment lids were difficult to open, and he would sometimes drop the whole container on the floor while trying to pop them open. Soon he got so frustrated with it that he stopped using it.

3. *The system is not easily accessible.* One reason for an organization system is to neaten up a space, which often means putting the system out of sight, such as in a closet or drawer. But if it is tucked away too thoroughly, it can lose its usefulness. A patient of mine who had a large extended family bought a special organizer that stored greeting cards and had a built-in calendar to remind her of important family events to commemorate. She put the organizer inside one of her bottom drawers, behind her billing paperwork—where she either forgot to refer to it or had trouble digging it out. She ended up missing several important family birthdays and discarded the organizer.

4. *The system does not capitalize on the user's strengths.* Whether or not you realize it, you have preferences for how you like information to be presented. You may find it easier to pay attention to visual than to auditory information (e.g., a colorful sign will grab your attention more than a sound alarm). You may prefer nonverbal over verbal information (e.g., pictures over words). You might respond well to tactile cues over visual or sound information (e.g., prefer the vibrate mode over the ringtone on your cell phone). If your ability to notice and remember pictures were much stronger than your ability to remember words, how do you think you'd do with a filing system that has folders all one color with nothing but words on the labels? Unfortunately, most of us learn organizational strategies from others or try to use systems designed by a manufacturer even when they don't take advantage of our own individual strengths. Your father's system for filing his bills, your Uncle Ted's system for organizing his tools, or your grandmother's system for storing her spices may not necessarily work for you.

5. *There is no set time to do maintenance tasks.* It's easy to get caught up in spending money (sometimes a lot of money) on filing systems, shelving systems, drawer organizers, pill boxes, and numerous other amazing gadgets designed to help you get organized. The trouble is that these structural tools don't maintain themselves. If you don't regularly refer to the system, put things away in their proper place, and discard items you no longer need, even the fanciest physical structure will be useless.

Tips for Organizational Success

Here are some tips to help you avoid organizational pitfalls.

1. *Keep it simple.* Focus on only one area you want to improve and try not to address too many things at once. If a messy bathroom were interfering with your daily grooming routine, you might think you had to organize the entire room before feeling some relief. Instead, you could pick one shelf or drawer as your "daily grooming" area and focus only on setting up that space to work well for you. The rest of the bathroom would still be important but would not have to be done all at once. Similarly, a cluttered space at work that was causing you to turn in assignments late wouldn't have to be overhauled; instead you could clean up the top of the desk or a top drawer to make it functional for everyday use.

2. *Choose tools that are very easy to use.* If you were organizing a bathroom or office area, you would not use a drawer that tends to stick or a shelf that is wobbly. Instead you would choose a drawer or cabinet that is easy to open. Any containers used in your system should also be easy to open and close.

3. *Make sure your system is easily accessible.* The personal grooming area discussed above shouldn't be a shelf on the bottom of an out-of-the-way closet, and your organized office space shouldn't be the rear area of a bottom file drawer. You'd want a shelf or drawer within arm's length when you are standing at your bathroom sink or sitting at your desk.

4. *Design it to tap your strengths.* Think about the mode you prefer when processing information—this is what we call your thinking style. Which sensory modality is your preferred "channel"? Which is prone to grab your attention and help you remember? Worksheet 16 on page 134 will help you figure out which is your favorite channel. Your organizational system is most likely to work if you set it up to tune in to your favorite channel—or, better yet, *multiple* strong channels.

5. *Schedule a regular time to maintain it.* If you have difficulty with the executive functions, a thinking difference described in Chapter 2, you will need to pay special attention to the three activities involved in maintenance: regularly checking the system, putting things away or stocking it, and removing things you no longer need.

Notes

Tips for Organizational Success

✓ Keep it simple.

✓ Choose tools that are very easy to use.

✓ Make sure your system is easily accessible.

✓ Design the system to tap your strengths.

✓ Schedule a regular time for maintenance:

☐ Check it

☐ Put away or replace needed items

☐ Remove and discard unnecessary items

In the bathroom example, you would look at it every day, use what is there for your grooming routine, take notice of things that are running low (e.g., toothpaste, shaving cream, lip balm), replace things that have run out, and discard empty containers or things you are no longer using (e.g., if you switched to a new type of razor, discard or store elsewhere the one you are not using every day). For an office space, you would need to check it every day and make sure it is stocked with all the office supplies you use daily (e.g., rubber bands, staples, paper clips, pens, Post-It notepads). Don't wait until you run out of something to refill it—that may lead to interruptions of your work flow; rather you would want to make sure it is stocked before you begin your work each day. You may need to set up reminders in your schedule (techniques for scheduling are covered next) to cue you to do your routine maintenance. The Organizational Checklist on page 135 can be a useful setup and maintenance tool.

Scheduling Techniques

Scheduling techniques are another set of strategies that should be considered first when you're struggling with *thinking* differences, particularly executive function problems related to planning and time management. Most people rely on a schedule of some sort to guide them through the day, week, month, and year. Even following a budget falls into this category as it requires you to plan and schedule the use of your money. As a person with an ASD, you may have thinking differences that make it particularly difficult to plan ahead and also to adopt new routines. If you are struggling with these types of issues, you may not be following any

My Favorite Channels

Use this worksheet to assess your thinking style—your best means of *paying attention* and *remembering* information.

1. When you take in new information, do you pay more attention to things that you (circle one)

 see   hear   touch/feel   depends

2. When you have to remember something, are you more likely to remember things you (circle one)

 saw   heard   touched/felt   depends

3. When you take in new information, do you pay more attention to (circle one)

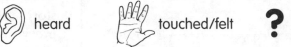 words   nonverbal info   depends

4. When you have to remember something, are you more likely to remember things as (circle one)

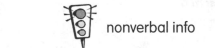 words   nonverbal info   depends

SUMMARY

Look at your answers to questions 1 and 3 to fill in the blanks:

My favorite channels for new information are _____ and _____.

Look at your answers to questions 2 and 4 to fill in the blanks:

My favorite channels for remembering things are _____ and _____.

Organizational Checklist

Use this when cleaning out and organizing a small personal space that is used every day, like a purse, backpack, briefcase, book bag. These tricks are meant to keep the space easy to use, ensure that you always have essential things on hand, and prevent those things from getting lost.

☐ Empty the space and spread the contents out on a clear work surface.

☐ Sort the items into these piles:

- I use this every day
- I use this once a week
- I use this once a month
- I have not used this in over one month
- This is garbage

☐ Is there anything you need at least weekly that is missing from the piles? Get it and add it to the right pile.

☐ Put the items away as follows:

- I use this every day → Place in a pocket that is easily accessible. → Keep a second one in an out-of-the-way place in the space as a backup.
- I use this once a week → Place it in a slightly less accessible space.
- I use this once a month → Place it in the space, but out of the way.
- I have not used this in over one month → Throw it out or store it at home.
- This is garbage → Throw it away.

☐ Go through this space once a week in the same way—build it into your schedule.

schedule at all, or you may be trying to follow one that is not really functioning for you. Some of the scheduling techniques described here include points you may recognize from the section on organizational techniques. That's because in many ways scheduling *is* an organizational technique, only you are organizing your time instead of your space. The main objectives of a schedule are to:

1. structure your time and create consistency in your life
2. help you plan the use of your time to ensure key tasks will get done
3. remind you to follow through with planned tasks and commitments and avoid conflicts (e.g., promising to be in two different places at the same time)

Being able to design and follow a schedule that matches your own thinking style (favorite channels) is crucial for you to be able to manage daily tasks that may be stressful for you. Some examples of scheduling techniques are:

- using a monthly calendar to write down important appointments and social activities
- using a weekly calendar to write down your work schedule
- using a daily checklist to write down key tasks for the day along with the times at which they will be completed
- using an electronic calendar (in your computer, PDA, or smart phone) to keep track of appointments and commitments
- using a calendar to ensure a regular sleep schedule
- using a calendar to ensure that you schedule pleasant events
- using a budget worksheet to plan and schedule the use of your money

As with organizational techniques, you may feel frustrated by having tried scheduling techniques that haven't worked for you. Here, too, there are common pitfalls that you can learn to avoid.

Why Schedules Fail

Schedules fail for many of the same reasons organizational systems fail, so some of the following points will be familiar to you.

1. *The schedule is too complicated or ambitious.* Sometimes people try to enter too much information, which makes the schedule hard to follow. Also, if you try to put more tasks in a day than you really have time to complete, you are setting yourself up for frustration and disappointment.

2. *The scheduling device is not easily accessible or is too easy to lose.* Whether using a paper or electronic calendar, keeping it where it's not at your fingertips is a common mistake. So is choosing a device that's easy to leave behind or lose. Keeping your schedule on a laptop computer will be effective only if you have your laptop whenever you make time commitments. On the other hand, if a pocket-sized book that seemed handy because you could tuck it into a pocket repeatedly gets lost, it's also of little use to you.

3. *The scheduling device does not capitalize on the user's strengths.* Look back at the "My Favorite Channels" worksheet that you filled out for the organization section. If you have a preference for taking in and remembering information using sound and nonverbal types of cues, for instance, none of the dozens of paper calendars and books in every stationery store is likely to work for you. But if you need verbal, visual reminders, it won't make much sense to use a PDA or smart phone that gives you audible reminders.

4. *There is no system for regularly checking and updating the schedule or calendar.* If you don't interact with your calendar regularly, it obviously won't remind you of appointments when you need a cue, and you won't add important dates to it.

Tips for Scheduling Success

To avoid common pitfalls, follow these guidelines for your schedule.

1. *Keep it simple.* Don't clog your schedule with commitments you can remember without it or with tasks you perform automatically, like getting dressed or brushing your teeth. Also try not to commit to too many things in one day. How do you know how much is too much? Base it on your past experiences, not on what someone else is pressuring you to do. For example, one patient of mine who has some chronic medical problems would always get very stressed if he had more than one doctor's appointment within a week. He had the habit of accepting the first appointment offered to him by a given receptionist, not realizing he could choose if he asked for options. Once he began carrying a calendar with him to all appointments, he could more easily ensure that he did not allow his appointments to be made too close together.

2. *Make it accessible.* Whether you are using a paper or electronic schedule, make sure you keep it nearby when you'll need it—and secure so it won't get lost. For the way your space is set up, are you most likely to see it if you keep it on your desk or night table, hanging on a wall, on your computer screen, in your phone, in your book bag, or in your briefcase?

3. *Choose a format that matches your strengths.* Look back at the "My Favorite Channels" worksheet that you filled out for the organization section. Use your answers to look up the best types of tools for you on the "Tools for My Favorite Channels" guide on the next page. Based on that, would you be better served by an electronic calendar or schedule, like the ones that can be found on a computer, PDA, or smartphone? Or would you find it easier to look at a paper calendar? If so, is it better if it is a single sheet of paper or in a booklet format? Whether it is electronic or paper, do you find it easiest to look at one day at a time, one week at a time, or the whole month at one time? Do you prefer to use pictures and colors to highlight important commitments and appointments? Do you need to set alarms to remind yourself to check the schedule? If so, are you best off with a nonverbal sound (beep or ring), a prerecorded spoken message, or a written message (e.g., programming your phone to send you a text message at a given time)? Remember as you answer each of these questions, you have to make this work for you in your own way. Don't automatically try to set it up the way someone else you know has his or hers set up. What works for another person may not work for you and vice versa.

4. *Build in a regular time for maintenance.* Remember that your schedule will only work as well as the user does in terms of upkeep. Try to set aside a time of day when you will look over your schedule. At that time, note any changes that may have arisen and double-check what you have to do during that week. Also, be vigilant about entering new information as you get it. For my patient who had

TOOLS FOR MY FAVORITE CHANNELS	Verbal		Nonverbal	
Sight	Written notes/ signs/text messages		Pictures and colors	
Sound	Spoken messages		Sound alarms	
Touch	N/A		Vibrating alarms	

Notes

<u>Tips for Scheduling Success</u>

✓ Keep it simple.

✓ Make sure your system is easily accessible.

✓ Choose a format that taps your strengths.

✓ Build in a regular time for maintenance:

☐ Check it

☐ Update it

trouble scheduling his doctor's appointments, taking the calendar along worked so much better than waiting until he got home to enter the new appointments. Even though the receptionists would always give him appointment cards, transferring the information from the card to the calendar after he got home was an extra step that he often forgot to take.

Relaxation Techniques

Relaxation techniques should be considered when your stressful situations seem to involve *emotional* and *sensory/movement* differences. Stress involves the mind and the body. People on the spectrum are more prone than others to have problems related to overarousal. As mentioned before, your body can become very tense and stay that way for prolonged periods, which is not good for your mental or physical health. *You need to have strategies* for bringing down the physical tension that can come from prolonged emotional arousal. You may find that you should just keep doing some of the things you already do to relax yourself or do them more often. Or you might find some of the ideas in the next few paragraphs helpful. Remember, though, that just because these ideas work for some other people there is no guarantee that they'll work for you. What is relaxing is a very individual experience. If any of these activities lead you to feel calmer, they are good ideas for you. Don't consider anything that would cause you stress or would be unpleasant (e.g., you would not choose to watch sports if you hate sports). Keep in mind that your goal should always be to help your body become calm, not just your mind.

Formal Arousal-Reducing Techniques

In the 40 years since they were first used to help patients with anxiety disorders, formal relaxation techniques have had many different applications and many specific exercises have been developed. These approaches are usually based on scripts that are read to you by a therapist and recorded onto a listening device so you can practice at home. You can also buy tapes and CDs that have a prerecorded voice instructing you through the exercises. The three types of formal arousal-reducing techniques are described briefly here, and the Resources at the back of the book list several references and recordings that you can choose from to find the approach that works best for you. Each of these types of exercises can be helpful alone, but they are often combined for maximum benefit.

BREATHING EXERCISES

Based on the idea that anxiety is perpetuated by maladaptive breathing patterns, these relaxation approaches are designed to help you focus on how you are breathing. Some exercises help you use your belly muscles (diaphragm) to breathe because you take deeper breaths that are more conducive to relaxation than the shallower breaths that come from chest breathing and sometimes contribute to an increase in anxiety. Other exercises are geared toward simply slowing the rate of your breathing. Breathing exercises alone can be helpful, or they can also enhance the effectiveness of the approaches described next.

PROGRESSIVE MUSCLE RELAXATION EXERCISES

The tension associated with anxiety and anger can be found throughout your body, particularly in your muscles. Progressive muscle relaxation exercises teach you how to become more aware of and release the tension in particular muscles to put your muscles in a state of relaxation. There are many protocols for doing this, and you have to try a few of them out before you can settle on the one that helps you the most. All of the approaches categorize the muscles into key groups and then walk you through the process of locating tension and then letting it go. Some of them do this by having you deliberately tense each muscle group to become more aware of what tension feels like. Here is what a segment of such a protocol might look like:

"Tense the muscles in your right hand by making a fist. After you have made a fist, try to tighten it even further. Pay attention to how the muscles feel as you hold your hand in a tense position. After a few seconds, release the fist and let your hand go back into a resting position. Pay attention to how the muscles feel right now. Notice the difference between the feeling you had when it was tense and the feeling you have right now in that hand. Now tense the hand again. Make another fist. Hold it as tight as you can and notice how it feels. After a few seconds, let it go again. Notice once again how different your hand feels now."

This type of approach, alternating tension with relaxation, will take you through all of the muscles in your body, grouped into categories such as these:

- hands and arms
- arms and shoulders
- shoulders and neck
- jaw
- face and nose
- stomach
- legs and feet

Other progressive muscle relaxation approaches, called "passive" protocols, will also take you through all of the muscles but do not include the step of deliberately tensing the muscles before relaxing them. So, for example, they may just direct you to notice and release the tension in your hand muscles but would not ask you to make the fist first.

VISUALIZATION EXERCISES

These approaches are also called "guided imagery" exercises. These also have the objective of decreasing tension in the body, but they guide you to think about all types of pleasant images and sensations, using your imagination. While your body parts may be mentioned in the scripts, there is less of a focus on the muscles per se and more on the overall pleasant sensations that can bring about relaxation. So, for example, you might be directed to close your eyes and think about a special place that you have found relaxing. You would be asked to picture yourself in that place, taking in all parts of that experience through your senses, using your imagination. You may also be asked to imagine your body as some type of empty vessel (like a vase or a jar) that is being filled up with a warm or soothing liquid, which is one common theme in these types of exercises.

Pleasant sensations are a highly subjective business. Even neurotypical people differ from one another in the types of sensations they find soothing or pleasing. As a person on the spectrum, your own sensory system, as you learned in Chapter 5, may be unique. Therefore, these types of visualization exercises have the potential to be very helpful if the right sensory image is captured for you, but some may be highly unpleasant as well. You would need to sample a few of these, or create your own, to find one that has a soothing effect on you.

Formal Mindfulness Techniques

Mindfulness is a term that refers to a set of practices that have evolved over thousands of years to help people notice and accept the present. Rooted in ancient cultures and religions and integrated into mental health treatment only recently, it encompasses various techniques that people can practice to bring their attention into the present moment and away from the past or the future. *Mindfulness* practices will be described in more detail under thinking techniques in this chapter, but I mention them here because of their calming value. These techniques differ from the arousal-reducing strategies described above in that they simply ask you to notice things but *not to try to change* them. The only thing you are directed to do is to modify the way you are using your *attention*. So, for example, where the breathing exercises above will teach you to change how you breathe, mindfulness exercises will simply help you *notice* your breath. The objective is not to relax you per se, but when people practice mindfulness exercises on a regular basis they tend to approach their lives in an overall calmer state. There are two ways you can build these practices into your life:

MEDITATION

This can take many forms, both secular and religious in nature. The objective of all meditation practices is to help you learn to use your attention in new ways to notice and accept the things that are happening inside your body, mind, and environment in the present moment and without judgment. You can find exercises as short as 5 minutes and as long as several days, depending on how much time you can invest. You may already practice meditation of some sort, which may include prayers if you are an active participant in your religion. You can find many books and audio recordings to guide you through meditation practices, and a sampling can be found in the Resources at the end of the book.

YOGA

Yoga really is a type of meditation practice, but it has a very active physical component, where exercises are geared toward having you focus and attend to what is happening in your body. It has the added benefit of physical exercise and can help you improve your physical condition. The resources at the back of the book list books, CDs, and DVDs that I have selected with people on the spectrum in mind. Also, you may consider taking a few classes to find out if this is a viable tool for you. I suggest starting with a simple continuing education class at your local library, high school, or community center so that your monetary investment can be kept to a minimum. Yoga is not enjoyable for everyone, so you want to be able to test it out without spending too much. While there are specialized yoga centers you can join, they often charge high membership fees and require commitments to terms that are not beneficial unless you are sure that yoga is a good practice for you.

Informal Self-Soothing Techniques

These techniques involve the use of a pleasant activity to enhance positive mood, reduce tension, or distract you during moments of extremely high anxiety. As a person on the spectrum, you may have a special interest or activity that you already use to reduce tension. People with ASDs often have a preferred activity that they spend a lot of free time pursuing. You do need to exercise caution when using your special interest because, if used to an extreme, it can become an unhealthy escape tactic—one you turn to so as to avoid something unpleasant in your life that does need your attention (e.g., a car enthusiast who spends hours surfing the Internet looking for car parts to avoid doing his banking and budgeting). With that said, your interest or hobby really can serve as a self-soothing, mood-enhancing tool if exercised thoughtfully.

PLEASANT EVENTS

Examples of pleasant activities that you can do without much planning or commitment are:

- listening to music
- taking a walk
- hiking through a natural setting
- walking through a public garden
- painting
- making something from clay
- playing with a dog
- planting something outside
- writing in a journal
- taking a warm bath
- drawing
- petting a cat
- watching your favorite sport
- watching a movie
- reading a book on your favorite subject

COMPANION ANIMALS

While owning an animal is not an option or desire for every reader, the idea is being mentioned here because there is a growing body of research to support the benefits of owning a pet. It certainly requires a bigger commitment than the ideas in the previous list (e.g., watching a movie), but the anxiety-reducing effects that pets can have for people on the spectrum has been documented. Whether you are interested in tiny fish, large horses, or any of the creatures that come in the sizes in between, caring for your pet and letting your pet care for you can be a very useful relaxation technique for many people on the spectrum.

Emotion Regulation Techniques

Emotion regulation techniques should be considered when your stressful situations seem to involve *social* or *emotional* ASD differences. In Chapter 4 you learned about the emotional differences that people on the spectrum are prone to and the ways in which those differences can contribute to problems. You may not be aware of emotions as you experience them, or may not be able to easily put a label on the feeling you're having. Likewise, you may have observed that you either overreact or underreact to important events that occur in your day-to-day life. These emotion regulation difficulties can be addressed if you can teach yourself to be more aware of the nature and purpose of the feelings you are having. Because these strategies are being applied during problem solving, I am going to focus only on the unpleasant emotions, as they are most likely to cause problems if not regulated effectively. To address your emotion regulation difficulties, you need to have the skills to:

- recognize that you are upset and to what degree
- label the emotion involved
- identify the purpose of that emotion or the need being signaled by it

- accept your emotion without judgment
- attend to relevant things in the environment that may help you address your need
- take action to address your need

You may refer back to Chapter 4 to review the basic emotions and the reasons human beings have them. The worksheet called "Understanding My Emotions" on the next page was designed to guide you through these processes after an upsetting event. These skills take a lot of practice, so you may choose to discuss your worksheet with someone you trust the first few times you fill it out. These are complex operations that are not yet automatic for you, so the help of a trusted second opinion can be invaluable as you work on this type of exercise.

Thinking Techniques

Thinking techniques make up a set of strategies that should be considered when you're having problems with *thinking*, *social*, or *emotional* differences. Chapter 2 discussed the thinking differences you may have and the ways they can contribute to problems and strengths. Two types of problems were discussed: problems with the *management* of information (i.e., executive functions) and with the *interpretation* of information. The techniques already described for environmental modification, organizing, and scheduling all address the management problems, so they will not be covered here. This section will focus on the techniques that can be most helpful with the problematic interpretation of information that people on the spectrum are prone to. Remember, these tendencies contribute to some of your strengths, but they can also contribute to a great deal of stress for you. They are:

- a tendency to look at details more than the whole
- a tendency to see things in an all-or-nothing fashion; things are black or white, all good or all bad, and there is very little attention to dimensions or "shades of gray"

Understanding My Emotions

For use when evaluating an upsetting event.

Fill this out soon after an event during which you found yourself very upset.

_____

Date and time of event: _____

1. Briefly describe the event: *I was upset when* _____

_____

2. Now look at the words, pictures, and synonyms below. On the top row are the basic negative emotions, and underneath are some common words that have similar meanings. Which of these emotions do you suspect was involved in your reaction to the event? Circle the relevant emotion. You can circle more than one.

Sadness	Anger	Fear
Depressed	Enraged	Terrified
Miserable	Annoyed	Anxious
Devastated	Frustrated	Tense
Down	Irritated	Nervous

3. *I felt* _____, *which may be a signal that I needed something.*

4. *Maybe I needed* _____

5. *Feeling* _____ *is a natural part of life and I accept that I felt that way.*

6. Now think about what was around you that may have helped you meet your need. This could be an object or a person. *I could have used* _____

_____

to help me meet my need.

7. *In circumstances like these, I may* _____
    to address my need.

The two most helpful approaches for these types of thinking habits are *mindfulness* techniques and *dimensional* thinking techniques.

Mindfulness Techniques

Introduced on page 141, *mindfulness* is a term that refers to an approach to life that involves a multitude of habits you can learn to help you *notice* and *accept* things about your present moment. It is quite a broad term that encompasses the ancient prayer and meditation practices of several world religions, as well as some secular exercises that can be found in modern-day motivational and mental-health-promoting techniques. The assumption behind all of these approaches is that when human beings focus their attention on past or future events and make judgments about those events, they cause themselves to suffer. People tend to spend so much time thinking about something that has already happened (e.g., obsessing about some action that you did or didn't take, ruminating in a guilty way about something you did or didn't say) or about things that have not happened yet (e.g., worrying about an upcoming family gathering, fretting about a scheduled exam) because they are trying to avoid or suppress a painful feeling. Related to that is a desire to control things over which we have no control. While it's natural for people to want to escape painful situations and emotions, when people follow those urges, they ironically cause themselves to feel even more pain in the long run. Mindfulness allows you to stay in the present *even when* it involves uncomfortable or unpleasant feelings. This does not come naturally to human beings, so it is fitting that the exercises involved are called "practices." To be able to stay in the present and accept what is there for what it is, people need to train themselves and then practice, practice, practice.

Mindfulness techniques can be helpful to you because, as noted several times in this book, people with ASDs have difficulty regulating the focus of their attention. You may have difficulty *shifting* your attention from one thing to the next, and you also may have a tendency to focus intently on a detail in a given scenario, which can cause you to miss other important details or to miss the big picture. If you think of your attention ability as a tool, mindfulness practices help you put conscious effort into experimenting with new uses for that tool.

Imagine that your attention ability is a pair of glasses. Let's say you've worn the same pair of glasses every day for many years. You are so accustomed to them that you're not even conscious of their presence on your face. They work the same way for you every day, and you take for granted the way you see the world around you through the lenses. One day you decide to experiment with looking through them in a different way. You become curious about how images would appear if you took them off and held them a few inches away from your face or put them on upside down. They are still the same old familiar glasses, but you found some new ways to look through them and, as a result, noticed the world around you in a different way. Mindfulness exercises direct you to do the very same thing with your attention. Your attention is an old familiar tool that has been with you for your entire life. You're accustomed to how you use it, and like your pair of glasses, it shapes how you see your world. Because you won't be trading in your brain for a new one, you have no choice but to use the one you have, yet you can experiment with new ways to play around with your attention tools. That is precisely what mindfulness exercises direct you to do. See the examples below for some short demonstrations of this concept.

Short Mindfulness Exercises

Think of these exercises as experiments with your attention tools. Each one gives you an opportunity to focus your attention in a slightly different way on something that has always been part of you. There is no right or wrong way to feel or think. Some may seem odd or meaningless to you, while others may be interesting and curious. Try them all and give yourself a moment to process each one, spending about 10 seconds on each. You can do them all in one sitting or try them at different times. Remember, there is no right or wrong way to do this.

Sit in a chair that is comfortable for you. Starting with the first statement, read it and then close your eyes for 10 seconds while thinking about what you read. Repeat that procedure for each of the statements.

Imagine the space between your eyes.

Notice the point where your back touches the chair.

Imagine the space within your mouth.

Notice where your arms come into contact with the chair.

Notice the air on your cheeks.

Imagine the distance between your right earlobe and your right shoulder.

Notice the point on each foot where it comes into contact with the floor.

Another reason mindfulness exercises can be helpful to people on the spectrum is that they foster *acceptance*. As mentioned in Chapter 2, people with ASDs can be prone to negative self-talk. This often involves harsh judgments of themselves and/or other people and contributes to problems with anxiety, anger, and depression. In my practice, the four most common things that I see my patients struggle to accept, without judgment, are that (1) their brains work differently; (2) no one person can do everything well—all people have things that they can't do; (3) living life includes making mistakes; and (4) the experience of negative emotion is a natural part of life.

Accepting something means you are noticing it, acknowledging it, and *not* judging, avoiding, or suppressing it. Acceptance also does *not* mean you are condoning or ignoring something that is harmful to you. While this phrase is probably overused these days, accepting something means being able to say "It is what it is" and truly believing that.

ACCEPTING THAT THE ASD BRAIN WORKS DIFFERENTLY FROM THE NEUROTYPICAL BRAIN

It's very common for people on the spectrum to label their ASD characteristics as defects or signs of inferiority. Many have, unfortunately, been given this idea by others (e.g., unkind peers, misinformed professionals). Some of my patients have reported to me that they always assumed that all people thought the way they did, and realizing, usually as adults, that their minds really did work differently came as a surprise. Accepting that your mind works differently and not judging that to be good or bad is a crucial ingredient for a healthy life on the spectrum.

ACCEPTING THAT SOME THINGS CAN'T BE DONE

Many people on the spectrum put a great deal of pressure on themselves to be able to do anything and then feel ashamed and frustrated whenever they encounter an obstacle. This attitude is a by-product of the pressure our society puts on all of us. Unfortunately, we live in a culture where people are expected to "multitask" all day long, be able to do anything at any time, and apply an "I can" attitude toward everything. But realistically, no one can do everything. There are plenty of things I could not do no matter how much I "put my mind to it" (e.g., be a brain surgeon, play tennis, cook something edible). What makes any of us—on the spectrum or not—successful is recognizing what we're really good at, *simultaneously* recognizing what we really can't do, and choosing not to waste time on the latter. Remember the definition of intelligence and success I have been using throughout this book: success comes from capitalizing on your strengths *and* compensating for your weaknesses. To be able to do that, you have to accept those weaknesses—not to judge them, but to simply plan ways around them.

Through the years of work with my patients, I have adopted a phrase that I use very often: "*Can't* is not a four-letter word." This is certainly true literally: the apostrophe adds a fifth element to the four letters. But it is the symbolic meaning that is more important to me and my patients. The idiom *four-letter word* describes a curse word that is offensive. In the "can-do" culture we live in, some people respond to the phrase "I can't" as if it were a curse. Yet to meet a challenge and say "I can," you have to choose *not* to do something else at the same time.

This book is all about positive approaches to your life, and I am hoping you will take from it a sense that you *can* meet your goals. However, to be able to do that, you must be able to identify and accept which things you *can't* do, simply to avoid wasting precious resources on efforts that will bring you nothing but frustration. A good example of using your resources wisely is *not* choosing organizational and scheduling systems that don't fit your style. That means being able to say, "I can't do it that way" and to say so without judgment.

ACCEPTING MISTAKES

Because of the "all or nothing" thinking style that is prevalent in people with ASDs, perfectionism is a common source of pressure and anxiety. Many of my patients have told me that they believe they should not make mistakes; making errors is a sign of weakness and should not be tolerated. Some believe their mistakes result directly from having an ASD and that neurotypical people do not make as many mistakes. Accepting that all people make mistakes and that it's impossible to live a life free of errors is a necessary step toward success. Once you accept that mistakes are inevitable for all adult humans, you will be able to address them more effectively when they occur.

ACCEPTING THAT NEGATIVE EMOTION IS A NATURAL PART OF LIFE

Perhaps the most difficult thing to accept for people on the spectrum (and some neurotypical people, too) is that painful emotions are natural, have a purpose, and cannot be avoided. As illustrated in Chapter 4, getting upset *about* being upset is a common trap that prolongs suffering. When you notice and accept a painful emotion, it tends to pass on its own, kind of like a storm cloud. But if you don't accept the emotion when it occurs, you're likely to engage in thinking and behavior that perpetuate the painful state and prevent it from running its natural course. As counterintuitive as it seems, accepting unpleasant emotions allows them to go away more quickly.

Acceptance Phrases for People on the Spectrum

- "I accept that my brain works differently."
- "I accept that there are things I can't do, just as there are things I can."
- "I accept that mistakes are an inevitable part of life."
- "I accept that painful emotions are natural and serve a purpose."

Techniques for Dimensional Thinking

As mentioned several times before, your thoughts have a very powerful influence over how you feel and behave at any moment. You may remember in Chapter 2 learning about the "internal voice" or "commentator" who is narrating everything that is happening to you. Sometimes that voice can say things that are unproductive or damaging, but you may not always be tuned in to it enough to realize it. In the previous discussion on mindfulness and acceptance, the judgmental voice was mentioned. For people on the spectrum the most common pitfall of their internal voice is dichotomous, or "black and white," thinking. The most useful techniques for you, if you find you are prone to it, are those that help you think in "shades of gray." Rather than putting everything into one box or another, you can learn to measure things along a continuum or in a dimensional way. This is useful when challenging the negative self-talk that is causing problems in your day-to-day life.

You've already been introduced to dimensional thinking techniques in three of the problem-solving steps, although I didn't use that term when I described the steps:

■ In Step 5 you use a scale to rate the feasibility of a solution you came up with during brainstorming. Using a scale of 0 to 4 prevents the tendency to evaluate ideas with "all-or-nothing" thinking, where everything is judged as either "a stupid idea" or "a fantastic idea." Seeing your ideas in "shades of gray" can prevent you from discarding an idea that has promise and could be refined to work or from putting all your resources into an idea that looks great on the surface but has flaws to be resolved.

■ In Step 7 you can track your progress by using a rating scale; for example, rate your daily emotions or feelings on a scale of 0 to 10 to prevent yourself from judging your day as either "horrible" or "wonderful"—assessments that don't permit much learning from your experiences.

■ And in Step 8 you use a scale of 0 to 100% to rate your overall success with your problem solving. Avoiding concluding either "I was a total failure" or "I was a total success" can again help you learn from your experience. In virtually all human efforts, there is something that we've done right and something we could do better, and recognizing those can help us continue to achieve our goals.

If you don't find numeric scales with this type of linear layout appealing, you can measure dimensions using a picture of a pie chart, thermometer, or measuring cup or flask as examples.

Understanding Other People

These techniques should be applied when you're having problems with your *social* differences. In Chapter 3 you learned all about social cognition. Strategies that help you make better guesses about the thoughts, feelings, intentions, and/or motives of the people around you include:

■ learning new ways to *pay attention* to people around you
■ knowing how to *learn about* a person in your life

Paying Attention to Other People

Each time you interact with other people, no matter what the reason, you'll be most successful if you can effectively pay attention to them. You probably already pay attention to others in some ways. But to do so *effectively* means taking in the type of information needed to respond adaptively, and this is where people on the spectrum often have social difficulties. Appropriate use of *eye contact* and *searching for the right clues* are two strategies that can help.

EFFECTIVE USE OF EYE CONTACT

One of the many myths about ASDs that I have encountered in my years of this work is that people on the spectrum make *no eye contact*. Not true! Most of my patients do make eye contact to varying degrees, and a total lack of eye contact is not even a requirement to meet the criteria for a diagnosis of AS or autism. So, why so much talk about this issue? Because people on the spectrum have difficulty *using* their eye contact effectively during social interactions. They also have difficulty *observing* how other people are using their eye contact.

There are three main purposes for looking at the eyes of other people during social interactions:

1. to let the other person know you are paying attention without having to use words
2. to find out what the other person is looking at (which tells you what he or she is paying attention to)
3. to monitor changes in the other person's face

Many factors can interfere with using your eyes during an interaction:

■ Eye contact may intensify anxiety about social interaction.
■ Sensory issues can make eye contact aversive or unpleasant.
■ Believing that eye contact is not important can dissuade you from using it.
■ Overusing eye contact, or staring, can make other people uncomfortable and cause them to withdraw.

Whichever obstacles you experience, the exercise on the facing page can reduce your discomfort by helping you learn to make well-timed momentary glances. You will need a trusted partner (friend, family member) to do this exercise with you.

Eye Punctuation: Exercise for Effective Eye Contact

Ask a trusted person to help you with this exercise. Pick a short paragraph from a newspaper, magazine, or book and give it to your partner. Give your partner a copy of these instructions as well. Both of you should then sit down in a comfortable place and each silently read through the entire set of instructions once before beginning.

This is a visualization exercise that promotes active and dynamic eye contact. It will give you ways to use not too much, not too little, but just the right amount. You may already be using quick glances and momentary eye contact during interactions. Here you will learn to pay more attention to how you are doing that and to fine-tune that practice.

Think about how punctuation is used in written work, especially commas (,) and periods(.). Commas mark *pauses*, and periods mark *endings*. Both represent a break in the flow of speech, which are good times to use your eyes.

1. Close your eyes and have your partner begin reading the passage you chose. As you hear the words, imagine the words being written or typed on a page. Picture in your mind where you would put a comma or a period as you hear the passage being read.

2. Now open your eyes and have your partner read the passage again. This time, briefly make eye contact with your partner at the point where you think there should be a comma or a period (pause). You do not have to continue looking at your partner. Hold the look for only a few seconds at each punctuation point.

3. Now say something to your partner and try to imagine where the punctuation marks would be as you talk. Give your partner a glance at each of those points. If you can't think of something to say, just tell your partner what you think about doing this exercise.

How did it feel to do this exercise? Did it feel awkward or unnatural? Many people feel that way because it is, indeed, awkward and unnatural at first. But with repeated practice, like anything new you learn, it will get easier. And you may notice quickly that you get a positive response from the other person because you're letting him or her know you're listening, checking in frequently enough to monitor the attention and changing facial expressions of the other person.

SEARCHING FOR THE RIGHT CLUES

When you look at the faces of other people to monitor changes, what exactly are you supposed to be looking for? Mainly, you should be looking at:

1. where the other person's eyes are looking
2. what kind of facial expression the other person has

Following are clues you might want to think about when interacting with and watching the eyes of another person.

Where Is Your Partner Looking?	What Is the Clue?
The other person is looking back at you.	The other person is paying attention to you.
The other person is not looking at you.	The other person is not paying attention to you.
The other person is looking at somebody or something else.	The other person is paying attention to and thinking about the person or object he/she is looking at.

Facial expressions are not always easy to figure out, especially because people on the spectrum sometimes have difficulty reading the basic emotions conveyed. In many cases, however, you could be missing the emotions of others simply because you are not looking at their faces. Here is another clue sheet that can help.

What Is Your Partner Doing with His or Her Face?	What Is the Clue?
No expression	The other person is feeling no strong emotion at that moment—neutral.
Frowning	The other person is concentrating on something OR is annoyed OR angry.
Smiling	The other person is happy.
Opening eyes extra wide	The other person is surprised OR scared.
Looking down with straight or downturned mouth	The other person is sad OR worried OR tired.

Learning about Other People

To interact successfully with people, you need not only to be able to read them in the moment, but also to collect information on them that you can store for future use. The type of information you collect about someone and how you then use those facts depend on the nature of your relationship and your reason for interacting with that person. Following are some strategies for *defining the type of* relationship you have with a person, *collecting and storing information* about a person, and using the stored information to guide your behavior while with that person.

DEFINING A RELATIONSHIP

Each person you encounter from day to day falls into one of the following categories in relation to you:

- Stranger
- Acquaintance
- Relative (grandparent, cousin, aunt, uncle)
- Immediate family member (parent, sibling, or child)
- Friend
- Romantic partner (boyfriend, girlfriend, spouse)

It's important to know where a person stands in your life because it determines how much and what type of information you may have or seek about him or her. These different types of people play different roles in your life, and the *boundaries* of the relationship vary greatly depending on how *close* you are to the individual in question. *Boundaries* refer to the rules that tell you what is OK versus what is not OK to do and say with a given person. The boundaries that exist between you and a stranger sitting next to you on a bus are different from the boundaries between you and your mother, for example, starting with the amount and type of information you have about the person.

Your role is to be aware of where the boundaries are so that you can better understand the other person's expectations of you. For instance, a person you are not close with would not expect you to ask a lot of personal questions, but someone who does consider you close *would* expect you to ask personal questions. If you ask too many personal questions of someone who does not know you very well, you will be perceived as being intrusive or "nosy." On the other hand, if you fail to ask enough questions about someone who is close, you will be perceived as aloof, indifferent, or uncaring. People on the spectrum struggle to understand boundaries and expectations in relationships because these "rules" and "contracts" are mostly *unwritten* and *unspoken*. My patients often say they find this whole business very confusing: how do neurotypical people just seem to know these rules? The fact that the very same behavior can be considered rude with one person and desirable with another is intimidating if you don't know how to tell the difference. How do you know how close you are to someone? How do you know what the boundaries might be? There is no single way to answer those questions. However, you can evaluate every relationship you have along several dimensions to get a better idea of how close you are to the person.

Generally speaking, the six types of people listed above appear in order of least to most close; a stranger is the least close to you, while a romantic partner would be the most close to you. However, the categories in between could vary from case to case. For example, you may feel closer to one of your cousins than to any of your friends or even your siblings. You could feel closer to an uncle than to one of your parents, or closer to a friend than to your sibling. Regardless of the exact order in your life, the diagram below illustrates that the amount of information you do have or should have about the person varies with the level of closeness.

At this point, you may be wondering exactly what *closeness* is and how to measure it. We often use the term to describe the depth of connection between two people, but that's not much more concrete than the word itself. Closeness refers to a combination of factors that determine how attached you are to a person as well as how important you perceive that person to be in your life. You can use the following four dimensions to evaluate your relationship with each person in your life. Be sure, however, to use *all* the dimensions to get an accurate estimation of how close you two are—closeness is complicated enough that omitting a dimension will give you only a partial picture.

Closeness	Type of Relationship	Amount of Information You Have about the Person
Not Close At All	stranger	None
	acquaintance	
	relative	
	immediate family	
	friend	
Extremely Close	romantic partner	Very Much

Defining relationships.

1. *How much time have you spent with the person?* You may have known this person for years but do not see the person very often (e.g., an uncle who you see only for holidays). Or you may see this person every day but for only a few minutes at a time (e.g., the man who sells you coffee every morning at the newspaper stand). Or you may have spent a lot of time with this person in the past but now don't see him or her very often (e.g., a parent who raised you but now lives in another state).

2. *How much do you rely on the person?* To what extent do you need something from this person? How much would you be affected if you suddenly lost contact with this person? What you need could be very tangible (e.g., help with the grocery shopping or house chores) or could be less tangible, such as emotional support (e.g., someone to listen to you and/or give you advice).

3. *How much do you and this person share in terms of common interests?* Do you enjoy the same leisure activities (playing a sport, going to the movies, etc.)? Do you have interests in common that contribute to your conversations (science, politics, books you've read, etc.)?

4. *How much do you enjoy the company of the person?* To what extent do you have fun and feel pleasant emotions when you are with this person?

Each person in your life, whether a taxi driver you met once, a friend who lives in another state, or your mother with whom you live, will have a different "profile" of closeness depending on your answers to these four questions. Try using the following rankings to answer each of the four questions for someone you know.

None	Almost None	Some	A Lot	Maximum Amount
0	1	2	3	4

Then add up the total of the four answers. Now pick someone else you know and perform the same rankings. How did the totals compare for the two people? If you used, for example, your best friend and then your favorite cashier at the grocery store, you probably found that your total was higher for your friend, meaning you have a closer relationship with that person than with the cashier. That may surprise you if you greatly enjoy seeing the cashier when you shop because she smiles and jokes with you and you feel confident that she likes you. But it gives you an idea that the boundaries between you and the cashier are different from those between you and your best friend. Again, the boundaries define the rules of what is appropriate to do and say with the person. These rules definitely apply to collecting information about a person.

COLLECTING AND STORING INFORMATION

Knowing the nature of your relationship with someone else is important for two reasons: (1) because it tells you how much and what type of information you need to collect about the person to *maintain* a good relationship—whether it's an acquaintance, a friendship, or a family bond—and (2) because it tells you where the boundaries lie between you and the other person even if you personally would like to *change* the nature of the relationship. The challenge for all of us—ASDs or no ASDs—is that relationships are always two-way streets, and that means the wishes of the other person are just as important as our own. This is why effectively paying attention to people, as described above, is so valuable; it helps you make better guesses about what the other person's wishes are. While the guessing or social inference process is very complex and can be addressed optimally in collaboration with a therapist (e.g., behavioral therapist or speech–language pathologist), some of the basic concepts will be presented here.

As mentioned, the closer you are, the more information you have. To complicate matters, the closer you *want* to be to someone, the more information you will need to collect. If you want an acquaintance to become a friend, or a friend to become a romantic partner, for example, then you need to learn more about the person. Why is it important to learn more about the people in your life? One reason is that it *makes people feel good about you if they think you want to learn about them*. No two people are alike, and most people appreciate it when someone takes an interest in learning about them as individuals. This applies not only to conversations you have with acquaintances and new friends, but also to people you have known for a long time, like your immediate family members or old friends. When people feel good about you, your day-to-day interactions with them are likely to be more pleasant and more productive. Relationships characterized by mutual goodwill can go a long way toward reducing the stress in your life. You can strengthen bonds with the people you are already close with, or if you're dealing with someone you want to be closer to, making the effort to get to know the person better can lead him or her to like you more.

Another reason to learn more about people is that it *allows you to discriminate between those you like and those you don't like*. On that two-way relationship street, you could encounter people who want to become closer to you, in which case it's important to learn about them so you know whether you want to spend more time with them. After all, your time is a resource that should be spent wisely.

The three best methods for gathering information about people in whom you are interested are:

- asking direct questions and listening to the answers
- observing things they do
- listening to what they say to you or to others

Remember, the effort you will put into these activities depends on the level of closeness you have or desire to have with the person in whom you are showing interest. On one hand, people feel good when you remember unique things about them, especially if they like you and feel comfortable with you. On the other hand, people do not like to be asked too much about themselves if they don't yet know you or feel comfortable with you. This is why it's important to know how close you are to the person right now. The less you know someone, the more "superficial" the information you seek should be. The closer you are to the person, the more freely you can ask questions, about a wider variety of personal matters. But this is a tough judgment call, because people's relationships evolve, and these shifts are rarely announced or even made explicit between the two people. You probably know that your best friend was at one time a stranger to you; maybe he or she became a friend very quickly, or maybe you progressed slowly from acquaintance to close friendship. I would bet, however, that neither of you can pinpoint the day when your relationship took on a new status.

Learning about other people supplies you with the facts you need to:

1. start or sustain a conversation with the person, either right now or at a later date

2. express interest in and/or concern for the person by focusing on topics you know he or she cares about

3. assess whether you like the person and whether you want to continue interacting with him or her in the future

---

If you are ever in doubt about whether a particular person is a stranger, acquaintance, a friend, or even a potential romantic partner, you can always use the rating scale to ask the four questions on page 155 about the person. In fact you can do this repeatedly for the same person over time, a very helpful "reality check" when you're not sure where a particular relationship stands.

Following are some guidelines for the types of information you should seek about a person based on the nature of your current relationship—the level of closeness between you. For handy reference, these guidelines are summed up in the diagram on the next page.

With Strangers or New Acquaintances. Limit your questions to the **immediate shared situation.** You two were probably brought together by circumstances, not by choice, and barely know each other. So, for example, if you are stuck together on a long grocery line, sitting next to each other in a crowded waiting room, or on some public transportation together (bus, train, or airplane), you may want to get to know the person just well enough to pass the time together. Limiting your questions to immediate issues lowers the risk that you could make the other person uncomfortable. So you may ask about what brought him or her there, where he or she is headed, or what his or her opinion is about the immediate situation (about the store you are in, the plane you are on, etc). Through this process you may also discover that the person is likable, and if so, may have the potential to become an acquaintance if you were to encounter each other again.

With Acquaintances. You can feel free to explore the **person's superficial facts** after you have started to get to know each other and no longer think of each other as pure strangers. You may seek information about specific matters such as hobbies, interests, school, or work, but still steer clear of his or her personal life.

With Friends. Once someone has become a friend (or in cases where another, closer relationship has been formed, such as when you gain new in-laws due to a marriage), you can start to ask questions about the **person's personal life**. This includes queries about home, family, and background, such as how many children or siblings the person has, who lives at home, and where the person grew up. Still, however, you should limit yourself to who is in the person's family and stay away from asking about conflicts, divorce, or deaths in the family—anything that might be painful to the person. Do be prepared for the other person to mention such things, but it is up to that person to decide to broach those topics; you would not ask about it at this stage.

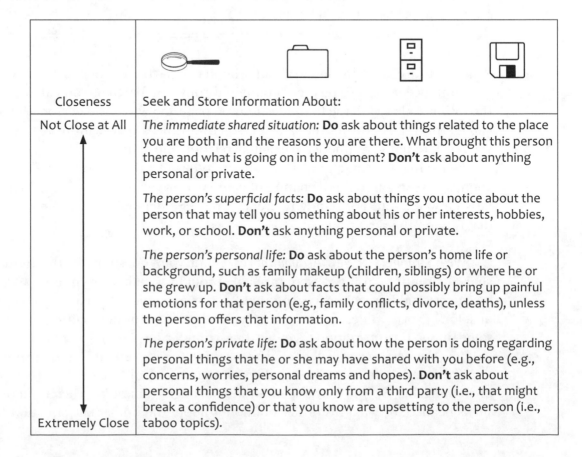

Closeness	Seek and Store Information About:
Not Close at All ↕ Extremely Close	*The immediate shared situation:* **Do** ask about things related to the place you are both in and the reasons you are there. What brought this person there and what is going on in the moment? **Don't** ask about anything personal or private.
	The person's superficial facts: **Do** ask about things you notice about the person that may tell you something about his or her interests, hobbies, work, or school. **Don't** ask anything personal or private.
	The person's personal life: **Do** ask about the person's home life or background, such as family makeup (children, siblings) or where he or she grew up. **Don't** ask about facts that could possibly bring up painful emotions for that person (e.g., family conflicts, divorce, deaths), unless the person offers that information.
	The person's private life: **Do** ask about how the person is doing regarding personal things that he or she may have shared with you before (e.g., concerns, worries, personal dreams and hopes). **Don't** ask about personal things that you know only from a third party (i.e., that might break a confidence) or that you know are upsetting to the person (i.e., taboo topics).

With Close Friends, Relatives, Immediate Family, and Romantic Partners. Strictly with those you know very well, you can ask about the **person's private life**, which involves more intimate details that people don't feel comfortable sharing unless they know and trust the other person well. These might include concerns, worries, personal dreams and hopes, or painful memories of some sort. Asking about such matters after the person has brought them up with you is usually considered a caring gesture. So, for example, if a close friend told you that she was very nervous about seeing a long-lost brother at a family reunion, you should ask her about it after she comes back from the reunion to see how it went for her. This shows that you remembered a topic that was sensitive for her, and people usually take that as a sign that you care about them.

Communication Techniques

Whether you are struggling with a *thinking, social, emotional,* or *sensory/movement* difference, sooner or later you are going to have to communicate with somebody else about it. So communication techniques are needed for all the types of differences you may be having difficulty with. The "Understanding Other People" section you just read focused on one part of the two-way communication process, where you are the *receiver* of information about another person. This section focuses on the other direction—your role as the *giver* of information.

Communication skills involve a broad range of behaviors, many of which are best taught by a speech–language pathologist or a behavioral psychologist because they are learned best with live practice and coaching. Chapter 14 gives you guidelines for seeking out those services. Here you'll find some basic strategies that you can try on your own to make some situations more manageable for you.

One place you can start is with giving information about yourself within a relationship, either new or old. When you're getting to know someone and that person asks you questions to learn more about you, follow the same guidelines in answering as for asking (see the chart on the previous page). If you'd characterize the person as an acquaintance, for example, when asked what you do for a living or whether you're in school, describe what you do (or study), where, and whom you work for (or where you're attending school) as you like. But resist any urge to bring in personal details such as that you hate your job or your professor, even if you do, or that your spouse wishes you made more money. Even if you love your job, remember that someone you just met probably isn't interested in hearing what you do in depth throughout your work or school day, so keep it brief.

Another thing that people on the spectrum struggle with is expressing their needs and desires to others. Even if you are a very talkative and outgoing person, you may find it difficult to let other people know about the key things you want and need from them. Some examples include:

■ asking someone to turn a light on or off because it is bothering you
■ asking someone to lower or turn off a noisy TV or radio because it is bothering you

- asking someone to accommodate a scheduling need you have
- asking for clarification of something you were told but either did not understand or do not remember
- asking for help on a task that is overwhelming to you
- saying "no" to a request that is made for something you do not want to do
- expressing your disagreement with someone who is in authority
- telling someone that he or she did something that was hurtful or upsetting to you
- asking someone to stop doing something that is hurtful or upsetting to you

Because of a combination of the thinking, social, emotional, and sensory differences discussed in Part I, you may struggle with expressing your needs and desires in any of these ways:

- You may have trouble recognizing or identifying a need when it arises.
- You may find it difficult to access the words or phrases to describe the need to another person.
- Anxiety over communicating may leave you overaroused, further hindering your expressive communication.
- Engaging in negative self-talk or judgmental thinking might interfere with your ability to express your need to someone else (e.g., "I don't have the right to ask for this accommodation" or "If I tell this person to stop what he is doing, he may get mad at me").

Two strategies—an exercise for *identifying a need* and a formula for *assertive expression*—can help.

IDENTIFYING A NEED

Before you can tell somebody what you need, you have to be able to recognize your emotions and understand what they are signaling. Only then can you involve other people in helping you solve your problem. You need to be able to complete this formula for preparing to express a need:

I feel _____; therefore, I need _____.

Yet you know that having an ASD can make it difficult to *recognize* your own internal mental state, *recognize* that distress can signal a need to initiate a change in the environment, and *translate* those feelings and thoughts into words. So you need some strategy or tool to help you put your current, distressing internal state and your desired state into words. One tool that I often recommend to my patients is called *Talk Blocks® for Work* (Innovative Interactions, 2000). Although this set of blocks was designed for use in the workplace, I find it useful to adults on the spectrum for many situations in which they have responsibilities and must interface with other people. It's a set of six blocks, each with a picture and phrase on each of the six sides. Three blocks are red, to symbolize *feelings*, and three blocks are blue, to symbolize *needs*. Each subset of blocks gives you eighteen choices to help you to access the words that best describe your internal state or subjective experience. The red feeling blocks contain these words:

Angry	Undervalued
Appreciated	Anxious
Exhausted	Bored
Happy	Motivated
Pressured	Focused
Impatient	Overwhelmed
Productive	Excited
Frustrated	Successful
Irritable	Disappointed

The blue need blocks contain these phrases:

To be listened to	To take a break
No interruptions	Solutions
Time alone	To listen
More information	To have fun
Nourishment	To laugh
To talk	To be patient
More support	To calm down
To assert myself	To stop and think
To set some limits	To take a deep breath

Each time you find yourself in distress because of a dilemma or conflict in any situation, you can use these blocks by yourself or with the help of a trusted other person. Simply spread the blocks out on a clear work surface (desk or table). Starting with the red ones, pick them up one by one and look at all the sides until you find the word(s) that best describe how you are feeling. You will be surprised at how doing this can help you identify a feeling that you had not yet clarified in your own mind.

After choosing the feeling word(s), take the blue blocks and ask yourself what you think you would *need* to help you with the feeling(s) identified with the red blocks. In other words, which of the phrases on the blue blocks best describes something that you think would alleviate your distress? Once you have done that, you can string together the red with the blue words to complete the formula for expressing a need. For example:

I FEEL *anxious*; therefore, I NEED *more information*.

I FEEL *overwhelmed*; therefore, I NEED *to take a break*.

The diagram below shows you pictures of the actual blocks used to formulate these sentences.

If you don't want to acquire the blocks, you can do this on paper as if you were using a worksheet. I prefer the blocks because they stimulate more than one channel (visual, tactile, verbal, and nonverbal), maximizing the chances that you will be able to identify your internal state.

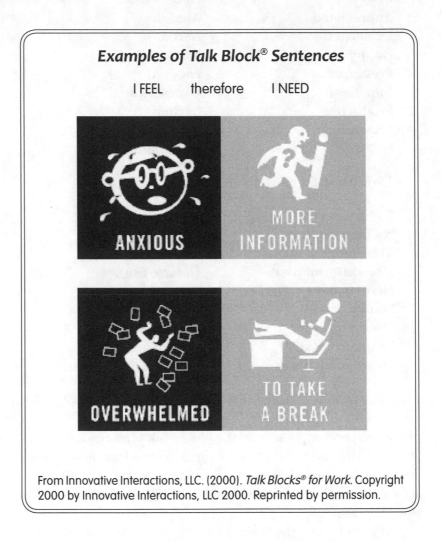

Examples of Talk Block® Sentences

I FEEL   therefore   I NEED

ANXIOUS

MORE INFORMATION

OVERWHELMED

TO TAKE A BREAK

From Innovative Interactions, LLC. (2000). *Talk Blocks® for Work.* Copyright 2000 by Innovative Interactions, LLC 2000. Reprinted by permission.

ASSERTIVE EXPRESSION

Unfortunately, being sure of your feelings and needs isn't always enough to make you feel comfortable telling someone else about them, especially if you're going to ask the other person to change his or her behavior or you're expressing disagreement. Fortunately, there's a formula that can help you express your need without feeling intimidated. There are four key ingredients to an effective assertive statement. They are clear and objective descriptions of:

1. your feeling
2. the other person's behavior that contributed to your feeling
3. the consequences of that behavior for you
4. your request

Here's how to lay this out in a statement:

I feel/felt _(your feeling)_ **when you** _(other person's behavior)_ **because** _(consequences of other's behavior)_ **, so I am asking you to** _(your request)_ **.**

You can use information from your Talk Blocks for some of these ingredients. *Your feeling* can come from the red blocks, and *your request* can come from the blue blocks. When you are describing the other person's behavior, remember not to use hostile or insulting remarks. It may be hard to avoid them if you're angry with the person, but a good way around it is to stick to what the person *did* and avoid talking about what the person *is*. So, for example, if you were angry because your roommate plays loud music at night when you're trying to read, you would say, "you play your music very loud at night" instead of "You're an inconsiderate jerk for playing your music so loud." Let's see how this looks in a complete assertive statement:

I feel _frustrated_ **when you** _play your music very loud at night_ **because** _I cannot concentrate on my reading_ **, so I am asking you to** _play the music at a lower volume, please_ .

■   ■   ■

The chapters that follow show you how to address issues that are causing you distress in specific domains of your life. Each chapter follows the same format but varies in the examples used. The problem-solving approach introduced in this chapter will always be your starting point. Then, depending on which of your ASD differences seem to be contributing to the problem, you can choose any one or a combination of the strategies described in this chapter to improve the situation by alleviating your distress. Feel free to skip ahead to any one of the chapters that seems most relevant to the part of your life you are struggling with. No matter how you go about doing that, I suggest you read Chapter 14 when you are finished.

Locate the ASD difference that you suspect is affecting your problem the most on the top of the chart. Then look down that column to find the dots, which lead you to corresponding strategies for addressing that problem.

STRATEGIES	Thinking	Social	Emotional	Sensory/ Movement
Environmental Modifications	*			*
Organizational Techniques	*			
Scheduling Techniques	*			
Relaxation Techniques			*	*
Emotion Regulation Techniques		*	*	
Thinking Techniques	*	*	*	
Techniques to Understand Other People		*		
Communication Techniques	*	*	*	*

Cheat sheet of solutions for ASD differences.

7

At Home

Your day begins and ends at home. Wherever you live, this place can and should help you feel secure, safe, and content. If you are to function successfully in the outside world, your home must support and rejuvenate you every day; it needs to be a place where you can "recharge your batteries." Nevertheless, people on the spectrum often report that their most troublesome problems are related to home life. Due to the thinking, social, emotional, and sensory/movement differences that are part of the autism spectrum, you may be vulnerable to a whole host of challenges managing the tasks and activities involved in living in an apartment or house, with or without other people. This chapter will help you identify the obstacles you are facing functioning in your own home. You will identify which of your differences are playing a role in those problems and use that information to choose and implement solutions.

In Chapter 1 you were introduced to three people who were having different kinds of problems at home, and their issues will be used as examples throughout this chapter.

Blanca is the graduate student in marine biology who is having problems with her sleep *schedule*; she is waking up earlier than she wants and is not getting enough rest, which leaves her tired all day. She's also having trouble *organizing her space*. Her messy room makes it hard for her to find what she needs for school, so she feels very pressured as she gets ready to leave for campus in the morning.

Henry, the 29-year-old college graduate who has been unemployed for 6 years, is having problems with *managing time*, believing he's not very productive during the day, particularly with his job search. He is also having problems *getting along* with his father; they often argue when they're at home together in the evening.

Charles, the 52-year-old teacher, is having trouble meeting the *needs of others*, specifically difficulty conversing with his son at a time of day when he is most tense and needs his own space.

As you well know, keeping up with the responsibilities of owning or renting and possibly sharing a house or apartment can sometimes feel like too much to handle. If filling out the clock worksheet in Chapter 1 revealed that the most stressful times of your day were spent at home, your home life must be causing you problems that are worth addressing. What exactly are those problems? Defining the problem is the first step in the problem-solving approach you learned in Chapter 6. Fill out the checklists in Worksheets 19 and 20 to begin the process. Each list includes problems that are common among people on the spectrum but also leaves blank spaces for you to fill in if you're having other problems at home.

WORKSHEET 19

My Problems at Home
Managing Personal Responsibilities

Check off (✓) the statements that sound familiar to you or reflect experiences you frequently have in your life at home. If you have a problem related to managing personal responsibilities that does not appear on this list, fill it in on one of the blanks at the bottom of the list.

- ☐ I can't keep my space organized.

- ☐ I am always losing things.

- ☐ I have trouble keeping up with the cleaning.

- ☐ I have trouble managing my time.

- ☐ I procrastinate on tasks I have to do around the house.

- ☐ I can't fall asleep at night, and I stay up later than I want to.

- ☐ I can't wake up when I am supposed to—I sleep through my alarm.

- ☐ I have difficulty sleeping and wake up a lot during the night and early morning.

- ☐ I have trouble paying my bills on time.

- ☐ I have too much debt.

- ☐ I don't know how to handle household repairs when they are needed.

- ☐ I can't seem to prepare food on my own.

- ☐ _____

- ☐ _____

- ☐ _____

My Problems at Home
Getting Along with the Other People
in My Home

If you live alone, you can skip this worksheet. Otherwise, list the person(s) who live in your home with you.

I live with _____   _____

_____   _____

_____   _____

Check off (✓) the statements that sound familiar to you or reflect experiences you frequently have in your life at home. Fill in the blank with the name of the person who is involved with any problem you check off. If you have a problem with the person(s) you live with that does appear on this list, fill it in on one of the blanks at the bottom of the list.

☐ _____ doesn't give me enough privacy.

☐ _____ makes too much noise.

☐ _____ is always picking on me.

☐ _____ has guests too often—I don't like to mingle so often.

☐ I have a lot of arguments with _____.

☐ _____ gets mad at me a lot because I procrastinate.

☐ _____ gets annoyed about my sleeping habits.

☐ _____ is constantly hounding me to clean.

☐ _____ is always watching TV when I want to see my own show.

☐ _____ does not understand that I need time alone.

☐ _____

☐ _____

☐ _____

Problem Solving

If you identified more than one problem at home, you will need to choose one to work on first; you can then repeat the eight-step problem-solving process for the other problems at a later time. As mentioned in Chapter 6, it makes sense to start out working on the issue that's causing you and/or the people around you the most distress. Worksheet 21 can help you figure out which one that is. Rate the level of distress caused by each problem and then pick the one with the highest score to tackle first. You can return to the others later, in order of most to least distress. It can also be helpful to talk over this prioritizing with a trusted person in your life.

The next few pages will guide you through steps for solving the problem you just identified. For each step you will be asked to write your answers in the question box. Each box will give you instructions, and then I'll show you how *Blanca* (who was used as an example for the clock worksheet in Chapter 1) filled out the box.

WORKSHEET 21

Choosing Which Problem
to Work On First

You don't need to use this worksheet if you checked off only one problem on Worksheets 19 and 20. Otherwise, list the problems you checked in the first column below. Then use the rating scale to estimate the amount of stress the issue is causing you and/or the people around you.

How much distress is this problem causing in my life?

Almost None	Some	Moderate Amount	A Lot	Extreme
1	2	3	4	5

Problem   **Distress Rating**

_____   _____

_____   _____

_____   _____

_____   _____

Step 1: Identify and Define Your Problem at Home

What is bothering you at home? You've already done this first step if you filled out Worksheets 19–21. Write the problem you have chosen to work on first in the box.

Step 1: Identify and Define Your Problem at Home

What is bothering you at home?

The problem that is bothering me most at home is:

_____

_____

_____

Example. **Blanca** had identified more than one home-based problem and used Worksheet 21 to choose which one to work on first.

Example from Blanca
WORKSHEET 21

Choosing Which Problem to Work On First

How much distress is this problem causing in my life?

Almost None	Some	Moderate Amount	A Lot	Extreme
1	2	3	4	5

Problem	Distress Rating
I am always running late in the morning	5
I can't keep my room organized	4
I have difficulty sleeping	3

Example. After choosing her first-priority problem, **Blanca** filled out her Step 1 question box this way:

Step 1: Identify and Define Your Problem at Home

The problem that is bothering me most at home is:

I am always running late in the morning when I am trying to get ready to

leave for class.

Step 2: Define Your Goal

What would you like to see change to minimize the problem you identified at home? What would need to be different for you to feel less bothered by the problem? The goal you lay out is simply the opposite of the problem you listed. List your goal in the box. If you need an example, look at Blanca's box. Notice how she stated her goal as the opposite of her problem. Leaving on time is the opposite of running late. Phrasing the goal in a positive, affirmative way is setting the stage for an action plan as well as a way to measure progress.

Step 2: Define Your Goal

What would you like to see change to minimize the problem you identified at home? The goal you lay out is simply the opposite of the problem you listed.

To feel less stressed by this problem, I would like to:

Example. **Blanca's** goal is shown next.

Step 2: Define Your Goal

To feel less stressed by this problem, I would like to:

Leave on time every day that I have to go to campus

Step 3: Identify the Obstacles in the Way of Your Achieving the Goal

What is getting in the way of your goal? The next step is to identify obstacles to meeting your goal. Here it is particularly important to consider your ASD characteristics as hidden players in your problem. As you go through this step, you may rely on the information you were given in Part I of this book about your ASD differences. As you think about the problem you listed above, look at the chart on page 173 called "ASD Differences That Can Contribute to Problems at Home." Read through that chart with your own problem in mind and also consider the following questions.

Thinking Differences

How might my *executive functioning* issues be contributing to my problems at home? For example, do I have difficulty planning, which causes me to procrastinate on my cleaning tasks? Do I find it hard to concentrate on more than one task at time, causing me to get very few things done each day? How might my *negative self-talk* be playing a role in my problems at home? What am I saying to myself that is putting more pressure on me? Could I be engaging in perfectionistic thinking, all-or-nothing thinking, or catastrophic thinking? For example, do I set up unrealistic expectations for myself, like "I must clean out the entire basement in one day or else I am a failure?"

Social Differences

How might my *social perception* be contributing to my problems at home? Is it possible that I sometimes misunderstand what my family member or roommate is trying to tell me? For example, I still can't tell when my mother wants me to help her and when she doesn't. Is it possible that this person is not communicating clearly enough about what he or she expects from me? For example, I believe I am doing what my roommate has asked of me, but he still keeps getting annoyed at me, and I don't know why. How might my *social/communication skills* be contributing to problems at home? Is my problem caused partly by my not knowing what to say or do when dealing with my family member or roommate? For example, my roommate keeps waking me up when he makes noise getting ready for work, and I don't know how to make him stop.

Emotional Differences

How could my emotional reactions be affecting my home life? Do I have difficulty *regulating* my emotions? Do I have difficulty *identifying* my feelings or *asking for help* when I am upset? Do I take too long to calm down after an upsetting incident? Am I overreacting or underreacting to things that happen in the home?

Sensory and Movement Differences

How might my sensory issues be contributing to my problems at home? Am I *oversensitive* or *undersensitive* to certain types of light, sound, smell, taste, or touch? For example, do I avoid family activities because they're too noisy? How might my *movement* and *coordination* issues be contributing to my problems at home? For example, do I feel awkward or have difficulty using tools or utensils?

Now fill out the question box, but try hard not to think about other problems you have besides the one you chose for this exercise.

Step 3: Identify the Obstacles in the Way of Your Achieving the Goal

What is getting in the way of your goal? Remember to focus *only* on the problem and goal you wrote down in Steps 1 and 2. First circle the category(ies) of ASD differences you suspect are involved in this problem:

Thinking   **Social**   **Emotional**   **Sensory/Movement**

I believe these differences are contributing in this way:

_____

_____

_____

_____

_____

Example. ***Blanca*** filled out her Step 3 question box as it appears on page 174:

Differences →	Thinking	Social	Emotional	Sensory/Movement
Problems Managing the Tasks and Responsibilities at Home	• *Attention regulation* difficulties can make it hard to complete chores and tasks • Difficulties *organizing information* make it hard to organize your personal spaces • Difficulties with *goal setting and planning* make it hard to design schedules, budgets, and "to-do" lists in your personal life • *Working memory* difficulties make it hard to do more than one task at a time in your home • *Focusing on detail* but ignoring the "big picture" may cause you to overlook important household issues • *Dichotomous, all-or-nothing* thinking can cause undue pressure and anxiety around household tasks	• Your unique style of processing *language* may lead you to miss others' expectations about your responsibilities around the home • Your difficulty *initiating conversations* may interfere with your ability to ask for help on tasks you find difficult to complete	• *Your difficulty recognizing and identifying negative emotions* that you are feeling can interfere with your awareness that you are struggling with tasks and may need a change (e.g., anxiety, anger) • *Your difficulty regulating your negative emotions* related to household tasks can contribute to your experience of getting extremely overwhelmed by the pressures involved	• *Hypersensitivity* to noise, light, smell, taste, or touch can interfere with certain types of household responsibilities (e.g., vacuum noise may be excruciating to you; chemicals and cleaning products could have smells that are unbearable to you) • *Hyposensitivity* (underresponsive sense) can interfere with picking up on cues to clean (e.g., may not smell the spoiled food in the fridge) • *Fine motor problems* (coordinated handwork) could affect tasks like cooking, laundry, repairs, operating electronic equipment, handwriting tasks • *Gross motor problems* (coordinated whole-body movement) could affect some chores (using a heavy vacuum, operating a lawnmower)
Problems with the Other People Who Live in Your Home	• People you live with may be affected adversely by your difficulties managing tasks and responsibilities that are due to your thinking differences (e.g., unequal distribution of work) • People you live with may be resentful or frustrated if they are affected and worse if they don't understand why	• You may not notice or properly *interpret the cues* from people about cooperative tasks • You may not *mind-read* what the others are expecting from you around the house • You may be perceived by others in your home as uncaring or aloof because of the way you *experience and express empathy* • The *unique way you process and express language* can contribute to misunderstandings with the people you live with and make it hard to assert yourself • Your difficulty with *conversation skills* may interfere with making positive connections with the people you live with	• *Your difficulty recognizing and identifying negative emotions* that you are feeling can contribute to your problems communicating to others in your home about your needs • *Your difficulty regulating your negative emotions* related to household tasks can put you at risk for having dramatic outbursts, which may be aggravating or intimidating to others in your home and will create further obstacles to communication; the quality of these relationships will be affected adversely.	• *Hypersensitivities* can cause problems with other people if they are unknowingly doing things that are unpleasant to you (playing music, wearing strong perfume, using friendly touch or hugs) • *Fine or gross motor problems* can be obstacles to many types of cooperative leisure activities like games or sports, giving you fewer opportunities to spend enjoyable time with others in your household

ASD differences that can contribute to problems at home.

> ### Step 3: Identify the Obstacles in the Way of Your Achieving the Goal
>
> (Thinking)   Social   (Emotional)   Sensory/Movement
>
> I believe these differences are contributing in this way:
>
> _My thinking differences make it hard for me to organize my stuff. I run_
> _late because my things are not organized and I spend time looking for them._
> _My emotional differences make it hard for me to manage my anxiety—I get so_
> _upset in the morning that I can't focus on looking for my stuff._
> _____

When you filled out your sheet, did you circle more than one area of ASD differences? Blanca indicated that both her thinking (executive functioning) and emotional differences were playing a role in her rushed and stressful mornings. This demonstrates an important point: sometimes an issue that seems like a single problem may really have several causes.

Step 4: List Several Possible Solutions to Address the Obstacle(s)

What are the possible solutions for the obstacles? Try to list as many ideas as possible. Remember that this is the step some people call "brainstorming." Generate as many possibilities as come to mind without inhibition. Don't judge or evaluate any idea—just write it down no matter how weird or silly it seems. In Step 5 you will weed through them and discard any that are not useful, so no harm can be done.

Look at the Cheat Sheet at the end of Chapter 6. This chart lists which solutions may be best to try first to address which types of ASD differences. Find the ASD differences you circled on the top row of the Cheat Sheet. Then look along the column underneath each and find the dots. Each dot marks the row in which you will find a solution in the far left column of the chart. Those approaches should be considered first for your problem, and Chapter 6 provides you with the instructions and tools for each of those solutions. Also, try to consider your *strengths* as you complete this step because they also play an important role in your solutions. Refer back to Worksheets 3 and 4 in Chapter 1. Write your primary strengths in the blanks here so you can keep them in mind while you are generating solutions.

My strengths are: _____, _____, and _____.

Step 4: List Several Possible Solutions to Address the Obstacle(s)

What are the possible solutions for the obstacles? Now, considering all the solutions that you saw on the Cheat Sheet, and some you may think of on your own, list all the possibilities you can imagine to address the ASD differences involved in the problem you listed in Step 1. For the moment, ignore the score columns on the right.

I could try to:

List strategies below	Pro (+) score	Con (−) score	Total pro–con

Example. **Blanca** filled out her question box this way:

Step 4: List Several Possible Solutions to Address the Obstacle(s)

I could try to:

List strategies below	Pro (+) score	Con (−) score	Total pro–con
1) organize my room			
2) organize my book bag			
3) quit school			
4) change my class schedule			
5) change where I keep my book bag			
6) move on campus			

Notice that Blanca included everything on her list that came to mind, even things that may seem outrageous (e.g., quitting school). She used the Cheat Sheet to come up with ideas 1, 2, and 5. The rest of the ideas she came up with on her own. This is an example of "brainstorming." She cannot possibly do all the things on this list but will use the next step to figure out what is most useful to her.

Step 5: Consider the Consequences of Each Solution

What are the pros and cons of each solution? Now you will take each item on your list and put it to the test of how feasible it is or how helpful it will be toward achieving the goal you wrote down in Step 2. Use the question box to give each item a score.

Step 5: Consider the Consequences of Each Solution

What are the pros and cons of each solution? Look back at each item you wrote down in Step 4. Then assign each one a score. Score the benefit (Pro +) in terms of how likely that strategy is to get you closer to your goal. Score the disadvantage (Con –) in terms of the effort, cost, or damage involved in implementing it.

Pro (+) Scale

How likely is it to get me closer to my goal?

Very Unlikely	Pretty Unlikely	Hard to Tell	Somewhat Likely	Very Likely
0	1	2	3	4

Con (–) Scale

How much effort, cost, or damage would this strategy involve?

None	Almost None	Some	A Lot	Extreme
0	1	2	3	4

---

*Example. **Blanca** filled out her question box this way when she carried out Step 5 and rated each one of her solutions from Step 4:

Step 4: List Several Possible Solutions to Address the Obstacle(s)

I could try to:

List strategies below	Pro (+) score	Con (−) score	Total pro−con
1) organize my room	3	4	−1
2) organize my book bag	4	2	2
3) quit school	0	4	−4
4) change my class schedule	2	3	−1
5) change where I keep my book bag	4	1	3
6) move on campus	3	4	−1

Step 6: Choose the Best One(s) to Try Out First

Which solutions should you try first? Now that you've scored all of your options, choosing the one or two strategies to start with should be easy. Which of your options had the highest total score? According to your own rating, the highest score has the most benefit compared to the cost, effort, or damage it could involve.

Step 6: Choose the Best One(s) to Try Out First

Which solutions should you try first? Which of the strategies in Step 5 had the highest score? Pick the top one or two and write them down below:

_____

_____

Example. Notice that none of Blanca's solutions had a perfect "4" score. Her skepticism and apprehension about trying something new contributed to the "con" score on some of the ideas with the highest "pro" score. This is a normal feeling, and you may have the same type of reaction. In the end, you need not expect a "perfect" pro–con score of 4 to consider an option; you need only pick the ones with the highest score.

After going through this comparison of pros to cons, Blanca decided to try **organizing** her book bag and also to change where she kept it in her room. While cleaning her room seemed like a good idea at first, she realized it would take too much time and effort. Being such a daunting task, it was only likely to bring her a lot more anxiety. Organizing and placing the book bag seemed like something she could do that would not be overwhelming. She considered her primary strength to be her sense of *purpose*, and that figured into her confidence to try this plan.

Blanca filled out her question box this way:

Step 6: Choose the Best One(s) to Try First

Organize my book bag

Change where I keep my book bag

Step 7: Implement the Solution and Track Your Progress

Now try the solution and track your progress. Use the next question box to map out your plan.

Step 7: Implement the Solution and Track Your Progress

Now try the solution and track your progress. Here is how:

Where will I do it?

_____

When will I do it?

_____

What do I need to do it?

_____

How will I do it?

_____

_____

Who can help me, if needed?

_____

How will I keep track of my success? (Look at your goal and than pick a way to track it—either a running count or a rating scale.)

_____

_____

_____

Example. **Blanca** filled out her question box this way:

Step 7: Implement the Solution and Track Your Progress

Where will I do it?

In my room.

When will I do it?

This Saturday.

What do I need to do it?

My book bag, the Organizational Checklist, and about 1 hour free time.

How will I do it?

Go through the bag using organization checklist. Keep my bag next to my door.

Who can help me, if needed?

I will try it on my own first, but my mother would help if I got stuck.

How will I keep track of my success? (Look at your goal and then pick a way to track it—either a running count or a rating scale.)

My goal is to be able to leave on time, which is 8:30, each day. So I will keep a running count log of the times I leave each day. I will write the time I left on my calendar that I have hanging on my bedroom door.

Step 8: Evaluate the Solution to See If It Met Your Goal

Did the solution meet your goal, or do you need to use a different solution? At this point you have tried out your new solution and are ready to see if it helped you meet your goal. Use the question box to evaluate your progress.

Step 8: Evaluate the Solution to See If It Met Your Goal

Did the solution meet your goal, or do you need to use a different solution? Answer the following questions to figure this out:

What was my goal? (Copy this from Step 2.)

_____

How did I measure my progress? (data, log, or record)

_____

What do the data show with regard to my goal?

_____

How would I rate my success, on a scale of 0–100% success for meeting my goal?

I was _____% successful.

0	10	20	30	40	50	60	70	80	90	100
None		A Little			Moderate			A Lot		Total

What should I do based on this success rate? (fill in the box next to the best choice)

☐ **Celebrate and keep doing what I am doing!**

☐ **Celebrate success and also modify the plan toward further improvement.**

Example. **Blanca** filled out her question box this way:

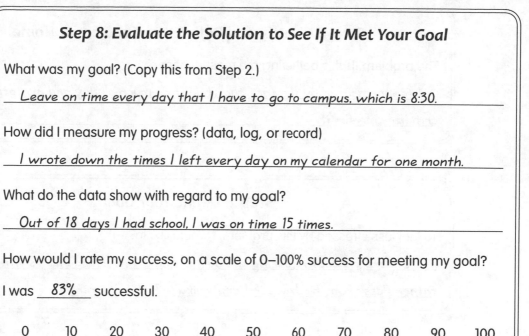

Step 8: Evaluate the Solution to See If It Met Your Goal

What was my goal? (Copy this from Step 2.)

Leave on time every day that I have to go to campus, which is 8:30.

How did I measure my progress? (data, log, or record)

I wrote down the times I left every day on my calendar for one month.

What do the data show with regard to my goal?

Out of 18 days I had school, I was on time 15 times.

How would I rate my success, on a scale of 0–100% success for meeting my goal?

I was ___83%___ successful.

0	10	20	30	40	50	60	70	80	90	100
None		A Little			Moderate			A Lot		Total

What should I do based on this success rate? (fill in the box next to the best choice)

☑ **Celebrate and keep doing what I am doing!**

☐ **Celebrate success and also modify the plan toward further improvement.**

Notice that Blanca considered herself successful even though she was not 100% consistent with her new goal. Nobody is going to have a perfect day every day. The important thing to realize is that she identified her problem, made a plan to try to improve it, and succeeded in making her home life much less stressful in the morning. You can use this problem-solving model for almost any problem you are having in your home.

Henry, introduced in Chapter 1 and mentioned again at the beginning of this chapter, approached his home-based problem using the problem-solving worksheet. Because he has been unemployed for several years, he struggles every day with the pressure of finding a job, but also has difficulty getting along with his father who is often critical of how he spends his day. Following are the question boxes he filled in.

Step 1: Identify and Define Your Problem at Home

The problem that is bothering me most at home is:

I feel pressured by the fact that I don't do much all day and my father criticizes me for it.

Step 2: Define Your Goal

To feel less stressed by this problem, I would like to:

Be more productive during the day and have fewer arguments with my father (less than the 3x/week I am having with him currently).

Step 3: Identify the Obstacles in the Way of Your Achieving the Goal

(**Thinking**) (**Social**) **Emotional** **Sensory/Movement**

I believe these differences are contributing in this way:

My thinking differences make it hard for me to make a schedule. My thinking differences also make me judge myself harshly. My social differences make it hard for me to communicate with my father about my struggles.

In the spirit of brainstorming, Henry wrote down all the ideas that came to his mind without judging any. He also used the Cheat Sheet from Chapter 6 to help him make the list of possible solutions. After listing them, he used the rating scale from the problem-solving sheet to weigh the pros and cons of each solution. The results of Steps 4 and 5 can be found in the box below.

Step 4: List Several Possible Solutions to Address the Obstacle(s)

I could try to:

List strategies below	Pro (+) score	Con (−) score	Total pro−con
1) stop looking for a job	0	3	−3
2) tell my father to go to hell	0	3	−3
3) make a schedule to follow at home	4	2	2
4) tell my father how he might help me	3	2	1
5) move out of my house into my own place	0	4	−4

In Step 6, Henry used the results of his evaluation to choose the two options with the highest pro–con score, which are highlighted in the box above. He then made a plan for how he would implement the solutions, using tools found in Chapter 6. His plan appears in the box for Step 7. He decided that his father might be able to help him design his *schedule*, so he planned to have a talk with his father that would help him carry out both strategies—telling his father how he could help and also designing a home schedule. Henry considered his primary strength in life to be *perseverance*, which he knew he could channel into any plan he might make.

Before doing this exercise, it had not occurred to Henry to make a schedule for his days at home because he assumed schedules were necessary only for working people. Now he realized that the structure would help him make better use of his time even though he wasn't working. He looked at several different kinds of schedules and datebooks and chose to use a "day at a glance" format that showed one day at a time. He designed his own template, which was very simple and he thought would be easy to use. It appears on the next two pages.

Henry was uncertain about what he should be filling in, so before approaching his father he spent a few days filling in exactly what he was doing with his time, as shown in the box below. Henry had thought he was doing absolutely nothing (black and white thinking), so he was surprised to see that, although there were several hours of the day that he could spend more productively, he was already making good use of some of his time—walking, checking job postings, running essential errands.

Daily Schedule		Day _____	Date _____
Time Blocks	**Activities**		**Done** ✓
9–10			
10–11			
11–12			
12–1			
1–2			
2–3			
3–4			
4–5			
5–6			
6–7			
7–8			
8–9			
9–10			

Henry's Daily Schedule		Day _Tuesday_	Date _March 2_
Time Blocks	**Activities**		**Done** ✓
9–10	Breakfast, e-mail		
10–11	Walk the dog		
11–12	E-mail, Internet surfing (random)		
12–1	Check job postings on Craigslist		
1–2	Internet surfing (random)		
2–3	Eat lunch		
3–4	Watch TV		
4–5	Watch TV		

Henry's Daily Schedule		Day _Tuesday_	Date _March 2_
Time Blocks	Activities		Done ✓
5–6	Watch TV		
6–7	Dad comes home, eat dinner		
7–8	Walk dog		
8–9	Grocery shopping for weekly household needs		
9–10	Watch TV, check e-mail		

Even with this evidence, Henry remained nervous about discussing time with his father. This is where the assertive statement formula came in handy. Henry used it to prepare to say the following to his dad.

ASSERTIVE STATEMENT FORMULA

I feel/felt __frustrated__ when you __criticize the way I spend time__ because __it does not help me be productive__, so I am asking you to __help me make a schedule and try not to criticize me__.

Step 7: Implement the Solution and Track Your Progress

Where will I do it?

__The kitchen table.__

When will I do it?

__Thursday evening.__

What do I need to do it?

__A blank Schedule Sheet, an Assertive Statement sheet.__

How will I do it?

__Prepare statement to use with father ahead of time, choose a schedule sheet that looks easy to use (find template online), ask father to sit with me after dinner to talk to me at the table, present idea to him, and ask him to help me.__

⇨

Who can help me, if needed?

My father.

How will I keep track of my success? (Look at your goal and then pick a way to track it—either a running count or a rating scale.)

I really have two goals that have to be tracked. I will measure my
productivity by counting up how many activities I complete compared to how
many I planned each day. I will also keep a tally of the number of arguments I
have with my father and compare it to the current rate of 3x/week by making
a tick mark on my schedule for each occurrence.

Henry's father seemed happy to be asked to help his son and promised not to be critical. He helped Henry replace some of his TV watching between 3:00 and 6:00 P.M. with other activities and gave him some pointers for improving his job search strategies. He also explained that he had been frustrated by Henry's apparent refusal to talk to him about these issues—that he was very worried about Henry and didn't know how to help him. Being given a chance to participate in the solution made his father feel less frustrated and less worried. Father and son agreed to try this new plan out for 2 weeks and then come back together to talk about how it went. Below are the results of the evaluation.

You can read more about how Henry changed his schedule and improved his job search in Chapter 8. But here the most important point is that until he went through all the problem-solving steps Henry didn't realize how anxious and stressed he was about the conflict with his father. He discovered he needed to address that first, and his problem solving helped him find some strategies to alleviate the pressure he was feeling at home.

Step 8: Evaluate the Solution to See If It Met Your Goal

What was my goal? Copy this from Step 2.

Be more productive and have less arguments with father.

How did I measure my progress? (data, log, or record)

I counted the number of completed vs. scheduled activities each day and kept
track of each argument I had with my father.

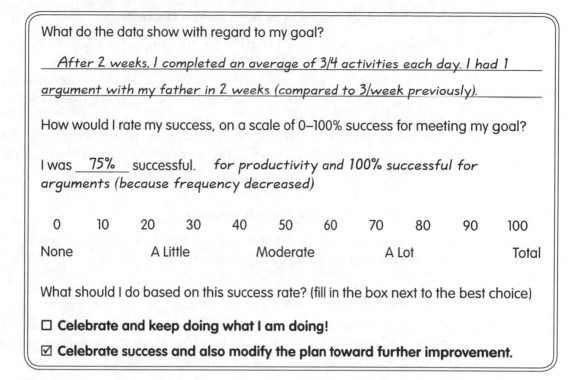

What do the data show with regard to my goal?

After 2 weeks, I completed an average of 3/4 activities each day. I had 1
argument with my father in 2 weeks (compared to 3/week previously).

How would I rate my success, on a scale of 0–100% success for meeting my goal?

I was __75%__ successful. _for productivity and 100% successful for_
arguments (because frequency decreased)

0	10	20	30	40	50	60	70	80	90	100
None		A Little			Moderate			A Lot		Total

What should I do based on this success rate? (fill in the box next to the best choice)

☐ **Celebrate and keep doing what I am doing!**

☑ **Celebrate success and also modify the plan toward further improvement.**

To give you one more example, here is how **Charles** used the eight steps to solve the problem of feeling too tense to interact with his son after they both got back from school in the afternoon. I've omitted the worksheet but described the process in Charles's own words:

Step 1: Identify and Define Your Problem

"I am bothered by my son's chatting when we both come home in the afternoon. I am tense from work and I find it hard to listen to him and answer him. I feel guilty because I may be hurting his feelings."

Step 2: Define Your Goal

"I would like to have a pleasant time with my son when we get home from school."

Step 3: Identify the Obstacles in the Way of Your Achieving the Goal

"I believe my *sensory* differences are contributing the most to this problem. It is very noisy at work, and coping with that takes a lot of effort. I'm successful but feel very tense after all of the hours of noise. My son's chatting feels like the 'last straw.'"

Step 4: List Several Possible Solutions to Address the Obstacle(s)

1. "Explore an after-school program for my son so he will not come straight home."
2. "Ask my wife to cut her work day short by two hours to come home early."
3. "Ask my wife to help us make an afternoon schedule that includes 'quiet time' for me when I get home."
4. "Listen to music with my son when we first get home because we both love it (I got this idea by looking at the Cheat Sheet—it made me think about relaxation techniques)."

Step 5: Consider the Consequences of Each Solution

"After evaluating the pros and cons of each solution, a combination of solutions 3 and 4 has the most benefit with the least cost."

Step 6: Choose the Best One(s) to Try Out First

"I'll ask my wife to help us make a schedule that includes 'iPod time' when we get home. I need only about 20 minutes to unwind. I consider my primary strength to be my *capacity for pleasure* (music), and my wife pointed out that I have a strong sense of *personal responsibility*, which is why I am working to make things better for my son when he is with me.

Step 7: Implement the Solution and Track Your Progress

"After discussing this with my wife, we introduced the idea of 'iPod time' to my son. We all agreed that when my son and I first come home from school we'll sit in the living room together listening to our iPods (we each have one, and we like different kinds of music). We agreed that we'll chat about my son's day after our iPod time. I will measure my success using a daily rating scale. Each weeknight I'll rate the degree to which I felt satisfied with the quality of time I spent with my son."

Step 8: Evaluate the Solution to See If It Met Your Goal

"After one month, I rated the quality of time between 7 and 10 every day. The low range (7) happened a few times when my son had some problem at school that he wanted to talk about right away. On average, I consider this solution 90% successful. Most days I feel so relaxed after my 20 minutes of music!"

A Word about Sleep Problems

Before ending this chapter on home-based problems, I want to leave you with some tips about healthy sleep habits. People on the spectrum commonly struggle with sleep difficulties of one kind or another. These range from sleeping too little (difficulty falling or staying asleep), to sleeping too much (difficulty waking up, long hours), erratic sleep patterns (too much one night, too little the next), or "night-owl syndrome" where one sleeps normally but the preferred sleep cycle is incongruent with conventional society (e.g., sleeping from 3:00 A.M. to 11:00 A.M.). Sleep is a complex human behavior, and problems in this area can be indicative of any number of medical (e.g., sleep apnea, thyroid disorders) or psychiatric (mood disorders) conditions. Poor sleep can be very disruptive and make problem solving less effective. If you have sleep problems, have an evaluation by a physician. Also try these tips for healthy sleep habits.

- Try to go to sleep at the same time every night. Pick a time that will not be affected by changes in your evening routine.
- Try to wake up at the same time every morning, regardless of your daytime schedule (try not to "sleep in" on the weekends).
- Don't get into bed until it's time to go to sleep. Avoid other activities in bed (e.g., using the laptop, watching TV, reading). Try to do all your evening activities any place but the bed.
- Do an environment check to see if any disruptive elements, such as light or noise, could be modified to promote sleep.
- If you are a "night owl" or an "early bird" by nature and your schedule permits it, try to make your sleep and wake-up times fit with your natural tendency. Consistency promotes healthy sleep.

8

At Work

Work is one of the greatest sources of pride and fulfillment for adults. Making an important contribution to others and maintaining financial independence are crucial to health, happiness, and self-confidence. Yet the majority of adults on the spectrum are either unemployed or underemployed (working at a job that does not tap their highest level of education or talent). This is one of the most devastating issues for my patients and their families. At best, you may be grappling with ongoing disappointment over lost opportunities to use your abilities and strengths productively. At worst, your lack of income may be severely restricting your housing and lifestyle choices. In the pages ahead, you'll find strategies that you can apply to improving your work situation.

If you read Chapter 7, you've already seen how **Henry** used the problem-solving steps to get along better with his father at home. Here you'll see how the 29-year-old unemployed college graduate addresses his difficulty with *planning and organizing* his job search and with *managing time*.

Margaret, the 61-year-old physician who works in a group medical practice, likes her career and work but has trouble participating in *conversations* and *connecting with her coworkers*.

Meredith, age 46, has a law degree but is an example of someone who is underemployed. Instead of using her degree, she works part-time at a nursery/home garden center and even in that job struggles to *multitask* work assignments and take care of her diabetes (discussed with health issues in Chapter 13).

Like these three people on the spectrum, you may be having difficulty finding or keeping a job or dealing with the multiple stressors that come with work life. If you identified times of day involving your work life as the most stressful when you filled out the clock worksheet in Chapter 1, this is an important chapter for you. Use the checklists in Worksheets 22–24 to begin the process of discovering how to manage your work life more effectively. These problems will look familiar to you as you already saw them in Chapter 1. Even if you have a job, make sure you look at all three sheets. Each sheet has a list of problems common among people on the spectrum but also leaves blank spaces at the bottom for you to fill in any other work-related problems.

My Problems with Work
Getting or Keeping a Satisfying Job

Check off (✓) the statements that sound familiar to you or reflect your experiences with unemployment or underemployment. If you have a problem related to getting or keeping a job that does not appear on this list, fill it in on one of the blanks at the bottom.

- ☐ I can't seem to find a job.
- ☐ I get so overwhelmed by the job search that I often avoid it altogether.
- ☐ I want to look for a job, but I don't know where to begin.
- ☐ I get so nervous on job interviews, and I never get called back.
- ☐ I often go on interviews that I think went well, but then I never hear back from the employer. I don't know what is going wrong.
- ☐ I can find only low-level jobs where I can't use my talents.
- ☐ I always do well at a new job, but eventually things fall apart and I get fired.
- ☐ I get bored really easily, and I have quit a lot of jobs in my life.
- ☐ I've given up on trying to work—I have stopped searching for jobs, but I worry because I don't have enough money to live on.
- ☐ _____
- ☐ _____
- ☐ _____

My Problems with Work
Getting Work Done on the Job

If you have a job now or had one in the past, check off (✓) the statements below that sound like experiences you have had while working. If you have a problem related to completing your work that does not appear on this list, fill it in on one of the blanks at the bottom.

- ☐ I can't seem to get everything done.
- ☐ I procrastinate.
- ☐ I never seem to have enough time.
- ☐ I make so many mistakes, over and over again.
- ☐ I can't get any work done when I am constantly interrupted.
- ☐ My desk is always a mess, and I can't find what I need.
- ☐ I have to have my work materials arranged a certain way, or I get thrown off.
- ☐ The schedule is too strenuous for me.
- ☐ I can't concentrate because my workspace is too noisy.
- ☐ I can't concentrate because the lighting bothers me.
- ☐ I hate telephone work; I have trouble following what the other person is saying.
- ☐ _____
- ☐ _____
- ☐ _____

WORKSHEET 24

My Problems with Work
Work Relationships

If you have a job now or had one in the past, check off (✓) the statements below that sound like your work experiences. Fill in the blanks with the name of the person involved with the problem you check off. If you have a problem with the person(s) you work with that does appear on this list, fill it in on one of the blanks at the bottom.

The people I deal with most at work are:

_____   _____

_____   _____

_____   _____

☐ _____ criticizes me all the time.

☐ I am worried that I am displeasing _____ (my supervisor).

☐ _____ has passed me over for promotion several times even though I deserve one.

☐ I get upset when customers or clients ask questions that I can't answer.

☐ I have a lot of arguments with _____.

☐ I can't seem to connect with _____.

☐ I have been told I am not a good team player.

☐ I am always getting irritated with _____.

☐ I have trouble sharing workspace because _____ keeps moving my stuff.

☐ I am afraid to ask _____ (supervisor) questions; he/she always looks too busy.

☐ _____ (supervisor) gets annoyed when I ask too many questions.

☐ _____

Problem Solving

If you identified more than one problem with work, you will need to choose one to address first; you can then repeat the eight-step problem-solving process for the other problems at a later time. As mentioned in Chapter 6, it makes sense to start out working on the issue that's causing you and/or the people around you the most distress. Worksheet 25 can help you figure out which one that is. Rate the level of distress caused by each problem and then pick the one with the highest score to tackle first. You can return to the others later, in order of most to least distress. It can also be helpful to talk over this prioritizing with a trusted person in your life.

The next few pages will guide you through the steps of solving the problem you just identified. For each step you will be asked to write your answers in the question box. Each box will give you instructions, and then I'll show you how *Henry* filled out the box.

WORKSHEET 25

Choosing Which Problem to Work on First

You don't need to use this worksheet if you checked off only one problem on Worksheets 22–24. Otherwise, list the problems you checked in the first column below. Then use this rating scale to estimate the amount of stress the issue is causing you and/or the people around you.

How much distress is this problem causing in my life?

Almost None	Some	Moderate Amount	A Lot	Extreme
1	2	3	4	5

Problem   **Distress Rating**

_____   _____

_____   _____

_____   _____

_____   _____

Step 1: Identify and Define Your Problem with Work

What is bothering you about work? You've already done this first step if you filled out Worksheets 22–24. Write the problem you have chosen to work on first in the box.

Step 1: Identify and Define Your Problem with Work

What is bothering you about work?

The problem that is bothering me most about work is:

_____

_____

_____

Example. **Henry** had identified two different problems with job seeking and used Worksheet 25 to choose which one to work on first.

Example from Henry

WORKSHEET 25

Choosing Which Problem
to Work on First

How much distress is this problem causing in my life?

Almost None	Some	Moderate Amount	A Lot	Extreme
1	2	3	4	5

Problem	Distress Rating
I get so overwhelmed by the job search I avoid it.	5
I have gone on interviews before, but never get called back.	4
_____	_____
_____	_____

Example. After choosing his first-priority problem, **Henry** filled out his Step 1 question box this way:

> ### *Step 1: Identify and Define Your Problem with Work*
>
> The problem that is bothering me most about work is:
>
> *I avoid job search activities because I am not sure what I should be doing and it makes me so nervous. I spend only an hour a day looking at postings on the Internet.*

Step 2: Define Your Goal

What would you like to see change to minimize the problem you identified with work? What would need to be different for you to feel less bothered by the problem? The goal you lay out is simply the opposite of the problem you listed. List your goal in the box below, and if you need an example, look at Henry's box. Notice how Henry stated the goal as the opposite of his problem. Spending more time is the opposite of avoiding the activity. Stating the goal in the affirmative gets Henry closer to an action plan and a way to measure progress.

> ### *Step 2: Define Your Goal*
>
> *What would you like to see change to minimize the problem you identified with work? The goal you lay out is simply the opposite of the problem you listed.*
>
> To feel less stressed by this problem, I would like to:
>
> _____
>
> _____

Example. **Henry's** goal is listed below.

> ### *Step 2: Define Your Goal*
>
> To feel less stressed by this problem, I would like to:
>
> *Spend at least two hours a day looking for a job*

Step 3: Identify the Obstacles in the Way of Your Achieving the Goal

What is getting in the way of your goal? The next step is to identify obstacles for meeting your goal. Here it is particularly important to consider your ASD characteristics as hidden players in your problem. As you go through this step, you may rely on the information you were given in Part I of this book about your ASD differences. As you think about the problem you listed above, look at the chart on page 199 called "ASD Differences That Can Contribute to Problems at Work." Read through that chart with your own problem in mind and also consider the questions below.

Thinking Differences

How might my *executive functioning* issues be contributing to my problems at work or finding work? For example, do I have difficulty planning, which causes me to procrastinate on my job search or work responsibilities? Do I find it hard to concentrate on more than one task at a time, causing me to get very few things done each day? Do I persist too long, repeating a strategy that is clearly not working because I have difficulty shifting to new strategies? How might my *negative self-talk* be contributing to my problems at work or finding work? What am I saying to myself that is putting more pressure on me? Could I be engaging in perfectionistic thinking, all-or-nothing thinking, or catastrophic thinking? For example, do I assume the worst will happen before an important activity? Do I expect perfection from myself and/or coworkers, which leads to frustration?

Social Differences

How might my *social perception* be contributing to my problems at work or finding work? Is it possible that I sometimes misunderstand what my coworkers or supervisors are trying to tell me? For example, do I still feel uncertain about what my boss expects from me? Am I still uncertain about how I should handle some aspects of a job interview? How might my *social/communication skills* be contributing to problems at work or finding work? Is it possible that coworkers, supervisors, or interviewers are not communicating clearly enough about what they expect and I don't know how to seek clarification? For example, I feel uncertain about when and how to ask my boss questions without annoying him or her. Is my problem caused partly by my not knowing what to say or do when dealing with coworkers, supervisors, or interviewers? For example, I don't know how I should handle it if there are moments of silence during a job interview. Or I don't know what to say if a coworker shares some personal information with me, like telling me what she did over the weekend.

Emotional Differences

How might my emotional reactions to things be affecting my problems at work or finding work? Do I have difficulty *regulating* my emotions? Do I take too long to calm down after an upsetting incident? Do I have difficulty *identifying* my feelings or *asking for help* when I am upset? Am I overreacting or underreacting to things that happen at work? Do I tend to avoid situations that cause me to feel too much anxiety or worry?

Sensory and Movement Differences

How might my sensory issues be contributing to my problems at work or finding work? Am I *oversensitive* or *undersensitive* to certain types of light, sound, smell, taste, or touch? Does my noisy work environment contribute to my avoiding work? How might my *movement* and *coordination* issues be contributing to my problems at work? For example, do I feel awkward and have difficulties using certain tools or devices? Is it possible that my hygiene is not acceptable to some people because my sensory/movement problems interfere with bathing or grooming?

Now fill out the question box, but try hard not to think about other problems you have besides the one you chose for this exercise.

Step 3: Identify the Obstacles in the Way of Your Achieving the Goal

What is getting in the way of your goal? Remember to focus *only* on the problem and goal you wrote in Steps 1 and 2. First circle the category(ies) of ASD differences you suspect are involved in this problem:

Thinking   **Social**   **Emotional**   **Sensory/Movement**

I believe these differences are contributing in this way:

_____

_____

_____

_____

_____

_____

Example. **Henry** filled out his Step 3 question box this way:

> ### Step 3: Identify the Obstacles in the Way of Your Achieving the Goal
>
> (Thinking)   Social   (Emotional)   Sensory/Movement
>
> I believe these differences are contributing in this way:
>
> _My thinking differences make it hard for me to make a good plan for job_
> _searching. I only know how to search Craigslist, but I don't know what else to_
> _do. Also, my résumé needs to be updated, but I am not sure how to do it. My_
> _emotional differences cause me to feel so nervous about all of this that I find_
> _it easier in the short run just to avoid it, but it makes me feel more_
> _depressed in the long run._

When you filled out your sheet, did you circle more than one area of ASD differences? Henry circled both thinking differences and emotional differences. This illustrates that sometimes a single issue can have several causes.

Step 4: List Several Possible Solutions to Address the Obstacle(s)

What are the possible solutions for the obstacles? Try to list as many ideas as possible. Remember that this is the step some people call "brainstorming." Generate as many possibilities as come to mind, without inhibition. Don't judge or evaluate any idea—just write it down no matter how weird or silly it seems. In Step 5 you will weed through them and discard any that are not useful, so no harm can be done.

Start by looking at the Cheat Sheet at the end of Chapter 6. Find the ASD difference that you circled on the top row of the Cheat Sheet. Then look down the column underneath each and find the dots. Each dot marks the row in which you will find a solution in the far left column. Those approaches should be considered first for your problem, and Chapter 6 provides you with the instructions and tools for each solution. Also, try to consider your *strengths* as you complete this step because they also play an important role in your solutions. Refer back to Worksheets 3 and 4 in Chapter 1. Write your primary strengths in the blanks here so you can keep them in mind while you are generating solutions.

My strengths are: _____, _____, and _____.

Differences →	Thinking	Social	Emotional	Sensory/Movement
Problems Getting or Keeping a Satisfying Job	• *Difficulties goal setting and planning* make it hard to plan and carry out the tasks involved in searching for a job • *Attention regulation difficulties* can make it hard to concentrate during an interview	• Your *unique style of processing language* may lead to difficulties managing a job interview • You may not notice or interpret cues or *mind-read* what others are expecting from you on a job interview	• Your difficulty *regulating your anxiety* can make job interviews very challenging • Your difficulty *regulating your emotions* can put you at risk for engaging in behaviors others would perceive as unusual (e.g., fidgeting, odd vocalizations or sounds) on a job interview	• Hypersensitivity to noise, light, smell, taste, or touch can interfere with your ability to concentrate during a job interview • *Fine motor problems* (coordinated handwork) could affect functions like handwriting in filling out an application • *Hypersensitivity or fine motor problems* can lead to poor hygiene
Problems Getting Work Done on the Job	• *Attention regulation difficulties* can make it hard to complete tasks • *Difficulties organizing information* make it hard to organize your personal spaces • *Working memory difficulties* make it hard to do more than one task at a time at work • *Focusing on detail but ignoring the "big picture"* may cause you to overlook important aspects of work assignments • *Dichotomous, all-or-nothing* thinking can cause undue pressure and anxiety around completing work tasks	• Your *unique style of processing language* may lead you to miss others' expectations about your work responsibilities • Your difficulty *initiating conversations* may interfere with your ability to ask for help on tasks you find difficult to complete • Any of your social differences can interfere with your ability to complete tasks that are done by a team	• Your difficulty *recognizing and identifying negative emotions* that you are feeling can interfere with your awareness that you are struggling with work assignments and may need a change (e.g., anxiety, anger) • Your difficulty *regulating your negative emotions* related to work can contribute to your experience of getting extremely overwhelmed by the pressures involved	• Hypersensitivity to noise, light, smell, taste, or touch can interfere with your ability to concentrate in the workplace • Hyposensitivity (underresponsive sense) can interfere with picking up on important cues in the workplace (e.g., signs, alarms) • *Fine motor problems* (coordinated handwork) could affect tasks like handwriting, typing, assembly work, use of hand tools, operating intricate electronic devices • *Gross motor* (coordinated whole-body movement) problems could affect some tasks (operating heavy equipment, moving large objects)
Problems with Work Relationships	• Supervisors may be frustrated if you have difficulty with your work assignments • Coworkers may be affected adversely by your difficulties managing tasks and responsibilities due to your thinking differences (e.g., unequal distribution of work) • Coworkers may be resentful if your work habits affect them adversely	• You may not notice or interpret cues or *mind-read* what others are expecting from you at work • You may be perceived by others as uncaring or aloof because of the way you *experience and express empathy* • The *unique way you process and express language* can contribute to misunderstandings with coworkers and supervisors; makes it hard to assert yourself • Your difficulty with *conversation skills* may interfere with making positive connections with coworkers	• Your difficulty *recognizing and identifying negative emotions* can contribute to problems communicating with supervisors or co-workers about your needs • Your difficulty *regulating your negative emotions* can also put you at risk for having anxious or angry outbursts, which may be disruptive in the workplace, leading to adverse effects on relationships at work	• *Hypersensitivities* can cause problems when others unknowingly doing things that are unpleasant to you (playing music, using strong perfume, using cleaning products with a strong smell, using friendly touch like a pat on the back or a handshake) • *Fine or gross motor problems* can be obstacles to many types of cooperative leisure activities that coworkers do during break time or at company events (e.g., like games or sports; fewer opportunities to make positive connections with coworkers) • *Hypersensitivity or fine motor problems* can lead to poor hygiene

ASD differences that can contribute to problems at work.

Step 4: List Several Possible Solutions to Address the Obstacle(s)

What are the possible solutions for the obstacles? Now, considering all the solutions you saw on the Cheat Sheet, and some you may think of on your own, list all the possibilities you can imagine to address the ASD differences involved in the problem you listed in Step 1. For the moment, ignore the score columns on the right.

I could try to:

List strategies below	Pro (+) score	Con (−) score	Total pro−con

Example. **Henry** filled out the question box this way:

Step 4: List Several Possible Solutions to Address the Obstacle(s)

I could try to:

List strategies below	Pro (+) score	Con (−) score	Total pro−con
1) stop looking for a job			
2) use thinking techniques to help my anxiety			
3) use some of my father's new ideas			
4) try to look at Craigslist more often			
5) use my new schedule to ensure 2 hours			
6) go back to school			

Notice that Henry included everything on his list that came to mind, even things that may seem outrageous or unlikely (e.g., stop searching, go back to school). He looked at the Cheat Sheet, which gave him ideas 2 and 5, and had already worked on some home-based problems with his father (see Chapter 7), which had led to some ideas for this work-related problem as well. This is an example of "brainstorming." Henry can't possibly do all the things on this list, but he'll be able to use the next step to figure out what is most useful to him.

Step 5: Consider the Consequences of Each Solution

What are the pros and cons of each solution? Now you will put each item on your list to the test of how feasible it is or how helpful it will be toward the goal you wrote down in Step 2. Use the question box to give each item a score.

Step 5: Consider the Consequences of Each Solution

What are the pros and cons of each solution? Look back at each item you wrote down in Step 4. Then assign each one a score. Score the benefit (Pro +) in terms of how likely that strategy is to get you closer to your goal. Score the disadvantage (Con –) in terms of the effort, cost, or damage involved in implementing it.

Pro (+) Scale

How likely is it to get me closer to my goal?

Very Unlikely	Pretty Unlikely	Hard to Tell	Somewhat Likely	Very Likely
0	1	2	3	4

Con (–) Scale

How much effort, cost, or damage would this strategy involve?

None	Almost None	Some	A Lot	Extreme
0	1	2	3	4

Example. ***Henry's*** answers appear in the next question box.

Step 4: List Several Possible Solutions to Address the Obstacle(s)

I could try to:

List strategies below	Pro (+) score	Con (−) score	Total pro–con
1) stop looking for a job	0	3	−3
2) use thinking techniques to help my anxiety	4	2	2
3) use some of my father's new ideas	3	1	2
4) try to look at Craigslist more often	1	1	0
5) use my new schedule to ensure 2 hours	4	2	2
6) go back to school	1	4	−3

Step 6: Choose the Best One(s) to Try Out First

Which solutions should you try first? Now that you've scored all of your options, choosing the one or two strategies to start with should be easy. Which of your options had the highest total score? According to your own rating, the highest score has the most benefit compared to the cost, effort, or damage it could involve. Notice that Henry ended up with three solutions, all tied with the same pro–con score. He feels anxious and even a little skeptical about trying his new strategies, which is why he assigned a "con" rating to even his best ideas. Feeling this way is perfectly natural, and you may experience the same type of reaction. In the end, you need not expect a "perfect" pro–con score of 4 to consider an option; you need only pick the ones with the highest score.

Step 6: Choose the Best One(s) to Try Out First

Which solutions should you try first? Which of the strategies in Step 5 had the highest score? Pick the top one or two and write them down below:

_____

_____

Example. **Henry** filled out the question box the following way. Notice he combined ideas 3 and 5 from Step 4 into one idea—using his father's ideas and applying scheduling techniques.

> ### Step 6: Choose the Best One(s) to Try Out First
>
> _Use thinking techniques to help my anxiety_
>
> _Use my father's ideas for search and schedule_

Step 7: Implement the Solution and Track Your Progress

Now try the solution and track your progress. Use the next question box to map out your plan.

> ### Step 7: Implement the Solution and Track Your Progress
>
> _Now try the solution and track your progress._ Here is how:
>
> Where will I do it?
>
> _____
>
> When will I do it?
>
> _____
>
> What do I need to do it?
>
> _____
>
> How will I do it?
>
> _____
>
> _____
>
> Who can help me, if needed?
>
> _____
>
> How will I keep track of my success? (Look at your goal and then pick a way to track it—either a running count or a rating scale.)
>
> _____
>
> _____

*Example. **Henry*** studied the ***thinking techniques*** in Chapter 6 and chose to use both ***mindfulness*** and ***dimensional*** thinking techniques to address his anxiety and avoidance. He became aware that he was judging himself harshly for his situation and was also thinking in black and white terms about his job search. The two most common examples of negative self-talk he discovered were: "I am a loser because I can't get my act together on my own to look for a job." "I am a total failure because I have not found a job in the 6 years since I graduated from college." Henry remembered to consider his primary strength, ***perseverance***, as an attribute that would help him implement his new plan.

Keep in mind that Henry had already addressed another home-based problem regarding his father, which was covered in Chapter 7 (using an assertive statement to approach his father for help), which led to the *scheduling* tools referred to in this plan.

Step 7: Implement the Solution and Track Your Progress

Where will I do it?

In my room at my desk

When will I do it?

Every morning

What do I need to do it?

My Schedule Sheet and my Job Search To-Do List

How will I do it?

Print a new schedule sheet each morning and use it as a checklist all day.

Who can help me, if needed?

My father, but only if I get stuck on something

How will I keep track of my success? (Look at your goal and then pick a way to track it—either a running count or a rating scale.)

My goal is to work for 2 hours each day on the job search. I will keep track of the number of days I complete 2 hours of job search activities.

Here is a schedule that Henry and his father designed that incorporated more time and strategies for job searching. The shaded items represent new things that were added to Henry's schedule after he sought help from his father (in Chapter 7).

Henry's Daily Schedule		Day _____ Date _____	
Time Blocks	**Activities**		**Done** ✓
9–10	Breakfast, e-mail, read Acceptance Phrases		
10–11	Walk the dog		
11–12	Work on an item from Job Search To-Do List		
12–1	Work on an item from Job Search To-Do List		
1–2	Internet surfing (random)		
2–3	Eat lunch		
3–4	Go to the Y to swim		
4–5	Errands for me or household		
5–6	Watch TV		
6–7	Dad comes home, eat dinner		
7–8	Walk dog		
8–9	Grocery shopping for weekly household needs		
9–10	Watch TV, check e-mail, Daily Rating of Success: _____		

Here are the "Acceptance Phrases" that Henry created after reading about acceptance in Chapter 6, to counteract his harsh judgments about himself.

<u>My Acceptance Phrases</u>

I accept that my brain works differently.

I accept that I need help to plan some things and that I don't have to do everything on my own.

I accept that my anxiety is a natural part of the job search.

Following are the "Job Search To-Do List" that Henry's father helped to create and the daily rating scale that Henry created to help himself address his all-or-nothing self-talk about being a "failure."

Job Search To-Do List

    1) Buy a current book on résumé writing

    2) Read the book on résumé writing

    3) Update résumé

    4) Check online job postings several times a week

    5) Do research online about professional job counselors

    6) Find out if job counseling may be offered by a government agency for people with an ASD diagnosis

    7) Make an appointment with a job counselor

    8) Meet with the job counselor

    9) Make a new to-do list with the help of the professional counselor

---

DAILY RATING OF SUCCESS

Today I felt *successful* to the following degree:

0	1	2	3	4	5	6	7	8	9	10
None		A Little			Moderate		A Lot			Extreme

Step 8: Evaluate the Solution to See If It Met Your Goal

Did the solution meet your goal, or do you need to use a different solution? At this point you have tried out your new solution and are ready to see if it helped you meet your goal. Use the question box below to evaluate your progress.

Step 8: Evaluate the Solution to See If It Met Your Goal

Did the solution meet your goal, or do you need to use a different solution? Answer the following questions to figure this out:

What was my goal? (Copy this from Step 2.)

_____

How did I measure my progress? (data, log, or record)

_____

What do the data show with regard to my goal?

_____

How would I rate my success, on a scale of 0–100% success for meeting my goal?

I was _____% successful.

0	10	20	30	40	50	60	70	80	90	100
None		A Little			Moderate			A Lot		Total

What should I do based on this success rate? (fill in the box next to the best choice)

☐ **Celebrate and keep doing what I am doing!**

☐ **Celebrate success and also modify the plan toward further improvement.**

Example. **Henry** filled out his question box this way after practicing his new schedule for 2 weeks.

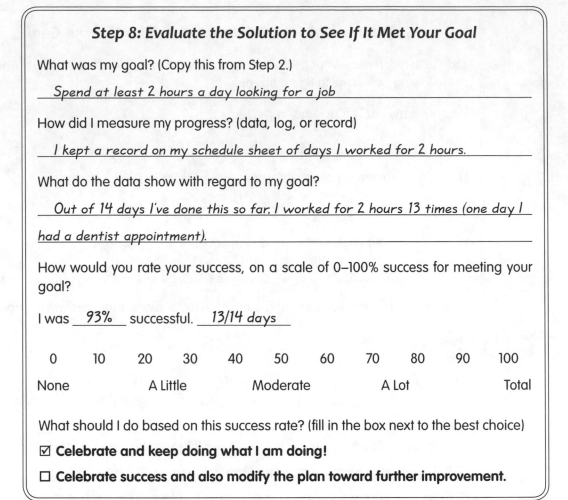

Step 8: Evaluate the Solution to See If It Met Your Goal

What was my goal? (Copy this from Step 2.)

Spend at least 2 hours a day looking for a job

How did I measure my progress? (data, log, or record)

I kept a record on my schedule sheet of days I worked for 2 hours.

What do the data show with regard to my goal?

Out of 14 days I've done this so far, I worked for 2 hours 13 times (one day I had a dentist appointment).

How would you rate your success, on a scale of 0–100% success for meeting your goal?

I was __93%__ successful. __13/14 days__

| 0 | 10 | 20 | 30 | 40 | 50 | 60 | 70 | 80 | 90 | 100 |
| None | | A Little | | Moderate | | | A Lot | | | Total |

What should I do based on this success rate? (fill in the box next to the best choice)

☑ **Celebrate and keep doing what I am doing!**

☐ **Celebrate success and also modify the plan toward further improvement.**

Notice that Henry considered himself successful even without 100% compliance—another excellent demonstration of dimensional thinking. The more Henry practices this new way of evaluating himself, the less he'll avoid looking for a job and the more willing he'll be to accept help.

Like Henry, *Margaret* used the problem-solving worksheet to tackle a work-related issue. Margaret wants to get along with her coworkers at the medical practice, but chatting with them during lunch as they expect robs her of the solitary relaxation time she needs. Following is the worksheet as she filled it in.

Step 1: Identify and Define Your Problem with Work

The problem that is bothering me most about work is:

I am frustrated because I do not like making small talk with coworkers, but I am concerned that I am not well liked by staff.

Step 2: Define Your Goal

To feel less stressed by this problem, I would like to:

Have more frequent social (non-work-related) interactions with staff while also having an opportunity to relax during my lunch-hour breaks.

Step 3: Identify the Obstacles in the Way of Your Achieving the Goal

Thinking   (**Social**)   (**Emotional**)   **Sensory/Movement**

I believe these differences are contributing in this way:

My social differences make it hard for me to make conversation with people I don't know very well. Also, my emotional differences contribute to a lot of tension at work, and I need quiet, restful time at lunch so I feel refreshed enough to complete my day's work.

For the next step, Margaret tried to think of as many solutions as possible, including ones that seemed unlikely to help. She used the Cheat Sheet at the end of Chapter 6 and also made up some solutions of her own. After listing them, she used the rating scale from the problem-solving sheet to weigh the pros and cons of each solution. The results of Steps 4 and 5 can be seen in the box below.

Step 4: List Several Possible Solutions to Address the Obstacle(s)

I could try to:

List strategies below	Pro (+) score	Con (−) score	Total pro–con
1) ignore my coworkers and office manager	0	4	−4
2) leave the group practice and go on my own	0	4	−4
3) use techniques to understand others	3	2	1
4) use relaxation techniques	4	1	3

In Step 6, Margaret used the results of her evaluation to pick the two options with the highest pro–con score, which are highlighted in the Step 4 box. Once again, the total scores are not a "perfect 4" because there is always some apprehension and effort that goes into trying anything new.

Margaret studied the ***techniques to understand other people*** found in Chapter 6 and was surprised that there could be so many levels of closeness with people. After examining the various definitions of relationships there, she decided that her coworkers should be *acquaintances* and they could have positive relationships without becoming close friends (another surprise and relief to her). She was also intrigued by the idea that people feel good when you try to learn and remember things about them—she had previously seen no purpose to "small talk," and its lack of structure made her very uncomfortable. With this new understanding, she knew that the objective of her small talk with coworkers would be to increase their comfort with her so that she would have more positive working relationships with them. Following the guidelines for gathering information about people that she found in Chapter 6 gave the activity enough structure in her mind to make it feel more comfortable.

At the same time, Margaret did not want to sacrifice the rest and relaxation that she needed at lunchtime, which led her to read about the ***relaxation techniques*** found in Chapter 6. Her solution was surprisingly simple. She had always loved walking and did so frequently during free time outside of work, but it had never occurred to her that she could use it as a relaxation technique at work. Luckily there was a nice park near the office. She reasoned that if she took a 15-minute walk at the beginning of her lunch break, she would have the time away from people that she so desperately needed after a busy morning of interacting with patients. She hoped that she would feel refreshed enough to spend the rest of the time in the lunchroom making small talk while she ate. She considered her primary strengths to be *perseverance* and *authenticity*, which added to her confidence that she could carry out her plan. Her implementation plan appears in the next box.

Step 7: Implement the Solution and Track Your Progress

Where will I do it?

  At work.

When will I do it?

  At lunchtime.

What do I need to do it?

  Comfortable walking shoes.

How will I do it?

  Begin my lunch hour with a 15-minute walk in the park across the street from my office. Then I will spend 30 minutes in the lunchroom, eating my lunch and trying to learn a little bit of information about each person who comes in.

Who can help me, if needed?

  I will try to implement this on my own but could discuss it with my office manager if I run into any problems.

How will I keep track of my success? (Look at your goal and then pick a way to track it—either a running count or a rating scale.)

  My goal involves two things. I will measure my relaxation by tracking how tense I feel before the walk and again after the walk each day. I will keep track of interactions with my coworkers by keeping a tally (e.g., ///) in my datebook of each time I learn one new fact about a person and each time I use a new fact in a later conversation with that person.

Here is the scale Margaret used to rate her level of tension before and after each lunchtime walk. Below that are the guidelines she followed for learning about her coworkers as acquaintances, which she took from reading Chapter 6.

RATING OF DAILY WALK

Before Walk: _____   **After Walk:** _____

I feel tense to the following degree:

0	1	2	3	4	5	6	7	8	9	10
None		A Little			Moderate			A Lot		Extreme

<u>My Guidelines for Learning about My Coworkers</u>

1) Gather information about them by:
   — asking direct questions about them and listening to the answers
   — observing things they do
   — listening to what they say to me or to others

2) Limit questions and comments to those reserved for acquaintances. Avoid questions about private life but do ask about
   — interests
   — hobbies
   — work
   — school

3) Remember to follow up on questions about this information during conversations I may have on another day

---

Margaret decided to try her new plan for 1 month before evaluating it. Her walks were successful in reducing her tension. She noticed that she still had moderate tension after the walk because she was nervous about going into the lunchroom, but it was still lower than before the walk. She found that it improved across the month. She managed to learn a lot of new things about her coworkers. For example, one of the medical technicians was going to school part-time to pursue a career as a physician's assistant. Once Margaret knew that about her, she made sure to ask her how things were going at school each time she found herself in the lunchroom with her. She also learned that the receptionist was a dog breeder on the side, which gave Margaret something to ask her about during lunchtime. Margaret also felt more comfortable when there were two or more people in the lunchroom making conversation, because she would simply listen to what they were saying, realizing that she could participate by just showing she was paying attention, but did not feel pressure to say something all of the time. This was another way for her to find out about their interests and hobbies. While Margaret did sometimes hear about topics she wasn't very interested in, she considered her goal of learning about others the rationale for paying attention. Her answers to the Step 8 questions appear below.

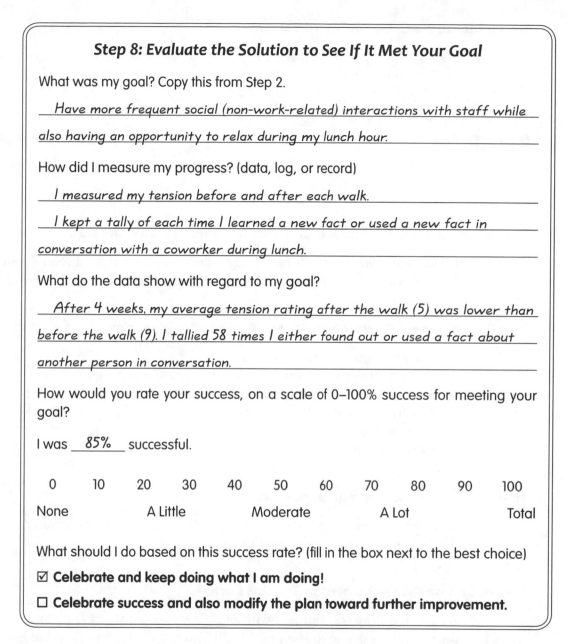

> ### *Step 8: Evaluate the Solution to See If It Met Your Goal*
>
> What was my goal? Copy this from Step 2.
>
> _Have more frequent social (non-work-related) interactions with staff while also having an opportunity to relax during my lunch hour._
>
> How did I measure my progress? (data, log, or record)
>
> _I measured my tension before and after each walk._
>
> _I kept a tally of each time I learned a new fact or used a new fact in conversation with a coworker during lunch._
>
> What do the data show with regard to my goal?
>
> _After 4 weeks, my average tension rating after the walk (5) was lower than before the walk (9). I tallied 58 times I either found out or used a fact about another person in conversation._
>
> How would you rate your success, on a scale of 0–100% success for meeting your goal?
>
> I was ___85%___ successful.
>
> | 0 | 10 | 20 | 30 | 40 | 50 | 60 | 70 | 80 | 90 | 100 |
> |---|----|----|----|----|----|----|----|----|----|-----|
> | None | | | A Little | | Moderate | | A Lot | | | Total |
>
> What should I do based on this success rate? (fill in the box next to the best choice)
>
> ☑ **Celebrate and keep doing what I am doing!**
>
> ☐ **Celebrate success and also modify the plan toward further improvement.**

Meredith is another person who used the problem-solving worksheet to improve her work life. Not only is she disappointed not to be using her law degree, but she's having enough trouble with her nursery/garden center job that she had to cut back to part-time and still goes home from her shifts completely exhausted, which she fears will damage her health over the long term since she's also struggling with managing her diabetes. Mostly, she has difficulty multitasking. None of her tasks is very hard, but she loses her focus and makes a lot of mistakes when she is responsible for more than one task at a time (e.g., waiting on a customer while also calculating inventory). Listed below are her problem-solving steps, in her own words.

Step 1: Identify and Define Your Problem

"I have difficulty concentrating when I have to do more than one task at a time. I would like to work full-time, but I feel so mentally exhausted after an 8-hour shift."

Step 2: Define Your Goal

"I would like to feel less mentally exhausted by my job so I can consider going back to full-time work."

Step 3: Identify the Obstacles in the Way of Your Achieving the Goal

"I believe my *thinking* differences are causing this problem. I read about executive function issues, and it explains why I have difficulty multitasking."

Step 4: List Several Possible Solutions to Address the Obstacle(s)

1. "Cut back on my hours even more."
2. "Ask my boss to help me reorganize my task assignments."
3. "Use scheduling techniques to plan my work day differently (got from Cheat Sheet)."
4. "Switch jobs."
5. "Quit the job and stay home."

Step 5: Consider the Consequences of Each Solution

"After evaluating the pros and cons of each solution, a combination of solutions 2 and 3 has the most benefit with the least cost."

Step 6: Choose the Best One(s) to Try Out First

"As a scheduling technique, I will set up my tasks so that I can complete one at a time before going to the next. I will also ask my boss to help me because he likes me and really wants me to come back full time. I believe that one of my strengths, *capacity for pleasure* (passion for plants and horticulture), is helping me here because that is why my boss likes me and is willing to help me."

Step 7: Implement the Solution and Track Your Progress

"I will write down all of my work tasks on a list. Then I will look at the number of hours I have in each work shift. I will plug the tasks into the time blocks and try to complete each one before moving to the next. Waiting on customers cannot be scheduled, of course, but I can try to schedule my other tasks at times when I know customer flow is slow. I will rate my feeling of mental exhaustion at the end of each day using a 0–10 rating scale. Currently, I would estimate my score to be, on average, 9. Because it will take a while to adjust to this new approach, I will try this out for 6 weeks before evaluating the plan.

*Today I felt **mentally exhausted** when I came home from work to the following degree:*										
0	1	2	3	4	5	6	7	8	9	10
None		A Little			Moderate		A Lot			Extreme

Step 8: Evaluate the Solution to See If It Met Your Goal

"After 6 weeks, my mental exhaustion was between 4 and 7 each day. The higher end of the range (7) happened more during the first 2 weeks of this new plan, and then the 4s and 5s were more frequent after I got used to it. On average, I consider this solution 95% successful. I am ready to try a full-time schedule again."

A Word about Disclosure

Many of my patients ask me if they should disclose their ASD diagnosis to their employer. Depending on your diagnosis and the extent to which your ASD differences have affected your work life, you may be considered a member of the class of people protected by the Americans with Disabilities Act (ADA, 1990). This law states that employers are not allowed to discriminate against a qualified potential employee on the basis of disability. Also, employers are required to make "reasonable accommodations" for any employee with a disability who is otherwise qualified to do the job. This law covers all types of disabilities, but disclosure and accommodation can be a very delicate issue for people with ASDs. ASDs are not obvious, like visual or other physical disabilities. Also, the needs of employees with ASDs will vary greatly from one person to the next. There is some further reading you can do on this subject in the resource list at the back of the book. Specifically, look for Stephen Shore's book *Ask and Tell: Self Advocacy and Disclosure for People on the Autism Spectrum*, listed under the section called Social Cognition and Social Understanding. Also, because this is a legal question, I advise you to consult an attorney specializing in disability law before disclosing to an employer. I always advise my patients to ask themselves the following questions and make sure they can come up with clear answers before moving forward on disclosure to any person. If you have difficulty answering these, you may want to discuss the issue with a trusted person who knows you well.

- Why do you want this person/your employer to know about your diagnosis?
- How do you think it will improve your relationship with this person/work life with your employer if this person knows about your diagnosis?
- Are you prepared to ask this person/your employer to support you in a different way or to accommodate you in specific ways?
- What are the risks of telling this person/your employer?
- If you are not sure about the risks because you do not know the person well, could you ask for an accommodation *without* revealing your diagnosis? (Meredith, e.g., asked her boss to help her modify her workday without revealing the diagnosis, and he complied.)

9

At School

People on the spectrum can have their best and worst experiences in educational settings. Those with AS and HFA often have the benefit of superior intelligence, which means academic success may come easily and can be a great source of pride. Yet some ASD differences can compromise learning in certain subject areas and/or in some types of environments. In addition, school environments are often great sources of social stimulation and opportunities to make friends, which can create a lot of pressure for someone with social differences. Unfortunately, many adults on the spectrum live with traumatic memories of being bullied at school, which can continue to make life on a college campus or vocational training school stressful, even many years later. A common complaint from many of my patients is that the transition from high school to college is more challenging than expected.

In Chapter 1 you were introduced to three people who were having different school-related problems. Once of them, **Blanca**, realized the cause of her problem (being late for class) was rooted in her home, so her issue has already been addressed in Chapter 7.

You met **Arnold** in Chapter 1. The 18-year-old college freshman is having difficulty *initiating conversations*, not only with his two roommates but with other students too. Arnold used Worksheet 14 in Chapter 6 to determine that his roommate problem was more urgent than the broader problem of making friends, so he tackled the roommate issue as an education-related problem first; you can read how he pursued the goal of making friends at college in Chapter 11.

Twenty-year-old **Jake**, also introduced in Chapter 1, hasn't been able to explain to his parents that he dropped out of community college because of a significant *fear of driving* (which will be addressed in Chapter 10) as well as a *difficulty identifying his need for help* and *extreme anxiety about asking for help*. Meanwhile, he's living back at home and working at a grocery store.

Liz, age 34, lives in an apartment program that has trained staff available to residents to help with various tasks of daily living. She goes to a vocational training center to prepare her for a clerical office job. Her peers in the program have a wide range of disabilities, and some of the more obvious impairments of others make her feel uncomfortable. Her *negative self-talk* about her own diagnosis as well as her *difficulty recognizing and expressing her emotions* contributes to frequent angry outbursts. Her supervisor says she's ready for a certificate of completion from the program but that the "meltdowns" are delaying the process.

If the time of day you identified as most stressful on the clock worksheet in Chapter 1 was associated with school, you may recognize the problems listed in Worksheets 26 and 27, which were enumerated in Chapter 1 as well. Each check-

---

WORKSHEET 26

My Problems with School
Performing the Work

Check off (✓) the statements below that sound familiar to you or reflect your experiences with school or vocational training. If you have a problem related to completing your work that does not appear on this list, fill it in on one of the blanks at the bottom.

☐ I can't seem to get everything done.

☐ I always run out of time.

☐ I start things at the last minute—I procrastinate too much.

☐ I find myself worrying about my grades all the time.

☐ The schedule is too strenuous for me.

☐ I can't stand sitting in the classroom.

☐ Sometimes I get so overwhelmed, but I have no clue where to get help.

☐ I would rather fail than go get help at the center for students with disabilities.

☐ I will stop going to class if I begin to struggle with a course.

☐ I have too many "withdrawals" or Fs on my transcript.

☐ I get bored easily with the work.

☐ I can't concentrate in the classroom if there is background noise.

☐ I can't concentrate in the classroom if the lighting bothers me.

☐ I can't seem to find a good space to study where I don't get distracted.

☐ I can't study when I keep getting interrupted.

☐ _____

☐ _____

My Problems with School
Relationships at School

Check off (✓) the statements below that sound familiar to you or reflect your experiences with school or vocational training. If you have a problem with the people at school that does not appear on this list, fill it in on one of the blanks at the bottom.

☐ I can't seem to get to know the other students.

☐ Other students bother me.

☐ I try to make friends, but other students are already in their own groups.

☐ I always end up in conflict with my professors or instructors.

☐ My professors or instructors get annoyed by the questions I ask in class.

☐ Other students get annoyed by the things I say in class discussions.

☐ I have been told I am too loud.

☐ I am afraid the professor or instructor will think I am stupid if I go for extra help.

☐ Other students taunt or tease me.

☐ I am in classes/groups with other students who have obvious disabilities, and that makes me feel uncomfortable.

☐ _____

☐ _____

list includes problems common to people on the spectrum, but also leaves blank spaces at the bottom for any other educational problems you have.

Problem Solving

If you discovered more than one problem with school, you will need to choose one to address first; you can then repeat the problem-solving steps for each of the other problems at a later time. As mentioned in Chapter 6, it makes sense to start working on the issue that is causing the most distress for you and/or the people around you. The exercise below can help you figure out which one that is. Rate the level of distress caused by each problem and then pick the one with the highest score to tackle first. You can return to the others later, in order of most to least distress. It can also be helpful to talk over this prioritizing with a trusted person in your life.

WORKSHEET 28

Choosing Which Problem
to Work on First

You don't need to use this worksheet if you checked off only one problem on Worksheets 26 and 27. Otherwise, list the problems you checked in the first column below. Then use this rating scale to estimate the amount of stress the issue is causing you and/or the people around you.

Almost None	Some	Moderate Amount	A Lot	Extreme
1	2	3	4	5

Problem   **Distress Rating**

_____   _____

_____   _____

_____   _____

_____   _____

The next few pages will guide you through the steps of solving the problem you just identified. For each step you will be asked to write your answers in the question box. Each box will give you instructions, and then I'll show you how **Arnold** filled out the box.

Step 1: Identify and Define Your Problem with School

What is bothering you about school? You've already done this first step if you filled out Worksheets 26–28. Write the problem you have chosen to work on first in the box.

Step 1: Identify and Define Your Problem with School

What is bothering me about school?

The problem that is bothering me most about school is:

_____

_____

_____

_____

Example. **Arnold** identified only one education-related problem and didn't need to use Worksheet 28. He filled out his Step 1 question box this way:

Step 1: Identify and Define Your Problem with School

The problem that is bothering me most about school is:

I am too shy to talk to my roommates when they hang out and have their

friends visit. I have not made any friends at college yet, and I have been here

for 2 months.

Step 2: Define Your Goal

What would you like to see change to minimize the problem you identified with school? What would need to be different for you to feel less bothered by the problem? The goal you lay out is simply the opposite of the problem you listed. List your goal in the box below, and if you need an example, look at Arnold's box. Notice how he took his problem and stated the goal as the opposite of his problem. Stating the goal in the affirmative gives Arnold something to act on and a means for measuring his success. After speaking to his mother and using Worksheet 14 on page 124, he decided to keep the goal simple and small. He originally wrote "Make at least one friend" but realized he first had to get comfortable just talking to his roommates.

Step 2: Define Your Goal

What would you like to see change to minimize the problem you identified with school? The goal you lay out is simply the opposite of the problem you listed.

To feel less stressed by this problem, I would like to:

_____

_____

---

*Example. **Arnold's** goal is shown below.*

Step 2: Define Your Goal

To feel less stressed by this problem, I would like to:

  Have some conversations with my roommates or other students on campus

---

Step 3: Identify the Obstacles in the Way of Your Achieving the Goal

What is getting in the way of your goal? Here it is particularly important to consider your ASD characteristics as key players in your problem. As you go through this step, you may rely on the information you were given in Part I of this book about your ASD differences. As you think about the problem you listed above, look at the chart on page 225 called "ASD Differences That Can Contribute to Problems at School." Read through that chart with your own problem in mind and also consider the following questions.

Thinking Differences

How might my *executive functioning* issues be contributing to my problems at school? For example, do I have difficulty planning, which causes me to procrastinate on my homework, studying, or projects? Do I find it hard to concentrate on more than one task at time, causing me to get very few things done each day? Do I persist too long, repeating a strategy that is clearly not working because I have difficulty shifting to new strategies? How could my *negative self-talk* be contributing to my problems with school? What am I saying to myself that is putting more pressure on me? Is it possible that I'm engaging in perfectionistic thinking, all-or-nothing thinking, or catastrophic thinking? For example, do I assume the worst will happen before an important activity? Do I expect perfection from myself and/or professors, instructors, or peers?

Social Differences

How might my *social perception* be contributing to my problems at school? Is it possible I sometimes misunderstand what my professors, instructors, or peers are trying to tell me? For example, do I still feel uncertain about what my professors or instructors expect from me? Am I still unsure how I should handle conversations with my peers? How might my *social/communication skills* be contributing to problems at school? Is it possible that professors, instructors, or peers are not communicating clearly enough about what they expect and I don't know how to seek clarification? For example, I feel uncertain about when and how to ask my professors or instructors questions without annoying them. Is my problem caused in part by my not knowing what to say or do when dealing with professors, instructors, or peers? For example, I don't know how I should handle it if I get to class before the professor and I am waiting in my seat with other students. Or I don't know what to say if a peer shares some personal information with me, like telling me what he has planned for the weekend.

Emotional Differences

How might my emotional reactions to things be affecting my problems at school? Do I have difficulty *regulating* my emotions? Do I take too long to calm down after an upsetting incident? Do I have difficulty *identifying* my feelings or *asking for help* when I am upset? Am I over- or underreacting to things that happen in the classroom or the dorm? Do I tend to avoid situations that cause me to feel too much anxiety or worry?

Sensory and Movement Differences

How might my sensory issues be contributing to my problems at school? Am I *oversensitive* or *undersensitive* to certain types of light, sound, smell, taste, or touch? For example, my dorm is noisy, and that contributes to my avoiding work. How might my *movement* and *coordination* issues be contributing to my problems with school? For example, I dread having to handwrite answers on tests because my penmanship is so poor. Is it possible that my hygiene is not acceptable to some people because my sensory/movement problems interfere with bathing or grooming?

Now fill out the question box, trying not to think about other problems you have besides the one you chose for this exercise.

Step 3: Identify the Obstacles in the Way of Your Achieving the Goal

What is getting in the way of your goal? Remember to focus *only* on the problem and goal you wrote down in Steps 1 and 2. First circle the category(ies) of ASD differences you suspect are involved in this problem:

Thinking   **Social**   **Emotional**   **Sensory/Movement**

I believe these differences are contributing in this way:

_____

_____

⇨

_____

_____

_____

Example. **Arnold** filled out his Step 3 question box in this way:

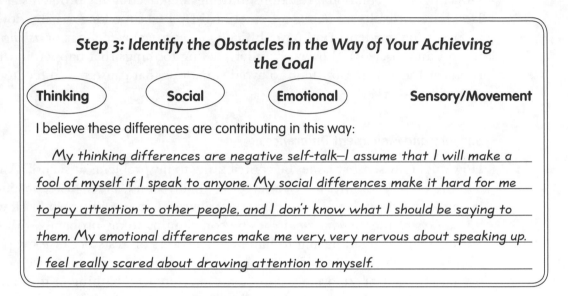

Step 3: Identify the Obstacles in the Way of Your Achieving the Goal

(Thinking)   (Social)   (Emotional)   Sensory/Movement

I believe these differences are contributing in this way:

My thinking differences are negative self-talk—I assume that I will make a fool of myself if I speak to anyone. My social differences make it hard for me to pay attention to other people, and I don't know what I should be saying to them. My emotional differences make me very, very nervous about speaking up. I feel really scared about drawing attention to myself.

When you filled out your sheet, did you circle more than one area of ASD differences? Arnold indicated that his shyness has three potential sources of difficulty: his thinking (negative self-talk), social (understanding other people and social communication), and emotional (anxiety) differences. This illustrates once again that often a single issue can have several causes.

Step 4: List Several Possible Solutions to Address the Obstacle(s)

What are the possible solutions for the obstacles? Try to list as many ideas as possible. Remember that this is the step some people call "brainstorming." Generate as many possibilities as come to mind, without inhibition. Don't judge or evaluate any idea—just write it down no matter how weird or silly it seems. In Step 5 you will weed through them and discard any that are not useful, so no harm can be done.

Start by looking at the Cheat Sheet at the end of Chapter 6. Find the ASD differences you circled on the top row of the Cheat Sheet. Then look along the column underneath each and find the dots. Each dot marks the row in which you will find a solution in the far left column of the chart. Those approaches should

Differences →	Thinking	Social	Emotional	Sensory/Movement
Problems Getting Work Done for School	• Attention regulation difficulties can make it hard to stay focused in the classroom or to complete tasks • Difficulties organizing information make it hard to organize your study spaces • Difficulties organizing information make it hard to plan your work and to think ahead • Working memory difficulties make it hard to do more than one task at a time for school • Focusing on detail but ignoring the "big picture" may cause you to overlook important aspects of assignments • Dichotomous, all-or-nothing thinking can cause undue pressure and anxiety around completing tasks	• Your unique style of processing language may lead you to miss your professors' or instructors' expectations about your assignments • Your difficulty initiating conversations may interfere with your ability to ask for help on tasks you do not understand or find difficult to complete • Any of your social differences can interfere with your ability to complete team or group projects	• Your difficulty recognizing and identifying negative emotions that you are feeling can interfere with your awareness that you are struggling with schoolwork and may need a change (e.g., anxiety, anger) • Your difficulty regulating your negative emotions related to schoolwork can contribute to your experience of getting extremely overwhelmed by the pressures involved	• Hypersensitivity to noise, light, smell, taste, or touch can interfere with your ability to concentrate on your studies • Hyposensitivity (underresponsive sense) can interfere with picking up on important cues in the school setting (e.g., signs, alarms) • Fine motor problems (coordinated handwork) could affect tasks like handwriting, typing, assembly work, use of hand tools, operating intricate electronic devices • Gross motor (coordinated whole-body movement) problems could affect some types of work (e.g., physical education class, physical labor in a vocational training program)
Problems with Relationships at School	• Professors or instructors may not be sympathetic if you have difficulty with your work assignments • Peers who rely on you (e.g., on a group project) may be affected adversely by your difficulties managing tasks and responsibilities (e.g., unequal distribution of work)	• You may not notice or interpret cues or mind-read what your professors or peers are expecting from you • You may be perceived by others as uncaring or aloof because of the way you experience and express empathy • The unique way you process and express language can contribute to misunderstandings with professors, instructors, or peers • The unique way you express language can make it hard to assert yourself with professors, instructors, or peers • Your difficulty with conversation skills may interfere with making positive connections with peers	• Your difficulty recognizing and identifying negative emotions can contribute to problems communicating with professors, instructors, or peers about your needs • Your difficulty regulating your negative emotions can also put you at risk for having anxious or angry outbursts, which may be disruptive on campus and can adversely affect your relationships with peers	• Hypersensitivities can cause problems when others unknowingly are doing things that are unpleasant to you (playing music, using strong perfume, using cleaning products with a strong smell, using friendly touch like a pat on the back or a handshake) • Fine or gross motor problems can be obstacles to many types of cooperative leisure activities that peers do during free time (e.g., games or sports; fewer opportunities to make positive connections with peers) • Hypersensitivity or fine motor problems can lead to poor hygiene

ASD differences that can contribute to problems at school.

be considered first, and Chapter 6 provides you with the instructions and tools for each of those solutions. Also, try to consider your *strengths* as you complete this step because they too play an important role in your solutions. Refer back to Worksheets 3 and 4 in Chapter 1. Write your primary strengths in the blanks here so you can keep them in mind while you are generating solutions.

My strengths are: _____, _____, and _____.

Step 4: List Several Possible Solutions to Address the Obstacle(s)

What are the possible solutions for the obstacles? Now, considering all the solutions you saw on the Cheat Sheet, and some you may think of on your own, list all the possibilities you can imagine to address the ASD differences involved in the problem you listed in Step 1. For the moment, ignore the score columns on the right.

I could try to:

List strategies below	Pro (+) score	Con (−) score	Total pro−con

---

*Example. **Arnold** filled out his question box the following way:*

Step 4: List Several Possible Solutions to Address the Obstacle(s)

I could try to:

List strategies below	Pro (+) score	Con (−) score	Total pro−con
1) leave my room when roommates are around			
2) use thinking techniques to help my anxiety			
3) use emotional regulation techniques for anxiety			
4) use techniques to understand others			
5) join an on-campus club that interests me			
6) stop trying to have friends—accept solitude			
7) go to campus counseling center for help			

Notice that Arnold listed everything that came to mind, including things that don't seem suitable (such as leaving the room when the roommates are there). He looked at the Cheat Sheet, which gave him ideas 2, 3, and 4. He also discussed this exercise with his mother on the phone, and together they came up with some of the other ideas. This is an example of "brainstorming." Arnold can't possibly do all the things on this list, but the next step will help him figure out what is most useful.

Step 5: Consider the Consequences of Each Solution

What are the pros and cons of each solution? Now you will take each item on your list and put it to the test of how feasible it is or how helpful it will be toward the goal you wrote down during Step 2. Use the question box to give each item a score.

Step 5: Consider the Consequences of Each Solution

What are the pros and cons of each solution? Look back at each item you wrote down in Step 4. Then assign each one a score. Score the benefit (Pro +) in terms of how likely that strategy is to get you closer to your goal. Score the disadvantage (Con −) in terms of the effort, cost, or damage involved in implementing it.

⇨

Pro (+) Scale

How likely is it to get me closer to my goal?

Very Unlikely	Pretty Unlikely	Hard to Tell	Somewhat Likely	Very Likely
0	1	2	3	4

Con (–) Scale

How much effort, cost, or damage would this strategy involve?

None	Almost None	Some	A Lot	Extreme
0	1	2	3	4

*Example. **Arnold's** answers in this question box appear below. He carried out Step 5 and rated each one of his solutions from Step 4.

Step 4: List Several Possible Solutions to Address the Obstacle(s)

I could try to:

List strategies below	Pro (+) score	Con (–) score	Total pro–con
1) leave my room when roommates are around	0	2	–2
2) use thinking techniques to help my anxiety	3	1	2
3) use emotional regulation techniques for anxiety	3	1	2
4) use techniques to understand others	4	2	2
5) join an on-campus club that interests me	3	2	1
6) stop trying to have friends—accept solitude	0	2	–2
7) go to campus counseling center for help	3	2	1

Step 6: Choose the Best One(s) to Try Out First

Which solutions should you try first? Now that you've scored all of your options, choosing the one or two strategies to start with should be easy. Which of your options had the highest total score? According to your own rating, the highest score has the most benefit compared to the cost, effort, or damage it could involve. Notice that Arnold ended up with three solutions, all with the same pro–con score. Even though he read about the techniques he will try, he believes they'll be difficult to learn and feels apprehensive about it. That's why he assigned a "con" rating even to the ones he gave a score of 4 for "pro." This is a perfectly natural reaction that you may have too. In the end, you need not expect a "perfect" pro–con score of 4 to consider an option; you need only pick the ones with the highest score compared to the others.

Step 6: Choose the Best One(s) to Try Out First

Which solutions should you try first? Which of the strategies in Step 5 had the highest score? Pick the top one or two and write them down below:

_____

_____

_____

Example. Arnold filled out his question box the following way, choosing ideas 2, 3, and 4. Ideas 5 and 7 also seemed good, but he decided, while discussing this with his mother, that it would be better not to try to do too much at once. Those options would be good to keep in mind to use after he tried his first three ideas.

Step 6: Choose the Best One(s) to Try Out First

Use thinking techniques to help my anxiety

Use emotional regulation techniques to help my anxiety

Use techniques to understand others to help my conversations

Step 7: Implement the Solution and Track Your Progress

Now try the solution and track your progress. Use the next question box to map out your plan.

Step 7: Implement the Solution and Track Your Progress

Now try the solution and track your progress. Here is how:

Where will I do it?

_____

When will I do it?

_____

What do I need to do it?

_____

How will I do it?

_____

_____

Who can help me, if needed?

_____

How will I keep track of my success? (Look at your goal and then pick a way to track it—either a running count or a rating scale.)

_____

_____

_____

Example. Arnold studied the *thinking techniques* in Chapter 6, which helped him become aware of the negative self-talk in which he was engaging. He realized that his "internal narrator" was often saying: "I will make a fool of myself if I say anything to my roommates" and "It is always best to avoid drawing attention to myself." These are examples of *catastrophizing* and *all-or-nothing* thinking. Although these statements were rooted in some bad experiences Arnold had in middle school, he realized that he did not have enough evidence to assume things would turn out this way in the present. In fact, if he were to use the *techniques to understand others*, he would be more confident that he would know what to say to his roommates, negating the assumption that he will make a fool of himself. Also, he realized that to address his goal he would *need* to draw attention to himself. Because that idea made his anxiety, as he put it, "go through the roof," he hoped that one of the *emotion regulation techniques* he read about would help him with that. Arnold and his mother also discussed his strengths. Despite his apprehension about the current problem, his mother shared with him her observation that he has always been characteristically *optimistic* and also can show *insight* about his problems when he is struggling; both of these would be assets in the current plan.

Step 7: Implement the Solution and Track Your Progress

Where will I do it?

In my dorm room

When will I do it?

Every evening

What do I need to do it?

Understanding my Emotions worksheet, my checklist for paying attention and learning about other people, and my anxiety rating scale

How will I do it?

Fill out the Emotions sheet once and then keep it on hand to read each day. Try to be part of roommates' conversations once a day by paying attention and offering one comment or question each day. Rate my anxiety afterward.

Who can help me, if needed?

My mother and possibly the counseling center on campus if I get really stuck

How will I keep track of my success? (Look at your goal and then pick a way to track it—either a running count or a rating scale.)

My goal is to converse more often than I am now (which is never). I will track the number of things I say each evening. I will also track my anxiety to see if it decreases over time.

Arnold used the Understanding My Emotions worksheet from Chapter 6 to help himself become more aware and accepting of his negative emotions, specifically the anxiety that has been such a big obstacle for him at college. Filling this out helped him see that his anxiety did serve a purpose, but what it was signaling to him now was not the same as what it had been signaling in the past. Understanding this did not eliminate the anxiety but rather helped him with his "anxiety *about* anxiety." He accepted that he would feel nervous when he tried to practice his new conversation approaches, and that made the whole prospect seem less threatening to him. He read through all the tips for paying attention to and learning about other people. He realized that he had often been so concerned about other people

---

Example from Arnold

WORSHEET 18

Understanding My Emotions

For use when evaluating an upsetting event. Fill this out soon after an event during which you found yourself very upset.

Date and time of event: _____ *Last night in the dorm room* _____

1. Briefly describe the event: I was upset when _____ *my roommates were talking and laughing and I wanted to join in.* _____

2. Now look at the words, pictures, and synonyms below. On the top row are the basic negative emotions, and underneath are some common words that have similar meanings. Which of these emotions do you suspect was involved in your reaction to the event? Circle the relevant emotion. You can circle more than one.

Sadness	Anger	Fear
Depressed	Enraged	Terrified
Miserable	Annoyed	Anxious
Devastated	Frustrated	Tense
Down	Irritated	Nervous

3. I felt _____ *terrified* _____, which may be a signal that I needed something.

4. Maybe I needed _____ *to hide. I did that in middle school, and it worked because my goal was to avoid the bullies. But now I need something different—I need to know what to say—I don't want to hide now.* _____

5. Feeling _____ *fear* _____ is a natural part of life, and I accept that I felt that way.

6. Now think about what was around you that may have helped you meet your need. This could be an object or a person. I could have used _____ *some guidance on what I should be doing and saying with my roommates* _____ to help me meet my need.

7. In circumstances like these, I may _____ *practice my new tips for paying attention to people to address my need.* _____

focusing on him that it had never occurred to him that he should be paying attention to them. By learning how to pay attention to others, he could become more occupied with that task and less preoccupied with removing himself from the center of others' attention. This idea came as a relief to him. He made a checklist of reminders for himself to refer to each day before his roommates came home, which appears below. His anxiety rating scale appears below that.

Checklist for Paying Attention to Other People

☐ *Look at the faces of the other people. Don't stare; just look often at each person.*

☐ *Look at faces to show I am paying attention without having to use words.*

☐ *Look at faces to find out what the other people are looking at (which tells you what they are paying attention to).*

☐ *Look at faces to monitor changes in expression.*

☐ *Gather information about their interests, hobbies, and classes by observing things they do.*

☐ *Gather information about their interests, hobbies, and classes by listening to what they are saying.*

☐ *Ask a question about the information you gathered.*

☐ *Make a comment about the information you gathered.*

DAILY RATING OF ANXIETY

Today I felt *fear when I talked to my roommates* to the following degree:

0	1	2	3	4	5	6	7	8	9	10
None		A Little			Moderate			A Lot		Extreme

Step 8: Evaluate the Solution to See If It Met Your Goal

Did the solution meet your goal, or do you need to use a different solution? At this point you have tried out your new solution and are ready to see if it helped you meet your goal. Use the question box to evaluate your progress.

Step 8: Evaluate the Solution to See If It Met Your Goal

Did the solution meet your goal, or do you need to use a different solution? Answer the following questions to figure this out:

What was my goal? (Copy this from Step 2.)

_____

How did I measure my progress? (data, log, or record)

_____

What do the data show with regard to my goal?

How would you rate your success, on a scale of 0–100% success for meeting your goal?

I was _____% successful.

0	10	20	30	40	50	60	70	80	90	100
None		A Little			Moderate			A Lot		Total

What should I do based on this success rate? (fill in the box next to the best choice)

☐ **Celebrate and keep doing what I am doing!**

☐ **Celebrate success and also modify the plan toward further improvement.**

Example. Arnold filled out his question box this way after practicing his new schedule for 2 weeks.

Step 8: Evaluate the Solution to See If It Met Your Goal

What was my goal? (Copy this from Step 2.)

Have some conversations with my roommates or other students on campus.

How did I measure my progress? (data, log, or record)

I kept a tally of times I said something and rated my anxiety every night.

What do the data show with regard to my goal?

In 2 weeks there were 12 nights that I was at home when my roommates

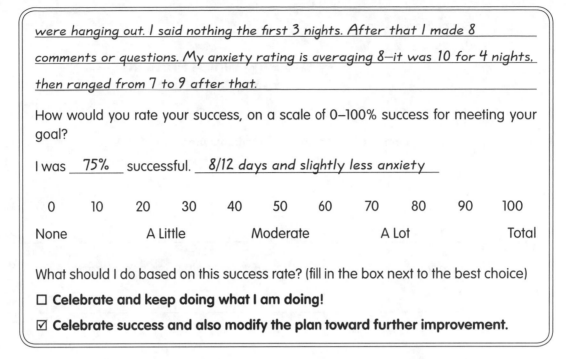

were hanging out. I said nothing the first 3 nights. After that I made 8 comments or questions. My anxiety rating is averaging 8—it was 10 for 4 nights, then ranged from 7 to 9 after that.

How would you rate your success, on a scale of 0–100% success for meeting your goal?

I was ___75%___ successful. ___8/12 days and slightly less anxiety___

0	10	20	30	40	50	60	70	80	90	100
None		A Little			Moderate		A Lot			Total

What should I do based on this success rate? (fill in the box next to the best choice)

☐ **Celebrate and keep doing what I am doing!**

☑ **Celebrate success and also modify the plan toward further improvement.**

Arnold was very surprised that he was able to make any comments at all. He felt proud of himself but was also very stressed out by this activity. He spoke to his mother every day on the phone about his progress, and she was very pleased as well. They both agreed that he could use the help of an on-campus counselor so that his stress would not interfere with his studies. He made an appointment with a counselor and planned to share his goals and materials with that person so that he could get some further assistance.

Jake used the problem-solving worksheet to address his *difficulties seeking help with schoolwork*. Despite the fact that he had never had academic problems in high school, in community college he ended up failing three courses and getting low grades in others and finally dropping out. Jake was ashamed of himself, and his parents had expressed a lot of anger toward him about his academic performance during the year he was struggling. Because the other reason he had quit college was his fear of driving, Jake used Worksheet 28 to prioritize, as shown on the next page. It turned out the driving problem was a higher priority for him, so he addressed that first, but that illustration is described in Chapter 10 as a community issue. Here I'll show you how he addressed the second problem.

Example from Jake
WORKSHEET 28

Choosing Which Problem to Work on First

How much distress is this problem causing in my life?

Almost None	Some	Moderate Amount	A Lot	Extreme
1	2	3	4	5

Problem	Distress Rating
Afraid to drive on the highways	5
I don't know whom or how to ask for help with schoolwork	4

Step 1: Identify and Define Your Problem with School

The problem that is bothering me most about school is:

I want to go back to school, but I need help with my work. This has never happened to me before, so I don't know what to do or whom to talk to.

Step 2: Define Your Goal

To feel less stressed by this problem, I would like to:

Tell my parents I want to go back and ask them to help me find help with my work.

Step 3: Identify the Obstacles in the Way of Your Achieving the Goal

Thinking   (Social)   (Emotional)   Sensory/Movement

I believe these differences are contributing in this way:

My social differences make it hard for me to tell people I need help. My

emotional differences make it hard for me to notice I am in trouble until it is

too late.

For the next step, Jake thought of as many solutions as he could, even ones that seemed silly to him. He used the Cheat Sheet from Chapter 6 and also made up some solutions of his own. After listing them, he used the rating scale from the problem-solving sheet to weigh the pros and cons of each solution. The results of Steps 4 and 5 can be found in the box below.

Step 4: List Several Possible Solutions to Address the Obstacle(s)

I could try to:

List strategies below	Pro (+) score	Con (−) score	Total pro–con
1) forget school and keep working at the store	0	4	−4
2) use communication techniques with parents	4	3	1
3) use thinking techniques to help anxiety	4	2	2
4) register for school on my own	0	4	−4

In Step 6, Jake used the results of his evaluation to pick the two options with the highest pro–con score, which are highlighted in the Step 4 box. Once again, the total scores are not a "perfect 4" because there is always some apprehension and effort that goes into trying anything new. Jake studied the *communication techniques* found in Chapter 6 and was very interested in the idea of the Talk Blocks, which provide a formula to use to identify a feeling and also a need. He could not do this spontaneously or independently when he was in college. However, by looking over the word lists he could recognize in this "multiple choice" format the words that described how he felt and what he needed when he was getting overwhelmed by the pressures of attending the community college. He ordered a set online and waited for them to arrive before he considered approaching his parents. Once he got them, he put together a few phrases he thought would work best for him. They were:

I feel *anxious*; therefore, I need *to talk*.

I feel *overwhelmed*; therefore, I need *more information*.

He planned to show his parents the Talk Blocks, tell them more about the things he had struggled with at school, then ask them to help him make a plan to go back to school with the idea he would get more help and support. He also looked over the ***thinking techniques*** in Chapter 6 and was helped by the ***acceptance*** phrases. Prior to reading this, he did not think it was acceptable to need or ask for help, especially because he had been so accustomed to success in school before he went to college. Realizing now that he had thinking differences because of his ASD, he found it more acceptable to ask for help because it did not mean that he was lazy or unmotivated. He was particularly helped by the phrase "I accept that my brain works differently" and then another he made up for himself: "I accept that I need help with some types of work." He also considered his primary strength to be his sense of ***purpose***. His dedication to being a student was indeed what caused him so much distress in the recent past but is also driving him to solve his problem now. His implementation plan appears in the next box.

Step 7: Implement the Solution and Track Your Progress

Where will I do it?

   At home

When will I do it?

   Sunday at lunchtime with Mom and Dad

What do I need to do it?

   Talk Blocks

How will I do it?

   Ask Mom and Dad to talk to me about school. Show them Talk Blocks and use them to tell them I want to go back to school.

Who can help me, if needed?

I will be asking Mom and Dad for help.

How will I keep track of my success? (Look at your goal and then pick a way to track it—either a running count or a rating scale.)

This is a one-time activity, so I will just measure my success with the 0–100% rating scale in Step 8.

Here is the evaluation Jake did after he met with his parents.

Step 8: Evaluate the Solution to See If It Met Your Goal

What was my goal? (Copy this from Step 2.)

Tell my parents I want to go back and ask them to help me find help with my work.

How did I measure my progress? (data, log, or record)

I used the rating scale on this sheet because it was a one-time thing.

What do the data show with regard to my goal?

I was nervous about the meeting, but my parents seemed glad to talk to me. They got excited about the Talk Blocks and repeated several times that they were surprised by what I had done. They agreed to let me go back to school and said they would get me a tutor. They would also help me get set up with the on-campus center for students with learning disabilities. I never thought I had a learning disability, but my ASD is sort of like one.

How would you rate your success, on a scale of 0–100% success for meeting your goal?

I was ___100%___ successful.

0	10	20	30	40	50	60	70	80	90	100
None		A Little			Moderate			A Lot		Total

⇨

> What should I do based on this success rate? (fill in the box next to the best choice)
>
> ☑ **Celebrate and keep doing what I am doing!**
>
> ☐ **Celebrate success and also modify the plan toward further improvement.**

Liz hopes to start looking for a clerical job in an office soon, but her supervisor is reluctant to let her graduate from the program because she is having frequent anger outbursts. Also a rehabilitation counselor, her supervisor helped her fill out the problem-solving worksheet to address this issue. Her answers to the individual questions for each step appear below, in her own words.

Step 1: Identify and Define Your Problem

"I don't like being placed with peers who have obvious disabilities. I don't think I belong here, and I really want to graduate so I can begin to work in an office. I get so frustrated about it that I scream and throw things sometimes."

Step 2: Define Your Goal

"I would like to stop having 'meltdowns' so I can graduate."

Step 3: Identify the Obstacles in the Way of Your Achieving the Goal

"I believe my *thinking* differences are causing part of the problem. I read about negative self-talk and discussed it with my supervisor, and I know I say a lot of bad things about disabled people—I realize I do this because I don't like the idea that my ASD is considered a disability. I also have *emotional* differences, which I discussed with my supervisor—I have difficulty identifying and expressing my negative emotions, and it is not until I 'blow up' that I realize I am mad."

Step 4: List Several Possible Solutions to Address the Obstacle(s)

1. "Stay at the vocational program permanently—forget working."
2. "Use thinking techniques to address negative self-talk (from Cheat Sheet)."
3. "Use emotion regulation techniques to deal with anger (from Cheat Sheet)."
4. "Use communication techniques to let others know when I need support (from Cheat Sheet)."
5. "Quit the vocational program and stay home."
6. "Ask my supervisor to keep me away from peers with disabilities."

Step 5: Consider the Consequences of Each Solution

"After evaluating the pros and cons of each solution with my supervisor, we decided a combination of solution 2, 3, and 4 has the most benefit with the least cost."

Step 6: Choose the Best One(s) to Try Out First

"As a thinking technique, I will challenge my negative self-talk about my own diagnosis by reading and learning more about ASDs. I will also learn to address all-or-nothing thinking about disabilities in general so I can be more tolerant of other people's differences. As an emotion regulation technique, I will fill out the Understanding My Emotions worksheet with my supervisor each time something upsets me in the program. As a communication technique, my supervisor will teach me to use Talk Blocks to let others know what I need before I 'blow.' My counselor and I agree that I have a strong sense of *personal responsibility*, which is going to help me stay on track with my new plan."

Step 7: Implement the Solution and Track Your Progress

"My supervisor will meet with me twice a week for 3 months to try out the new plan. We will keep a tally of the number of 'meltdowns' (incidents where I scream and throw things) I have in 3 months. Before this plan I have had an average of one meltdown per week in the program."

Step 8: Evaluate the Solution to See If It Met Your Goal

"In 3 months, I had four meltdowns. Three of them were in the first month, then only one in the second month. It has been about 6 weeks since I had one. I used my Understanding My Emotions worksheet after each meltdown. My supervisor is pleased, and I am also very happy because I might be going to work soon! I think this is 90% successful. We agreed to try this for 3 more months."

A Word about Transition and Self-Advocacy

As mentioned at the beginning of this chapter, the transition from high school to college can be very difficult for people on the spectrum. All too often I am referred a young person who is suffering the aftermath of what I have come to call the "freshman crash-and-burn"—a major crisis that occurs by winter vacation of the student's first semester at college. I use that unfortunate nickname to describe cases where a student starts college full time in the fall of the freshman year, and by Christmas vacation has suffered a major crisis. Often the crisis—academic (poor grades or failures), social (negative or traumatic experiences with peers), and/or psychiatric (episodes of severe anxiety or depression)—comes without warning for the parents but begins for the student within the first few weeks of the semester. Sometimes the catalyst is the drastic change in structure that comes with college and a need for more self-direction to meet academic demands. Other times disappointment can come when people on the spectrum and their families assume that the social difficulties encountered throughout middle school and high school will suddenly disappear in a new environment, such as a college campus. Unfortunately, that is often not what happens, and the strains of navigating a brand-new social landscape can be too much to handle without careful planning and assistance. Of course every case is different, but some common elements have emerged as I have listened to these stories during my years of practice. The case of *Jake* described in this chapter gives you an example of such a scenario. *Arnold*, also presented earlier, would have been at risk for this if he had not begun to work on his social difficulties. The risk factors for such a crisis include:

- Academic success in high school (which is structured) can mask the need for extra support in college
- Students who succeeded in high school with special education support and a good IEP (individualized education plan) may not take the steps necessary to carry accommodations over to the college campus
- Students who are not properly educated about their diagnosis and related differences may not know about avenues for help available on campus
- Students who have communication difficulties may not be prepared to ask for help when needed
- Students whose social difficulties appeared to improve in high school can regress because the student was used to one environment but gets overwhelmed by a dramatically different social world
- Students assume that their social difficulties will disappear once they leave high school behind

If you are still considering school or you are the parent of a child on the spectrum who is in middle or high school, take into consideration the following tips about transition for yourself or any student you are supporting:

- Become a self-advocate. This means you need to learn how to articulate your needs to others. If you're used to having your parents speak for you regarding educational needs, assume they can no longer do that when you are in college (even if they are continuing to provide you with emotional and financial support).
- If you had an IEP in high school, make sure you know what it said, what your diagnosis (classification) was, and what accommodations were written into it (e.g., extended test time, a scribe to take notes for you). Do not rely on your parents to communicate these issues on your behalf anymore.
- Don't assume you have to go to college, even if you are very bright and got good grades

in high school. There may be technical or trade schools offering programs that will be of more interest and use to you.

- When you are choosing colleges, make sure you schedule visits to the campuses and always include an appointment with the office that handles services for students with disabilities. These centers vary in name and extent of supports. Even if you don't think you need it, it is important to know what would be available to you if you were to hit some unexpected problems. Take along a copy of your IEP if you had one in high school.
- If you are already at a school, get connected with the office of student disability services on your campus. Once again, you may not think you need it, but having the name and phone number of a person you have already met can be a real lifeline if you encounter some trouble spots during a semester.
- Find out where the campus mental health center is located. As a proactive measure, make sure you learn what the protocol is for making an appointment so you will have it on hand if needed. It's a lot easier to find out about such things when you are *not* upset, which is why the proactive research can be so helpful; you will have the information on hand to use if you do become upset by some college-related problems.

10

In the Community

Your community can offer you some of the best opportunities to enjoy independence and make social connections. Far too many people on the spectrum, however, don't get the full benefit of what their city, town, or village has to offer. Some stay home to avoid anxiety-provoking situations, while others find their activities outside of home constricted by ASD differences. Whether you are, at the very least, shopping and running errands or, at the most, active in sports teams or leagues, clubs or religious congregations, these activities may be stressful for you for any number of reasons related to your ASD.

Twenty-five-year-old college-educated **Richard**, introduced in Chapter 1, drives himself to weekly appointments with a vocational counselor but doesn't leave home by himself otherwise because he has always relied on his mother to speak for him. He'd like to be able to run his own errands or use local resources like the library and gym but is apprehensive about talking to anyone he doesn't know since he has difficulty *initiating* interactions.

In Chapter 9 you saw how **Jake** used the problem-solving steps to address his issues with asking for help so he can try to go back to community college. In this chapter I'll show you how he used problem solving to deal with his *fear of driving*.

Jean, age 65, felt lonely and bored after recently being widowed and retiring from a 40-year career as a librarian, so she began volunteering at her church. She hopes to get to know other members of the congregation now that she's doing more than attending Sunday services, but she's having difficulty because she is not successfully *noticing and interpreting cues* from others about what is expected during various activities. She worries that she is not fitting in.

If the clock worksheet in Chapter 1 showed that your most stressful time of day is related to your community life, you'll find the problems listed in Worksheets 29 and 30 familiar; they were first listed in Chapter 1. Each sheet has a list of problems common to people on the spectrum but also leaves blank spaces at the bottom for you to fill in any other community-related problems you have.

WORKSHEET 29

My Problems in the Community
Getting Around and Managing Tasks

Check off (✓) the statements below that sound familiar or reflect your experiences with getting around or managing the nonsocial aspects of accessing the community. This includes experiences with car travel, public transportation, stores, and services as well as recreational and religious activities. If you have a problem with getting around that does not appear on this list, fill it in on one of the blanks at the bottom.

☐ I have had a lot of car accidents.

☐ I am too nervous to drive.

☐ I never seem to carry enough money with me.

☐ I am bothered by the lighting in some stores.

☐ I am afraid of elevators or escalators.

☐ I always seem to be dropping everything [my money, shopping items].

☐ I lose things a lot [wallet, purse, keys].

☐ I can't seem to figure out the bus/train schedule.

☐ I like to stick to routes that I know; otherwise I get lost.

☐ I get lost a lot, even going to places I have been before.

☐ I fumble when I try to buy my ticket using the automatic machine.

☐ I am bothered by the lighting in my gym.

☐ I love to swim, but I can't deal with the noisy community pool.

☐ I get too impatient while sitting through long religious services.

☐ There is too much background noise/echo in my church or temple.

☐ _____

☐ _____

Problem Solving

If you found that you have more than one problem with accessing your community, you'll need to choose one to address first; then you can repeat the problem-solving steps for each of the other problems at a later time. As mentioned in Chapter 6, it makes sense to start working on the issue that is causing the most distress for you and/or the people around you. The exercise in Worksheet 31 can help you figure

WORKSHEET 30

My Problems in the Community
People

Check off (✓) the statements below that sound familiar to you regarding experiences with the people around you while shopping, or using services such as the bank, post office, or library. Also consider attendance at gatherings related to fitness, hobbies, sports, or worship. If your problem does not appear on this list, fill it in on one of the blanks at the bottom.

☐ I feel nervous when I have to go to any public place.

☐ I get furious with other drivers.

☐ Public transportation (train/bus) is too crowded for me.

☐ I can't stand to have strangers bumping into me, even if by accident.

☐ I have had arguments with conductors on the train.

☐ I have had arguments with bus drivers.

☐ I am afraid to ask for directions.

☐ I have been told that my clothes are not right for the weather (I either wear too little for the cold or too much for the heat).

☐ I get thrown off if the bank teller asks me something I was not expecting.

☐ I get upset if a clerk seems rude.

☐ I don't like to ask for help when I can't find something at the library.

☐ I am always afraid the cashier is giving me the wrong change.

☐ I am afraid to ask for assistance or direction from store employees.

☐ I practically panic if a salesperson approaches me when I am browsing.

☐ I feel really uncomfortable talking to people at my church or temple.

☐ I feel really uncomfortable talking to people at my fitness center or gym.

☐ I get very nervous when I walk my dog and a stranger tries to talk to me.

☐ I have problems getting along with my sports teammates [e.g., bowling, softball, basketball].

☐ I belong to a club related to my hobby, but I don't enjoy it when people talk about anything other than the hobby.

☐ _____

☐ _____

out which one that is. Rate the level of distress caused by each problem and then pick the one with the highest score to tackle first. You can return to the others later, in order of most to least distress. It can also be helpful to talk over this prioritizing with a trusted person in your life.

The next few pages will guide you through the steps of solving the problem you just identified. For each step you will be asked to write your answers in the question boxes. Each box will give you instructions, and then I'll show you how Richard filled out the box.

Step 1: Identify and Define Your Problem Using Your Community

What is bothering you about going out and using your community? If you filled out Worksheets 29 and 30, you've already done this step. Write the problem you have chosen to work on first below.

WORKSHEET 31

Choosing Which Problem to Work on First

If you checked off only one problem on Worksheets 29 and 30, you don't need to use this worksheet. Otherwise, list the problems you checked in the first column below. Then use this rating scale to estimate the amount of stress the issue is causing you and/or the people around you.

How much distress is this problem causing in my life?

Almost None	Some	Moderate Amount	A Lot	Extreme
1	2	3	4	5

Problem   **Distress Rating**

_____   _____

_____   _____

_____   _____

_____   _____

> ### Step 1: Identify and Define Your Problem with Using Your Community
>
> *What is bothering you about going out and using your community?*
>
> The problem that is bothering me most about going out into my community is:
>
> _____
>
> _____
>
> _____

Example. **Richard** didn't need to use Worksheet 31 because he identified only one community problem. He filled out his Step 1 question box this way:

> ### Step 1: Identify and Define Your Problem with Using Your Community
>
> The problem that is bothering me most about going out into my community is:
>
> *I am afraid to talk to people I don't know, like the people who work in stores, the bank, the post office, and the gym. I am stuck at home all the time and too dependent on my mom to help me run errands.*

Step 2: Define Your Goal

What would you like to see change to minimize the problem you identified with going out into your community? What would need to be different for you to feel less bothered by the problem? The goal you lay out is simply the opposite of the problem you listed. List your goal in the box below, and if you need an example, look at Richard's box.

> ### Step 2: Define Your Goal
>
> *What would you like to see change to minimize the problem you identified with using your community?* The goal you lay out is simply the opposite of the problem you listed.
>
> To feel less stressed by this problem, I would like to:
>
> _____

Example. **Richard's** goal is listed below. Notice how he stated the goal as the opposite of his problem. Stating the goal in the affirmative gives Richard something to work toward and also lends itself to measuring success.

Step 2: Define Your Goal

To feel less stressed by this problem, I would like to:

Go on errands by myself and join a gym.

Step 3: Identify the Obstacles in the Way of Your Achieving the Goal

What is getting in the way of your goal? The next step is to identify obstacles to meeting your goal. Here it is particularly important to consider your ASD characteristics as hidden players in your problem. As you go through this step, you may rely on the information you were given in Part I of this book about your ASD differences. As you think about the problem you listed, look at the chart on page 252 called "ASD Differences That Can Contribute to Problems in the Community." Read through that chart with your own problem in mind and also consider the following questions.

Thinking Differences

How might my *executive functioning* issues be contributing to my problems in the community? For example, do I have difficulty organizing new information, which makes it hard for me to get oriented to new places? Do I get lost a lot? Do I find it hard to plan my errands efficiently? Does my focus and concentration difficulty cause me to have problems driving or using public transportation? Do I persist too long, repeating a strategy that is clearly not working because I have difficulty shifting to new strategies? How might my *negative self-talk* be contributing to my problems using the community? What am I saying to myself that is putting more pressure on me? Could I be engaging in perfectionistic thinking, all-or-nothing thinking, or catastrophic thinking that makes it harder for me to function outside my home? For example, do I assume the worst will happen before an important activity? Do I expect perfection from myself and/or store clerks or other members of my recreational or religious groups?

Social Differences

How might my *social perception* be contributing to my problems in the community? Is it possible that I sometimes misunderstand what clerks, salespeople, or other members of my recreational or religious groups are trying to tell me? For example, do I still feel uncertain about what my teammates or fellow club members expect from me? Am I still uncertain about how I should handle conversations with strangers at the store or acquaintances at my church or temple? How might my *social/communication skills* be contributing to problems in the community? Is it possible that clerks, salespeople, or fellow members of teams or groups are not communicating clearly enough about what they expect and I don't know how to seek clarification? For example, I feel uncertain about when and how to ask for help from a store clerk. I am unsure about when or how to start a conversation with someone at the gym. Is my problem caused partly by my not knowing what to say or do when dealing with another member of the community, whether a stranger or an acquaintance? For example, I don't know how to handle someone sitting next to me on the train beginning to talk to me. Or, I don't know what to say if a salesperson begins to talk to me when I'm browsing at a store.

Emotional Differences

How might my emotional reactions to things be affecting my problems in the community? Do I have difficulty *regulating* my emotions? Do I take too long to calm down after an upsetting incident? Am I overreacting or underreacting to things that happen in public places, like at a bank, in a store, or on the bus? Do I have difficulty *identifying* my feelings or *asking for help* when I am upset? Do I tend to avoid situations that cause me to feel too much anxiety or worry, such as driving by myself or running errands?

Sensory and Movement Differences

How might my sensory issues be contributing to my problems in the community? For example, my YMCA is noisy, and that contributes to my avoiding exercise. Am I *oversensitive* or *undersensitive* to certain types of light, sound, smell, taste, or touch? How might my *movement* and *coordination* issues be contributing to my problems using the community? For example, I was asked to join a church softball team, but I feel so clumsy and awkward when playing sports. Is it possible that my hygiene is not acceptable to some people because my sensory/movement problems interfere with bathing or grooming?

Now fill out the question box below, but try not to think about other problems you have besides the one you chose for this exercise.

Step 3: Identify the Obstacles in the Way of Your Achieving the Goal

What is getting in the way of your goal? Remember to focus *only* on the problem and goal you wrote down in Steps 1 and 2. First circle the category(ies) of ASD differences you suspect are involved in this problem:

Thinking   **Social**   **Emotional**   **Sensory/Movement**

I believe these differences are contributing in this way:

_____

_____

_____

_____

_____

_____

_____

Example. ***Richard*** filled out his Step 3 question box in this way:

Step 3: Identify the Obstacles in the Way of Your Achieving the Goal

Thinking   (**Social**)   (**Emotional**)   (**Sensory/Movement**)

I believe these differences are contributing in this way:

My social differences leave me with nothing to say—I literally do not have any idea about the right thing to do or say with strangers I have to talk to in stores, the bank, and the post office. I am so nervous about this that I am overwhelmed, and that makes me freeze (emotional differences). My sensory differences make me really sensitive to bright light, which only makes matters worse in public buildings.

Differences →	Thinking	Social	Emotional	Sensory/Movement
Problems Getting Around and Managing Tasks in the Community	• *Attention regulation* difficulties can make it hard to focus on driving tasks • *Difficulties organizing information* make it hard to find your way around new areas—may be prone to get lost • *Difficulties organizing information* make it hard to plan and carry out your errands in an efficient way • *Difficulties organizing information* make it hard to get oriented inside a store or public building	• You may not notice or interpret cues from strangers; difficulty with "unwritten rules" about where to sit on a train or bus, how to respond to a person sitting next to you • You may not notice or interpret cues from others that may help you find your way or get oriented	• Your difficulty *recognizing and identifying negative emotions* can contribute to inability to address an anxiety-provoking situation until it is overwhelming (e.g., on public transportation, in a store or public building) • Your difficulty *regulating your negative emotions* can contribute to extreme anger with other drivers or users of public transportation	• *Hypersensitivity* to noise, light, smell, taste, or touch can cause discomfort on public transportation • *Hypersensitivity* to noise, light, smell, taste, or touch can cause discomfort in stores and public buildings • *Hyposensitivity* (underresponsive sense) can interfere with picking up on important navigation cues, such as signs or signals • *Fine or gross motor problems* could affect confidence while driving
Problems With People in the Community	• *Attention regulation* difficulties can make it hard to coordinate your focus on other people during team activities or religious services • *All-or-nothing thinking* can make it difficult to interpret the rules of a group (sports team, club, or religious group)	• Your difficulty *initiating conversations* may interfere with your ability to ask for help if you need directions • The *unique way you process and express language* can contribute to misunderstandings with clerks, fellow customers, or members of recreational or religious groups • The *unique way you express language* can make it hard to assert yourself with strangers if needed (e.g., someone cuts in front of you in line) • Your difficulty with *conversation skills* may interfere with making positive connections with others in a club, team, or religious group • You may be perceived by others as uncaring or aloof because of the way you *experience and express empathy* • You may not notice or interpret cues or *mind-read*, making it difficult to know what others expect from you in a group	• Your difficulty *recognizing and identifying negative emotions* can prevent you from addressing the anxiety you may feel around other people in the community • Your difficulty *regulating your negative emotions* can contribute to anger with clerks, fellow customers, or members of recreation or religious groups • *Hyper- or hyposensitivity* to temperature can contribute to wearing clothes inappropriate for the weather—can make you stand out from others	• *Fine or gross motor problems* can be obstacles to many types of cooperative leisure activities (e.g., games or sports); may narrow your choice of activities • *Hypersensitivity or fine motor problems* can lead to poor hygiene and possible rejection by others

ASD differences that can contribute to problems in the community.

When you filled out your sheet, did you circle more than one area of ASD differences? Richard identified three potential sources of difficulty: his social (difficulty initiating interactions), emotional (anxiety), and sensory (sensitivity to bright light) differences. This illustrates once again that often a single issue can have several causes.

Step 4: List Several Possible Solutions to Address the Obstacle(s)

What are the possible solutions for the obstacles? Try to list as many ideas as possible. Remember that this is the step some people call "brainstorming." Generate as many possibilities as come to mind, without inhibition. Do not judge or evaluate any solution that comes to mind—just write it down no matter how weird or silly it seems. In Step 5 you will weed through them and discard any that are not useful, so no harm can be done.

Start by looking at the Cheat Sheet at the end of Chapter 6. Find the ASD difference that you circled on the top row of the Cheat Sheet. Then look along the column underneath each and find the dots. Each dot marks the row in which you will find a solution in the far left column of the chart. Those approaches should be considered first, and Chapter 6 provides you with the instructions and tools for each of those solutions. Also, try to consider your *strengths* as you complete this step because they also play an important role in your solutions. Refer back to Worksheets 3 and 4 in Chapter 1. Write your primary strengths in the blanks here so you can keep them in mind while you are generating solutions.

My strengths are: _____, _____, and _____.

Step 4: List Several Possible Solutions to Address the Obstacle(s)

What are the possible solutions for the obstacles? Now, considering all the solutions you saw on the Cheat Sheet, and some you may think of on your own, list all the possibilities you can imagine to address the ASD differences involved in the problem you listed in Step 1. For the moment, ignore the score columns on the right.

I could try to:

List strategies below	Pro (+) score	Con (−) score	Total pro−con

⇨

Example. ***Richard*** filled out his question box this way:

Step 4: List Several Possible Solutions to Address the Obstacle(s)

I could try to:

List strategies below	Pro (+) score	Con (−) score	Total pro–con
1) continue to stay home where it is safe			
2) practice communication techniques			
3) use mindfulness techniques for anxiety			
4) ask for the lights to be dimmed in each place			
5) wear tinted glasses to filter bothersome lights			
6) try to run errands without talking to others			

Notice that Richard listed everything that came to mind, even things that seem inappropriate (e.g., stay home). He looked at the Cheat Sheet, which gave him ideas 2, 3, and 5. He also decided to talk to his vocational counselor about his discomfort with talking to strangers because it could also eventually affect his work life (e.g., going on job interviews, interacting with coworkers), and she agreed to help him with his solutions. This is an example of "brainstorming." He cannot possibly do all the things on this list but will use the next step to figure out what is most useful to him.

Step 5: Consider the Consequences of Each Solution

What are the pros and cons of each solution? Now you will put each item on your list to the test of how feasible it is or how helpful it will be toward the goal you wrote down during Step 2. Use the question box below to give each item a score.

Step 5: Consider the Consequences of Each Solution

What are the pros and cons of each solution? Look back at each item you wrote down in Step 4. Then assign each one a score. Score the benefit (Pro +) in terms of how likely that strategy is to get you closer to your goal. Score the disadvantage (Con –) in terms of the effort, cost, or damage involved in implementing it.

Pro (+) Scale

How likely is it to get me closer to my goal?

Very Unlikely	Pretty Unlikely	Hard to Tell	Somewhat Likely	Very Likely
0	1	2	3	4

Con (–) Scale

How much effort, cost, or damage would this strategy involve?

None	Almost None	Some	A Lot	Extreme
0	1	2	3	4

Example. **Richard's** answers in this question box appear below. He carried out Step 5 and rated each one of his solutions from Step 4.

Step 4: List Several Possible Solutions to Address the Obstacle(s)

I could try to:

List strategies below	Pro (+) score	Con (–) score	Total pro–con
1) continue to stay home where it is safe	0	4	–4
2) practice communication techniques	4	3	1
3) use mindfulness techniques for anxiety	3	1	2
4) ask for the lights to be dimmed in each place	3	3	0
5) wear tinted glasses to filter bothersome lights	3	2	1
6) try to run errands without talking to others	2	3	–1

Step 6: Choose the Best One(s) to Try Out First

Which solutions should you try first? Now that you've scored all of your options, choosing the one or two strategies to start with should be easy. Which of your options had the highest total score? According to your own rating, the highest score has the most benefit compared to the cost, effort, or damage it could involve. Notice that Richard ended up with three solutions that seemed worthwhile to him, even though none of them had high pro–con scores. He believed his strategies had some promise, but he was nervous about learning something new and had some concerns about his ability to practice the new skills. That is why he assigned a "con" rating even to ideas he had chosen after looking at the strategies in Chapter 6. Being skeptical is natural; don't be surprised if you have some of the same feelings yourself. In the end, you need not expect a "perfect" pro–con score of 4 to consider an option; you need only pick the ones with the highest score compared to the others.

Step 6: Choose the Best One(s) to Try Out First

Which solutions should you try first? Which of the strategies in Step 5 had the highest score? Pick the top one or two and write them down below:

_____

_____

_____

---

*Example. **Richard** filled out his question box the following way, choosing ideas 2, 3, and 5.

Step 6: Choose the Best One(s) to Try Out First

Practice communication techniques for use with clerks/salespeople

Use thinking techniques to help with anxiety

Use environmental modification (tinted glasses) to help with lights

Step 7: Implement the Solution and Track Your Progress

Now try the solution and track your progress. Use the next question box to map out your plan.

Step 7: Implement the Solution and Track Your Progress

Now try the solution and track your progress. Here is how:

Where will I do it?

_____

When will I do it?

_____

What do I need to do it?

_____

How will I do it?

_____

_____

Who can help me, if needed?

_____

How will I keep track of my success? (Look at your goal and then pick a way to track it—either a running count or a rating scale.)

_____

_____

_____

---

*Example. **Richard** first studied the **communication techniques** in Chapter 6, which helped him focus on what he **needs** from each person he encounters in the community. With the help of his mother and his vocational counselor, he determined that the primary purpose of any conversation he has with clerks, salespeople, or staff at the gym should be related to the actual need that each of those people is fulfilling for him. He also looked at the *techniques to understand other people*, which helped him define everyone he would encounter on errands or at the gym as strangers or acquaintances, which alleviated some pressure he felt, as did coming up with scripts he could use with each person.

Richard also studied the *thinking techniques* in Chapter 6 and found the *mindfulness* approach of staying focused on the present very useful. Finally, reading about *environmental modifications* helped him come up with the idea of wearing tinted glasses in stores and public buildings. He and his counselor chose lightly tinted ones so others could see his eyes—opaque glasses worn indoors might make others feel uncomfortable.

Richard and his counselor also considered his primary strengths, which they agreed were his sense of *personal responsibility* and *perseverance*. These traits were motivating him to solve this problem and would be useful in the implementation of the plan he worked out in the question box following the Step 7 question box. Following the plan is a list of scripts he and his counselor designed. Each script has three main elements: a polite greeting, a request for the item or service he needs from that person, and a polite way to end the interaction. The box after that shows his mindfulness phrases, designed to help him focus on what is going on in the moment. Some of the phrases seem irrelevant to the task (e.g., notice the color of the clerk's shirt) but can help you keep your mind on the present, which can help to regulate anxiety. Finally you'll see Richard's anxiety scale.

Step 7: Implement the Solution and Track Your Progress

Where will I do it?

In a store, the bank, or the post office

When will I do it?

Twice a week

What do I need to do it?

Scripts for My Errands, Mindfulness Phrases, and my
Anxiety Rating scale

How will I do it?

Meet with my counselor once a week and go over Scripts. Pick two places
I will visit as practice. Review Scripts and Mindfulness Phrases before each
outing into community. Rate anxiety before and after each outing.

Who can help me, if needed?

My vocational counselor and my mother

How will I keep track of my success? (Look at your goal and then pick a way to track it—either a running count or a rating scale.)

My goal is to run two errands each week by myself. I will also track my anxiety to see if it decreases over time. I will practice with errands for 4 weeks before joining a gym. Once my anxiety is manageable to me (e.g., 5 or below on rating scale) I will work on joining a gym.

SCRIPTS FOR MY ERRANDS

<u>Bank Teller</u>

1. *Approach counter and remember Mindfulness Phrases.*
2. *Say "Hello," make brief eye contact, and smile.*
3. *Say "I would like to [deposit this check, withdraw, etc.], please."*
4. *Practice Mindfulness Phrases.*
5. *Listen to hear any questions teller may ask.*
6. *Watch for teller to hand you your receipt.*
7. *Listen for teller's ending phrase, which could be "Thank you," "Goodbye," "Have a nice day," or "Is there anything else I can help you with?"*
8. *If you hear nothing, look at teller's face for a nod or a smile, which is another way to end the interaction.*
9. *If you have another transaction to complete, go back to Step 3 and repeat.*
10. *If you have no other tasks, say "Thank you. Have a nice day."*

<u>Postal Clerk</u>

1. *Approach counter and remember Mindfulness Phrases.*
2. *Say "Hello," make brief eye contact, and smile.*
3. *Say "I would like to [mail this, buy stamps, etc.], please."*
4. *Practice Mindfulness Phrases.*
5. *Listen to hear any questions clerk may ask.*
6. *Watch for clerk to hand you your receipt.*
7. *Listen for clerk's ending phrase, which could be "Thank you," "Goodbye," "Have a nice day," or "Is there anything else I can help you with?"*
8. *If you hear nothing, look at clerk's face for a nod or a smile, which is another way to end the interaction.*
9. *If you have another transaction to complete, go back to Step 3 and repeat.*
10. *If you have no other tasks, say "Thank you. Have a nice day."*

<u>Grocery Store Clerk/Cashier</u>

1. *Approach checkout lane and remember Mindfulness Phrases.*
2. *Say "Hello," make brief eye contact, and smile.*
3. *Practice Mindfulness Phrases.*

⇨

4. *Listen to hear any questions cashier may ask.*
5. *Help cashier place your items in bags.*
6. *Listen for instructions from cashier about amount due.*
7. *Tell cashier how you will pay (cash, check, credit/debit card).*
8. *Listen for further instructions from cashier during payment.*
9. *Watch for cashier to hand you your change and/or receipt.*
10. *Listen for cashier's ending phrase, which could be "Thank you," "Goodbye," or "Have a nice day."*
11. *If you hear nothing, look at teller's face for a nod or a smile, which is another way to end the interaction.*
12. *Say "Thank you. Have a nice day."*

Pharmacist/Pharmacy Clerk

1. *Approach counter and remember Mindfulness Phrases.*
2. *Say "Hello," make brief eye contact, and smile.*
3. *Say "I would like to [fill, pickup] this prescription, please."*
4. *Practice Mindfulness Phrases.*
5. *Listen to hear any questions pharmacist/clerk may ask.*
6. *Watch for pharmacist/clerk to hand you your item(s) or listen for instructions on when to come back to pick up.*
7. *Listen for pharmacist/clerk's ending phrase, which could be "Thank you," "Goodbye," "Have a nice day," or "Is there anything else I can help you with?"*
8. *If you hear nothing, look at pharmacist/clerk's face for a nod or a smile, which is another way to end the interaction.*
9. *If you have another transaction to complete, go back to Step 3 and repeat.*
10. *If you have no other tasks, say "Thank you. Have a nice day."*

MINDFULNESS PHRASES—STAYING IN THE PRESENT ON MY ERRANDS

For every errand I will focus on the purpose of the visit to the store or service counter (e.g., to deposit a check, to buy stamps, to buy milk, to fill a prescription). During every encounter with a clerk or salesperson, I will focus on the person who is serving me. I will notice what is going on in the moment. I will say these things to *myself* (not out loud).

> *I will focus on why I came here.*
> *I will notice the color of the shirt on the person helping me.*
> *I will notice whether that person is wearing glasses.*
> *I will notice the person moving his/her arms and hands while serving me.*
> *I will notice if the person smiles.*
> *I will notice when the person hands something to me.*

DAILY RATING OF ANXIETY

Today I feel *anxiety about talking to clerks and salespeople* to the following degree:

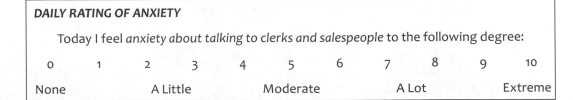

0	1	2	3	4	5	6	7	8	9	10
None		A Little			Moderate			A Lot		Extreme

Step 8: Evaluate the Solution to See If It Met Your Goal

Did the solution meet your goal, or do you need to use a different solution? At this point you've tried out your new solution and are ready to see if it helped you meet your goal. Use the question box to evaluate your progress.

    *Example. **Richard** filled out his question box this way after practicing his plan for 4 weeks.

Step 8: Evaluate the Solution to See If It Met Your Goal

What was my goal? (Copy this from Step 2.)

   Go on errands by myself and join a gym

How did I measure my progress? (data, log, or record)

   I kept a log of the errands I ran each week. I rated my anxiety before and after each errand.

What do the data show with regard to my goal?

   In 4 weeks I went on 10 errands (more than I planned). My anxiety was an average of 9 before each trip and 7 after. But the highest numbers came from the first 2 weeks. Last week my ratings before were an average of 8 and 6 after each errand.

How would you rate your success, on a scale of 0–100% success for meeting your goal?

I was __*100*__ % successful.   *because I did more than 2 errands each week. My anxiety went down, but I want to work on this more before joining a gym.*

0	10	20	30	40	50	60	70	80	90	100
None		A Little			Moderate			A Lot		Total

What should I do based on this success rate? (fill in the box next to the best choice)

☐ **Celebrate and keep doing what I am doing!**

☑ **Celebrate success and also modify the plan toward further improvement.**

    Richard was very pleased that he did more errands than planned. He was also happy that he had decided not to try to join a gym at the same time as starting to run errands, because even after 4 weeks of practice in the community his anxiety was quite high. He found the Mindfulness Phrases helpful but sometimes forgot to use them in crowded places, so his counselor helped him make a wallet-sized laminated card with the phrases on them so he could read them while on an errand if needed.

Now let's look at how *Jake* used problem solving to deal with his *fear of driving*. As shown in Chapter 9, Jake rated this problem a higher priority than his *difficulties seeking help with school work*, so he tackled the driving issue first.

Step 1: Identify and Define Your Problem with Using Your Community

The problem that is bothering me most about going out into my community is:

I am afraid to drive on highways. I have had my license for 2 years and I have not gotten any better at this.

Step 2: Define Your Goal

To feel less stressed by this problem, I would like to:

Be more confident driving on highways.

Step 3: Identify the Obstacles in the Way of Your Achieving the Goal

(Thinking)   Social   (Emotional)   Sensory/Movement

I believe these differences are contributing in this way:

My thinking differences make it hard for me to focus on the right things while driving and make me put pressure on myself to be a perfect driver. My emotional differences make me feel panicky when I drive on highways.

Next Jake "brainstormed" solutions and then weighed the pros and cons of each, shown in the box below.

Step 4: List Several Possible Solutions to Address the Obstacle(s)

I could try to:

List strategies below	Pro (+) score	Con (−) score	Total pro−con
1) keep taking back roads—avoid highways	0	4	−4
2) ask parents to give me more driving lessons	4	3	1
3) use emotion regulation techniques to help with fear	4	2	2
4) use thinking techniques to help with fear	4	2	2
5) take taxis to avoid driving	0	4	−4

In Step 6, Jake used the results of his evaluation to pick the three options with the highest pro–con score, which are highlighted in the Step 4 box. Notice that the total scores are not a "perfect 4" because he felt there was a lot of effort he would need to put into these options. For example, asking his parents for driving lessons seemed like a good idea on one hand, but he was very nervous about talking to them about this, which caused his "con" score on that item to be high. Studying the *emotion regulation techniques* found in Chapter 6 helped Jake tune in to the fact that his heart races and he sweats whenever he drives on highways, where he hadn't been aware before that anxiety and fear were his problem with driving. He decided to use the Understanding My Emotions worksheet on page 265 and then also to buy a relaxation CD to learn to relax before his driving lessons. He also looked over the *thinking techniques* in Chapter 6 and was helped by the *acceptance* phrase "I accept that my brain works differently" and then another he made up for himself, "I accept that I need some extra help with learning to drive." (He used acceptance phrases to help him accept needing help with schoolwork too.) Jake's sense of *purpose* is a strength that he considered important in solving both his school-based and community-based problems. His implementation plan appears in the next box.

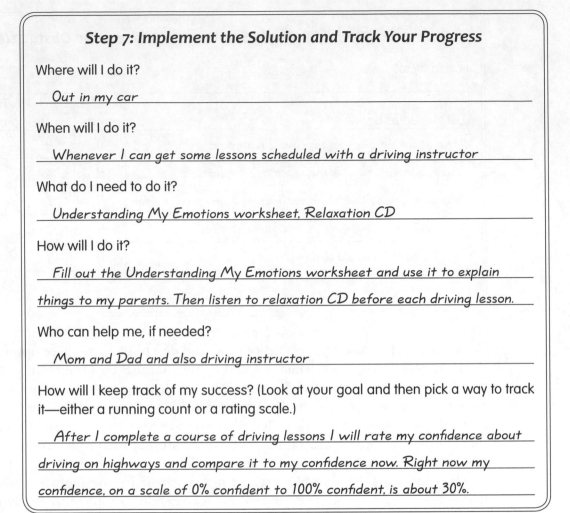

Step 7: Implement the Solution and Track Your Progress

Where will I do it?

Out in my car

When will I do it?

Whenever I can get some lessons scheduled with a driving instructor

What do I need to do it?

Understanding My Emotions worksheet, Relaxation CD

How will I do it?

Fill out the Understanding My Emotions worksheet and use it to explain things to my parents. Then listen to relaxation CD before each driving lesson.

Who can help me, if needed?

Mom and Dad and also driving instructor

How will I keep track of my success? (Look at your goal and then pick a way to track it—either a running count or a rating scale.)

After I complete a course of driving lessons I will rate my confidence about driving on highways and compare it to my confidence now. Right now my confidence, on a scale of 0% confident to 100% confident, is about 30%.

Here is Jake's confidence scale and the Understanding My Emotions worksheet follows:

CONFIDENCE RATING
How much confidence do you have about driving on highways?

0	10	20	30	40	50	60	70	80	90	100
None		A Little			Moderate			A Lot		Extreme

Example from Jake
WORKSHEET 18

Understanding My Emotions

For use when evaluating an upsetting event. Fill this out soon after an event during which you found yourself to be very upset.

Date and time of event: ___the last time I drove on a highway___

1) Briefly describe the event: I was upset when ___I had to merge or change lanes. The other cars whizzing by me were freaking me out.___

2) Now look at the words, pictures, and synonyms below. On the top row are the basic negative emotions and underneath are some common words that have similar meanings. Which of these emotions do you suspect was involved in your reaction to the event? Circle the relevant emotion. You can circle more than one.

Sadness	Anger	Fear
Depressed Miserable Devastated Down	Enraged Annoyed Frustrated Irritated	Terrified Anxious Tense Nervous

3) I felt ___terrified___, which may be a signal that I needed something.

4) Maybe I needed ___more practice before being on my own___.

5) Feeling ___fear___ is a natural part of life and I accept that I felt that way.

6) Now think about what was around you that may have helped you meet your need. This could be an object or a person. I could have used ___more coaching from someone___ to help me meet my need.

7) In circumstances like these, I may do ___more practice with an instructor___ to address my need.

Here is the evaluation Jake did after he completed a course of driving lessons.

Step 8: Evaluate the Solution to See If It Met Your Goal

What was my goal? (Copy this from Step 2.)

___Be more confident driving on highways.___

⇨

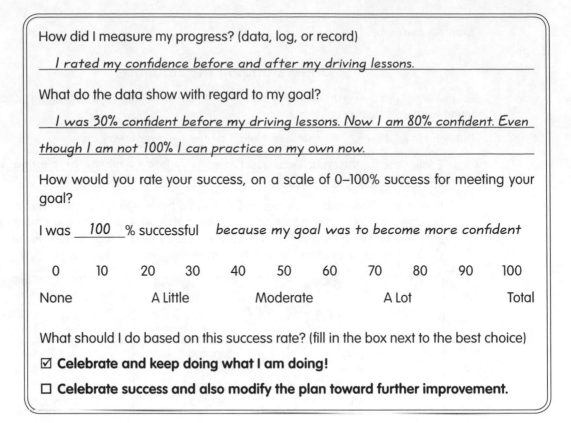

To give you one more illustration of problem solving for issues related to community life, without showing the entire worksheet, here are *Jean's* steps in her own words:

Step 1: Identify and Define Your Problem

"I don't feel comfortable during meetings and activities when I am volunteering at my church. I try to talk to people, but it seems like they are not interested in talking to me. I am disappointed because I had hoped to make connections with some people."

Step 2: Define Your Goal

"I would like get to know several people who are volunteering along with me."

Step 3: Identify the Obstacles in the Way of Your Achieving the Goal

"I believe my *social* differences are causing the problem. I was told many times during my years at the library that I talk too much. Recently at church I overheard a woman say something about me 'never stopping to take a breath.'"

Step 4: List Several Possible Solutions to Address the Obstacle(s)

1. "Drop out of all committees at the church."
2. "Keep trying to talk to people the same way I have been."
3. "Use techniques for understanding others to improve my conversation skills (got this idea from Cheat Sheet)."
4. "Tell these ladies on the committees that they also talk too much."

Step 5: Consider the Consequences of Each Solution

"After evaluating the pros and cons of each solution, I think number 3 is the only viable option."

Step 6: Choose the Best One(s) to Try Out First

"After reading about techniques for understanding others, I believe I need to pay more attention to other people. In all my years of working with people, I always assumed the best way to get to know someone is to talk. I have never been shy, and I assumed that was an asset. I still think it is an important part of my *optimism*, but it never occurred to me that listening to people is just as important as talking."

Step 7: Implement the Solution and Track Your Progress

"I am going to follow the guidelines for learning about others. Fortunately, I have a very good memory for details, so I'll be able to remember things people tell me without writing anything down. I will try this for about 6 weeks and then count how many people I've gotten to know. Right now I would say the number is zero."

Guidelines for Learning about Other People at Church

   1) Gather information about them by:

      — asking direct questions about them and listening to the answers

      — observing things they do

      — listening to what they say to you or to others

   2) Limit questions and comments to those reserved for acquaintances. Avoid questions about private life, but do ask about

      — interests

      — hobbies

                                               ⇨

> — work
>
> — other church activities
>
> 3) Remember to follow up on questions about this information during conversations you may have on another day

Step 8: Evaluate the Solution to See If It Met Your Goal

"After 6 weeks I have gotten to know three of the other ladies. They act more welcoming toward me when I arrive at meetings, and I now feel more connected to the church. I would rate my success at 80% because I'd like to get to know more people."

A Word about Strangers and Acquaintances

When you are out and about in the community, most of the people you encounter are either strangers or acquaintances. As discussed in Chapter 6, by definition you know nothing or very little about people who fall into those categories. On the one hand this can relieve social pressure because any interactions can be brief and superficial. On the other hand it makes their behavior relatively unpredictable.

Here are some safe assumptions to make about strangers and acquaintances out in the community:

- They will not automatically know that you have an ASD diagnosis.
- They have varying backgrounds, attitudes, and personalities that are unknown to you.
- You can't predict how they will respond to the behavioral differences that can come from having an ASD.
- You're a stranger to them to the same degree that they are strangers to you.

In this book I promote an attitude of self-acceptance and encourage you to be yourself, even if it means taking an unconventional approach to life. I believe your success and growth depend on your embracing your differences and using good communication to help the people close to you also understand and embrace your differences. But it's important to understand that the rules and goals are different with strangers. You can't expect people you don't know to accept you automatically. It's human nature to feel uncomfortable or even threatened by unusual or unconventional behavior from a stranger. Feeling uncomfortable or threatened can lead people to act defensive or even hostile. Therefore, it's important to protect your own safety in the community in these ways:

- Pay attention to your personal appearance when traveling in the community. Avoid habits that would make you stand out or draw attention to you. Good hygiene, a neat appearance, and weather-appropriate clothes can help you blend in when around strangers. If you're uncertain about your appearance, ask someone you know well and trust to give you feedback.

- Don't give a stranger feedback about how he or she looks.
- Avoid staring at strangers.
- If a conversation begins between you and a stranger, remember to follow the guidelines in Chapter 6 about the topics you should stick to.
- If you have specific wardrobe or accessory choices you must make to accommodate sensory problems, choose things that look conventional and don't make you stand out in a crowd. If you're uncertain, ask someone you know well and trust to give you feedback.
- Don't challenge a stranger about his or her unusual behavior.
- Don't give feedback to a stranger about his or her behavior unless the behavior is directed at you and is having a negative impact on you.

11

Building Friendships

Much of what has already been discussed in Part II of this book pertains to friendships. All the social skills and strategies illustrated are as necessary to making and keeping friends as they are to other relationships. And people form friendships in all settings: at home (such as when you and a roommate develop a closer relationship than one defined by simply sharing a residence), at work, at school, and in the community. If you've read the earlier chapters, you've seen *Margaret* learn to connect with coworkers at her group medical practice (Chapter 8), which may lead to a friendship or two. In Chapter 9, I described how *Arnold* learned to make conversation on campus toward the goal of making friends in college. And in Chapter 10 you saw how *Jean* began to make the friends she wanted to make at church.

You may be perfectly content to have few or no friends. Just because she's getting along better with the staff doesn't mean *Margaret* has to pursue friendships with anyone at the office. You can make a similar choice. But if you're like the many people on the spectrum I've met who feel dissatisfied with the number or quality of friendships they have, this chapter can help.

As you learned in Chapter 6, one of the greatest social difficulties that ASDs impose is confusion over how relationships are defined. If *Margaret* doesn't want to become closer to her coworkers, they will remain acquaintances rather than friends. The difference between an acquaintance and a friend is one of closeness, as measured on four dimensions:

- How much time have you spent with the person?
- How much do you rely on the person?
- How much do you and this person share in terms of common interests?
- How much do you enjoy the company of the person?

Using the scoring system that was included in the definition, a *friend* is a person to whom you would assign a fairly high score on all of these dimensions and who would do the same for you: it's someone you spend a lot of time with, where there is mutual reliance and trust, as well as common interests and mutual enjoyment of each other's company.

Fred is the 31-year-old single man described in Chapter 1 who works full time at a bank and lives alone in a studio apartment. Fred's good friend from high school shares his love of sports but is now threatening to stop going to a sports bar with Fred on Friday nights because he's tired of Fred's *anger outbursts* whenever he disagrees with Fred about some aspect of the game they're watching.

Arnold's problem solving in Chapter 9 was directed at learning to converse with his roommates, but in this chapter I'll show you how he addressed the broader problem of *making friends* on campus.

Sophie, age 26, is studying part-time to become a medical assistant. She lives at home with her parents and works full time as a receptionist at an outpatient physical therapy/sports medicine center. She likes her job because the environment is very friendly and relaxed; her bosses are warm toward all the people who work there. Sophie is very outgoing and enjoys chatting with a lot of different people. She has made several friends there. She and the other receptionist have become very friendly with a few of the patients who are frequent visitors to the center. They sometimes go to a bar or club together on weekends, but Sophie does the driving since she's the only one with a car, and recently she's started to worry that these people are more interested in having her drive than in being her friends. She is struggling with *social judgment* and the ability to discriminate between genuine friendship and casual acquaintanceship.

In Chapter 1, your clock worksheet may have indicated that you are stressed at a particular time of day because of a friendship issue. Worksheets 32 and 33 can help you identify and solve your friendship-related problems. The items on the checklists may look familiar, as they were listed first in Chapter 1. Each sheet has a list of problems common to people on the spectrum but also leaves blank spaces at the bottom for you to fill in any other friendship-related problems.

Problem Solving

If you found you have more than one problem with making or keeping friends, you will need to choose one to address first; you can then repeat the eight steps of problem solving for each of the other problems at a later time. As mentioned in Chapter 6, it makes sense to start working on the issue that is causing the most distress for you and/or the people around you. Worksheet 34 can help you figure out which one that is. Rate the level of distress caused by each problem and then pick the one with the highest score to tackle first. You can return to the others later, in order of most to least distress. It can also help to talk over this prioritizing with a trusted person in your life.

The next few pages will guide you through the steps of solving the problem you just identified. For each step you will be asked to write your answers in the

My Problems with Friendships
Making Friends

Check off (✓) the statements below that sound familiar or reflect your experiences with trying to meet new people and make friends. If you have a problem with making friends that does not appear on this list, fill it in on one of the blanks at the bottom.

☐ I can't seem to meet people who have my interests.

☐ I don't know where I should be looking for friends.

☐ I can't figure out which acquaintances could be good friends.

☐ I am intimidated by online social networking sites that many people use.

☐ I can't seem to make "small talk"—I can't keep a conversation going.

☐ I have been told I am aloof and people think I am rejecting them.

☐ I don't know how to join in when it looks like everyone knows each other.

☐ I have been told I talk too much.

☐ I am too shy—I would never start talking to someone I don't know.

☐ _____

☐ _____

From Living Well on the Spectrum by Valerie L. Gaus. Copyright 2011 by The Guilford Press.

My Problems with Friendships
Keeping Friends

Check off (✓) the statements below that sound familiar or reflect your experiences with the friends you already have. If your problem does not appear on this list, fill it in on one of the blanks at the bottom.

☐ I have been told I don't keep in touch with friends enough.

☐ I can't seem to make time to do things with my friends.

☐ I don't like to talk on the phone.

☐ I like to be with a friend one on one, but I don't like group gatherings.

☐ I don't know what to do when a friend is mad at me or vice versa.

☐ I don't like being pressured to do something I don't want to do.

☐ I am too afraid to say "no" when a friend asks a favor.

☐ Sometimes I think my friends are using me.

☐ I have been told I am too bossy or that I dominate the conversation.

☐ I have been told I act arrogant or like a "know-it-all."

☐ I have been told that I don't think of other people's feelings.

☐ _____

☐ _____

From Living Well on the Spectrum by Valerie L. Gaus. Copyright 2011 by The Guilford Press.

question box. Each box will give you instructions, and then I'll show you how *Fred* filled in the box.

Step 1: Identify and Define Your Problem with Friendships

What is bothering you about either making or keeping friends? If you filled out Worksheets 32–34, you've already done this step. Write the problem you've chosen to work on first below.

Step 1: Identify and Define Your Problem with Friendships

What is bothering you about your friendships?

The problem that is bothering me most about friendship is:

_____

_____

_____

Choosing Which Problem to Work on First

If you checked only one problem on Worksheets 32 and 33, you need not fill out this question box. Otherwise, list the problems you checked in the first column below. Then use this rating scale to estimate the amount of stress the issue is causing you and/or the people around you.

How much distress is this problem causing in my life?

Almost None	Some	Moderate Amount	A Lot	Extreme
1	2	3	4	5

Problem   **Distress Rating**

_____   _____

_____   _____

_____   _____

_____   _____

From Living Well on the Spectrum by Valerie L. Gaus. Copyright 2011 by The Guilford Press.

*Example. **Fred** identified only one friendship-related problem, so he didn't need to use Worksheet 34. He filled out his Step 1 question box this way:*

Step 1: Identify and Define Your Problem with Friendships

The problem that is bothering me most about friendship is:

My friend Jim told me he does not want to meet me on Friday nights anymore if I don't stop yelling at him in public.

Step 2: Define Your Goal

What would you like to see change to minimize the problem you identified with friendships? What would need to be different for you to feel less bothered by the problem? The goal you lay out is simply the opposite of the problem you listed. List your goal in the box below, and if you need an example, look at Fred's box. Notice how he stated the goal as the opposite of his problem. Stating the goal in the affirmative gives Fred something to work toward and also lends itself to measuring success.

Step 2: Define Your Goal

What would you like to see change to minimize the problem you identified with friendship? The goal you lay out is simply the opposite of the problem you listed.

To feel less stressed by this problem, I would like to:

_____

_____

---

*Example. **Fred's** goal appears next.*

Step 2: Define Your Goal

To feel less stressed by this problem, I would like to:

Stop yelling at my friend and continue meeting him on Friday nights to watch sports.

Step 3: Identify the Obstacles in the Way of Your Achieving the Goal

What is getting in the way of your goal? Here it is particularly important to consider your ASD characteristics as hidden players in your problem. As you go through this step, you may rely on the information you were given in Part I of this book about your ASD differences. As you think about the problem you listed, look at the chart on page 278 called "ASD Differences That Can Contribute to Problems with Friendships." Read through that chart with your own problem in mind and also consider the following questions.

Thinking Differences

How might my *executive functioning* issues be contributing to my problems making or keeping friends? For example, do I have attention problems that make it hard for me to focus on conversations or to keep up with what is going on in a group? Do I have difficulty organizing information, which makes it hard for me to stay on top of keeping in touch with friends? Does my difficulty with organization get in the way of scheduling time to get together with friends? Do I persist too long, repeating a strategy for making friends that is clearly not working because I have difficulty shifting to new strategies? How might my *negative self-talk* be contributing to my problems with friends? What am I saying to myself that is putting more pressure on me? Could I be engaging in perfectionistic thinking, all-or-nothing thinking, or catastrophic thinking that makes it hard to set realistic expectations for myself or my friends? For example, do I assume the worst will happen before I get together with people? Do I expect perfection from myself and/or my friends?

Social Differences

How might my *social perception* be contributing to my problems with making or keeping friends? Is it possible I sometimes misunderstand what acquaintances or friends are trying to tell me? For example, do I still feel uncertain about what an acquaintance expects of me? Do I find it hard to tell whether someone is trying to be my friend? Am I still uncertain about how I should handle conversations with acquaintances who could potentially become friends? How might my *social/commu-*

nication skills be contributing to problems making or keeping friends? Is it possible that acquaintances or friends are not communicating clearly enough about what they expect and I don't know how to seek clarification? For example, I feel uncertain about when and how to suggest getting together with someone I would like to be my friend. Is my problem caused in part by my not knowing what to say or do when dealing with someone who is already my friend? For example, I don't know how I should handle it if I think my friend is annoyed with me or vice versa. Or, I don't know what to say if a person I do not like is trying to become my friend.

Emotional Differences

How might my emotional reactions to things be affecting my problems with making or keeping friends? Do I have difficulty *regulating* my emotions? Do I take too long to calm down after an upsetting incident? Am I overreacting or underreacting to things that happen while I'm socializing? Do I have difficulty *identifying* my feelings or *asking for help* when I am upset? Do I tend to avoid situations that cause me to feel too much anxiety or worry, such as meeting a friend at a crowded or noisy place?

Sensory and Movement Differences

How might my sensory issues be contributing to my problems with making or keeping friends? Am I *oversensitive* or *undersensitive* to certain types of light, sound, smell, taste, or touch? For example, I can't hear what my friends are saying when we meet in bars or clubs because I can't screen out the background noise. How might my *movement* and *coordination* issues be contributing to my problems with making or keeping friends? For example, I love sports, but I am afraid to play on any team or league because I feel so clumsy—I don't want my friends to notice that. Is it possible that my hygiene is not acceptable to some people because my sensory/movement problems interfere with bathing or grooming?

Now fill out the question box below, but try not to think about problems you have besides the one you chose for this exercise.

Step 3: Identify the Obstacles in the Way of Your Achieving the Goal

What is getting in the way of your goal? Remember to focus *only* on the problem and goal you wrote down in Steps 1 and 2. First circle the category(ies) of ASD differences you suspect are involved in this problem:

Thinking   **Social**   **Emotional**   **Sensory/Movement**

I believe these differences are contributing in this way:

_____

_____

_____

_____

_____

_____

_____

Example. **Fred** filled out his Step 3 question box in this way:

Step 3: Identify the Obstacles in the Way of Your Achieving the Goal

(**Thinking**)   (**Social**)   (**Emotional**)   (**Sensory/Movement**)

I believe these differences are contributing in this way:

   All of the differences are involved. My thinking differences are negative self-talk about my friend disagreeing with me in front of other people. My social differences make me miss cues from other people in the bar when I am too loud. Also, I have difficulty communicating properly with my friend about any of this. My emotional differences make it hard for me to control my anger. My sensory differences are involved because I do not like crowds—they are loud and moving around so much it bothers me.

Differences →	Thinking	Social	Emotional	Sensory/Movement
Problems Making Friends	• *Attention regulation* difficulties may contribute to problems following conversations • Difficulties *organizing information* may make it hard to keep track of new acquaintances who are potential friends • *Catastrophic thinking* can lead you to assume the worst will happen in a social encounter, which affects your performance in a negative way • *All-or-nothing thinking* can lead you to hold unrealistic expectations for yourself or others during social interactions (e.g., perfectionism)	• You may not notice or interpret cues from others, leading to difficulty with "unwritten rules" about interacting in a group • You may have difficulty judging when an acquaintance is a potential friend • Your difficulty with *conversation skills* may interfere with making positive connections with others with whom you are acquainted • You may not notice or interpret cues or *mind-read*, making it difficult to know what others expect from you in a group • You may not notice or interpret cues or *mind-read*, making it difficult to know when others have negative intentions toward you; you may be overly trusting	• Your difficulty *recognizing and identifying negative emotions* can contribute to the inability to address anxiety you may feel around other people • Your *difficulty regulating* your negative emotions can contribute to anger toward others • Your attempts to *regulate strong emotions* may appear as behaviors that others would deem odd (movements, gestures)	• *Hypersensitivity to noise, light, smell, taste, or touch* can cause discomfort in some social settings (e.g., parties, bars, clubs) • *Hyper- or hyposensitivity to temperature* can contribute to wearing clothes not appropriate for the weather—can make you stand out to others • *Hypersensitivity or fine motor* problems can lead to poor hygiene and possible rejection by others • *Fine or gross motor problems* can be obstacles to many types of cooperative leisure activities (e.g., games or sports) that can be used to make friends; may narrow your choices of activities
Problems Keeping Friends Once You Have Them	• *Attention regulation* difficulties can make it hard to coordinate your focus on other people during social activities with friends • Difficulties *organizing information* may interfere with keeping in touch or scheduling enough time with friends • *All-or-nothing thinking* can make it difficult to interpret the rules of a group of friends	• The unique way you *process and express language* can contribute to misunderstandings with friends • The unique way you express language can make it hard to assert yourself with friends • You may be perceived by others as uncaring or aloof because of the way you *experience and express empathy* • You may not notice or interpret cues or *mind-read*, making it difficult to know what friends expect from you	• Your difficulty *recognizing and identifying negative emotions* can prevent you from addressing the anxiety you may feel in some interactions with friends • Your difficulty *regulating* your negative emotions can contribute to anger outbursts, which can alienate your friends	• *Hypersensitivity to noise, light, smell, taste, or touch* can cause discomfort in some social settings (e.g., parties, bars, clubs) • *Fine or gross motor problems* can be obstacles to many types of cooperative leisure activities (e.g., games or sports) in which your friends are active • *Hypersensitivity or fine motor* problems can lead to poor hygiene and possible rejection by others

ASD differences that can contribute to problems with friendships.

When you filled out your sheet, did you circle more than one area of ASD differences? In the example, Fred's problem has four potential sources of difficulty: his thinking (negative self-talk about disagreements), social (difficulty noticing cues from others), emotional (anger), and sensory (sensitivity to noise and movement of crowds) differences are playing a role in his anger outbursts in public. This illustrates once again that often a single issue can have several causes.

Step 4: List Several Possible Solutions to Address the Obstacle(s)

What are the possible solutions for the obstacles? Try to list as many ideas as possible. Remember that this is the step some people call "brainstorming." Generate as many possibilities as come to mind, without inhibition. Don't judge or evaluate any solution that comes to mind—just write it down no matter how weird or silly it seems. In Step 5 you will weed through them and discard any that are not useful, so no harm can be done.

Start by looking at the Cheat Sheet at the end of Chapter 6. Find the ASD difference that you circled on the top row of the Cheat Sheet. Then look along the column underneath each and find the dots. Each dot marks the row in which you will find a solution in the far left column of the chart. Those approaches should be considered first for your problem, and Chapter 6 provides you with the instructions and tools for each of those solutions. Also, try to consider your *strengths* as you complete this step because they also play an important role in your solutions. Refer back to Worksheets 3 and 4 in Chapter 1. Write your primary strengths in the blanks here so you can keep them in mind while you are generating solutions.

My strengths are: _____, _____, and _____.

Step 4: List Several Possible Solutions to Address the Obstacle(s)

What are the possible solutions for the obstacles? Now, considering all the solutions you saw on the Cheat Sheet, and some you may think of on your own, list all the possibilities you can imagine to address the ASD differences involved in the problem you listed in Step 1. For the moment, ignore the score columns on the right.

I could try to:

List strategies below	Pro (+) score	Con (−) score	Total pro–con

⇨

List strategies below	Pro (+) score	Con (−) score	Total pro–con

Example. **Fred** filled out his question box this way:

Step 4: List Several Possible Solutions to Address the Obstacle(s)

I could try to:

List strategies below	Pro (+) score	Con (−) score	Total pro–con
1) give up my friendship with Jim			
2) practice thinking techniques for self-talk			
3) use communication techniques with Jim			
4) use relaxation for my anger			
5) tell everyone at the bar to quiet down			
6) meet somewhere less crowded (environ. mod.)			

Fred listed everything that came to mind, even things that don't seem appropriate (e.g., give up the friendship). He looked at the Cheat Sheet, which gave him ideas 2, 3, 4, and 6. This is an example of "brainstorming." He cannot possibly do all the things on this list but will use the next step to figure out what is most useful to him.

Step 5: Consider the Consequences of Each Solution

What are the pros and cons of each solution? Now you will put each item on your list to the test of how feasible is it or how helpful it will be toward the goal you wrote down during Step 2. Use the question box below to give each item a score.

Step 5: Consider the Consequences of Each Solution

What are the pros and cons of each solution? Look back at each item you wrote down in Step 4. Then assign each one a score. Score the benefit (Pro +) in terms of how likely that strategy is to get you closer to your goal. Score the disadvantage (Con –) in terms of the effort, cost, or damage involved in implementing it.

Pro (+) Scale

How likely is it to get me closer to my goal?

Very Unlikely	Pretty Unlikely	Hard to Tell	Somewhat Likely	Very Likely
0	1	2	3	4

Con (–) Scale

How much effort, cost, or damage would this strategy involve?

None	Almost None	Some	A Lot	Extreme
0	1	2	3	4

*Example. **Fred's** answers in this question box appear below. He carried out Step 5 and rated each one of his solutions from Step 4.

Step 4: List Several Possible Solutions to Address the Obstacle(s)

I could try to:

List strategies below	Pro (+) score	Con (–) score	Total pro–con
1) give up my friendship with Jim	0	4	–4
2) practice thinking techniques for self-talk	4	3	1
3) use communication techniques with Jim	4	1	3
4) use relaxation for my anger	3	2	1
5) tell everyone at the bar to quiet down	3	3	0
6) meet somewhere less crowded (environ. mod.)	3	2	1

Step 6: Choose the Best One(s) to Try Out First

Which solutions should you try first? Now that you've scored all of your options, choosing the one or two strategies to start with should be easy. Which of your options had the highest total score? According to your own rating, the highest score has the most benefit compared to the cost, effort, or damage it could involve. Fred ended up with four solutions that seemed worthwhile. Notice that none of the ones he chose had very high pro–con scores. After reading about each strategy in Chapter 6, he believed that the solutions could work, but he was apprehensive about trying so many new things. That's why he assigned a "con" rating to all of his ideas, even the best ones. Some skepticism is natural when you're thinking about making changes, so don't be surprised if you have some of the same feelings. In the end, you need not expect a "perfect" pro–con score of 4 to consider an option; you need only pick the ones with the highest score.

Step 6: Choose the Best One(s) to Try Out First

Which solutions should you try first? Which of the strategies in Step 5 had the highest score? Pick the top one or two and write them down below:

_____

_____

_____

Example. Fred filled out his question box the following way, combining his solutions 2, 3, 4, and 6.

Step 6: Choose the Best One(s) to Try Out First

Use thinking techniques to change negative self-talk

Use relaxation techniques to help anger

Use communication techniques to ask Jim to meet in a quieter place

---

Step 7: Implement the Solution and Track Your Progress

Now try the solution and track your progress. Use the next question box to map out your plan.

Step 7: Implement the Solution and Track Your Progress

Now try the solution and track your progress. Here is how:

Where will I do it?

_____

When will I do it?

_____

What do I need to do it?

_____

How will I do it?

_____

_____

Who can help me, if needed?

_____

How will I keep track of my success? (Look at your goal and then pick a way to track it—either a running count or a rating scale.)

_____

_____

_____

Example. Fred studied the *thinking techniques* described in Chapter 6 and realized he was making an assumption about his friend for which he had no evidence. His self-talk about Jim's differing opinions about sports was:

"Jim is putting me down in front of other people."

Fred observed that he does not get so upset with Jim when they disagree on the phone or when they're not out in public. That realization, combined with the fact that he had once mentioned to Jim that he had been diagnosed with AS, made Fred feel Jim could possibly be a supporter. (See the end of Chapter 8, page 216, for some guidelines on disclosure.) So he studied the *communication techniques* in Chapter 6 to come up with a strategy for talking to Jim about changing where they meet to watch sports.

Fred also realized that feeling very tense from work and "keyed up" when he got to the bar was contributing to his getting angry so easily. **Relaxation** exercises between work and meeting Jim might also help, he decided. So he checked out a few relaxation CDs from the library and listened to all of them before picking one he liked. Then he purchased his own copy so he could have it on hand.

Fred considered his personal strengths to be *courage* and *capacity for pleasure*, because he was willing to face his problem and also rely on a friend that he may not have had in his life if not for his passionate love for sports. His plan is outlined below.

Step 7: Implement the Solution and Track Your Progress

Where will I do it?

At home.

When will I do it?

One evening on phone with Jim, then every Friday night.

What do I need to do it?

Assertive Statement to use with Jim, Relaxation CD to use after work.

How will I do it?

Call up Jim and tell him I am working on my anger problem. Use my Assertive Statement to ask him to change locations of some Friday night get-togethers. Practice relaxation exercises when I come home from work before meeting Jim (can also try it every night if it helps).

Who can help me, if needed?

Jim

How will I keep track of my success? (Look at your goal and then pick a way to track it—either a running count or a rating scale.)

My goal is to stop yelling and keep meeting Jim on Fridays to watch sports. I will simply count how many times I have an outburst after I start this plan. I will do it for 1 month before I decide whether it helped me. I can also ask Jim what he thinks after the month is over.

Fred drafted his assertive statement, which appears in the box below. He modified it slightly from the version found in Chapter 6 because he was not going to be addressing anything about Jim's behavior per se. He was simply explaining to Jim how the *situation* could be made easier for him.

ASSERTIVE STATEMENT FORMULA

I feel/felt _____tense_____ **when you** _____and I meet and talk sports at the bar_____
because _____I am sensitive to noisy crowds_____ , **so I am asking you to** _____meet me every other week at one of our own places to watch a game_____ .

Step 8: Evaluate the Solution to See If It Met Your Goal

Did the solution meet your goal, or do you need to use a different solution? At this point you have tried out your new solution and are ready to see if it helped you meet your goal. Use the question box below to evaluate your progress.

Step 8: Evaluate the Solution to See If It Met Your Goal

Did the solution meet your goal, or do you need to use a different solution? Answer the following questions to figure this out:

What was my goal? (Copy this from Step 2.)

_____

How did I measure my progress? (data, log, or record)

_____

What do the data show with regard to my goal?

_____

How would you rate your success, on a scale of 0–100% success for meeting your goal?

I was _____% successful.

0	10	20	30	40	50	60	70	80	90	100
None		A Little			Moderate		A Lot			Total

⇨

What should I do based on this success rate? (fill in the box next to the best choice)

☐ **Celebrate and keep doing what I am doing!**

☐ **Celebrate success and also modify the plan toward further improvement.**

Example. Fred filled out his question box this way after practicing his plan for 4 weeks.

Step 8: Evaluate the Solution to See If It Met Your Goal

What was my goal? (Copy this from Step 2.)

Stop yelling at my friend and continue meeting him on Friday nights to watch sports.

How did I measure my progress? (data, log, or record)

I counted how many times I yelled at my friend, and I double-checked with him, too.

What do the data show with regard to my goal?

I did not have any loud outbursts. One night Jim and I did have a disagreement about something that happened during a game we were watching, but I did not lose control. Jim agreed that I did not yell.

How would you rate your success, on a scale of 0–100% success for meeting your goal?

I was ___100___ % successful

0	10	20	30	40	50	60	70	80	90	100
None		A Little			Moderate			A Lot		Total

What should I do based on this success rate? (fill in the box next to the best choice)

☑ **Celebrate and keep doing what I am doing!**

☐ **Celebrate success and also modify the plan toward further improvement.**

Fred felt relieved after telling Jim about his solution. Jim said that he, too, would enjoy a break from the noisy bar. Fred's relaxation exercises were so helpful that he practiced them every night after work, not just on Fridays. Fred was also grateful that Jim was willing to help him out and valued the friendship as much as he did.

When **Arnold** went through the checklists in Chapter 1, he indicated a problem at school, with his roommates, and also with making friends in general. He used Worksheet 14 in Chapter 6 to decide that the problem that was more strictly school related—because it involved his relationship with his roommates in a dorm— was more urgent than the broader goal of making friends. That's why the problem-solving steps he took to start conversing with his roommates are described in Chapter 9. Here you'll see how he addressed the second problem, making friends.

The first problem-solving exercise Arnold did led him to begin working with a campus-based counselor he found at the university mental health center. Following are the problem-solving steps carried out with the help of his counselor.

Step 1: Identify and Define Your Problem with Friendships

The problem that is bothering me most about friendship is:

I have not made any friends at college yet, and I have been here for 2 months.

Step 2: Define Your Goal

To feel less stressed by this problem, I would like to:

Make one friend during this school year.

Step 3: Identify the Obstacles in the Way of Your Achieving the Goal

(Thinking)   (Social)   (Emotional)   Sensory/Movement

I believe these differences are contributing in this way:

My thinking differences are negative self-talk—I assume that I will make a fool of myself if I speak to anyone. My social differences make it hard for me to pay attention to other people, and I don't know what I should be saying to them. My emotional differences make me very, very nervous about speaking up. I feel really scared about drawing attention to myself.

Because Arnold had gone through the problem-solving steps once before (to address roommate issues as presented in Chapter 9), he found that some of his answers to the questions the second time around were similar to the first. For example, in Step 3, shown above, his ASD differences affected his ability to make friends in the same way they affected his ability to hold conversations with his roommates. When he completed Step 4, shown below, he took some solutions from his first sheet and included them here. Since he had already tried some of them (2–4) with his roommates, he mentioned here that he would continue to use them after he joined an on-campus club. He then consulted the Cheat Sheet again and discussed all the possibilities with his counselor. After listing them, he used the rating scale to weigh the pros and cons of each solution. The results of Steps 4 and 5 can be found in the following box.

Step 4: List Several Possible Solutions to Address the Obstacle(s)

I could try to:

List strategies below	Pro (+) score	Con (–) score	Total pro–con
1) stop trying to have friends—accept solitude	0	4	–4
2) join an on-campus club that interests me	4	3	1
3) continue using thinking techniques	4	1	3
4) continue to use emotional regulation techniques	4	1	3
5) continue to use techniques to understand others	4	1	3

In Step 6, Arnold used the results of his evaluation to pick the three options with the highest pro–con score, which are highlighted in the Step 4 box. Notice that the total scores are not a "perfect 4" because he felt that he would need to put a lot of effort into these options. His confidence in his *insight* and ability to use these techniques had increased since he had tried some of them once before, which is why the scores are slightly higher than they were when he went through this exercise the first time.

Step 7: Implement the Solution and Track Your Progress

Where will I do it?

On campus in the student activity center

When will I do it?

Whenever the club meets

What do I need to do it?

Understanding My Emotions worksheet, my Checklist for Paying Attention to Other People.

How will I do it?

Join the Computer Animation Club. Refer back to the Understanding My Emotions worksheet I had filled out before. Use the Checklist for Paying Attention to Other People while in the club.

Who can help me, if needed?

My counselor

How will I keep track of your success? (Look at your goal and then pick a way to track it—either a running count or a rating scale.)

After I attend club for a few meetings my counselor and I will decide who may be a possible friend to ask to meet for dinner or lunch or coffee outside of club time. If I meet with the same person several times and we enjoy each other's company, it will be considered a friendship.

Example from Arnold

Understanding My Emotions

For use when evaluating an upsetting event. Fill this out soon after an event during which you found yourself very upset.

Date and time of event: _____ At the first meeting of the Computer Animation Club_____.

1. Briefly describe the event: I was upset when _____ I went to the first club meeting and I was not sure how well I would fit in with the other people_____.

2. Now look at the words, pictures, and synonyms below. On the top row are the basic negative emotions, and underneath are some common words that have similar meanings. Which of these emotions do you suspect was involved in your reaction to the event? Circle the relevant emotion. You can circle more than one.

Sadness		Anger		Fear	
Depressed		Enraged		Terrified	
Miserable		Annoyed		Anxious	
Devastated		Frustrated		Tense	
Down		Irritated		Nervous	

3. I felt _____ nervous _____, which may be a signal that I needed something.

4. Maybe I needed _____ to hide. I did that in middle school, and it worked because my goal was to avoid the bullies. But now I need something different—I need to know what to say—I don't want to hide now_____.

5. Feeling _____ fear _____ is a natural part of life, and I accept that I felt that way.

6. Now think about what was around you that may have helped you meet your need. This could be an object or a person. I could have used _____ some guidance on what I should be doing and saying with my fellow club members _____ to help me meet my need.

7. In circumstances like these, I may _____ practice my new tips for paying attention to people _____ to address my need.

Checklist for Paying Attention to Other People

- ☐ Look at the faces of the other people. Don't stare; just look often at each person.

- ☐ Look at faces to show I am paying attention without having to use words.

- ☐ Look at faces to find out what the other person is looking at (which tells you what they are paying attention to).

- ☐ Look at faces to monitor changes in expression.

- ☐ Gather information about their interests, hobbies, classes by observing things they do.

- ☐ Gather information about their interests, hobbies, classes by listening to what they are saying.

- ☐ Ask a question about the information you gathered.

- ☐ Make a comment about the information you gathered.

Arnold's Understanding My Emotions worksheet and his Checklist for Paying Attention to Other People appear above. He used these tools for his roommates and also found them useful for his fellow club members.

Here is the evaluation Arnold did with his counselor at the end of the school year.

Step 8: Evaluate the Solution to See If It Met Your Goal

What was my goal? (Copy this from Step 2.)

Make one friend by the end of the school year.

How did I measure my progress? (data, log, or record)

I observed whether I had repeated outings with one person outside of club activities.

What do the data show with regard to my goal?

I made friends with two people from my club. We went to lunch and dinner many times and have exchanged contact information so we can keep in touch over the vacation.

⇨

How would you rate your success, on a scale of 0–100% success for meeting your goal?

I was ___100___ % successful

0	10	20	30	40	50	60	70	80	90	100
None		A Little			Moderate			A Lot		Total

What should I do based on this success rate? (fill in the box next to the best choice)

☑ **Celebrate and keep doing what I am doing!**

☐ **Celebrate success and also modify the plan toward further improvement.**

Twenty-six-year-old *Sophie*, introduced at the beginning of this chapter, is afraid that the people she's met at work that she goes out with on weekends don't want to be her friends; they just want her to give them all rides. Her suspicion was aroused when her car was in the shop for a few days and she found out later that two friends had gone out without her by taking the city bus to a movie theater. She is having difficulty making a good judgment about the people in her social life and deciding who may or may not be a genuine friend.

Without presenting the problem-solving sheet, here are her problem-solving steps, in her own words.

Step 1: Identify and Define Your Problem

"I think some of my friends might be using me. I am not sure how to tell who is a genuine friend and who is not."

Step 2: Define Your Goal

"I would like to figure out which of my friends is worth keeping and which ones are not genuine friends so I can assert myself with them and stop giving them rides."

Step 3: Identify the Obstacles in the Way of Your Achieving the Goal

"I believe my *social* differences are causing the problem. I cannot pick up the cues that would tell me who is really a friend and who may be using me. I had difficulty making those judgments all through high school as well."

Step 4: List Several Possible Solutions to Address the Obstacle(s)

1. "Quit my job so I can cut ties with all the people who claim to be my friends."
2. "Continue to drive everyone around and stop questioning it."
3. "Use techniques for defining relationships to help my judgment (got idea from Cheat Sheet)."
4. "Use communication techniques to be assertive when I don't want to drive (got idea from Cheat Sheet)."
5. "Tell the people I met at work that I'm through with them and to leave me alone."

Step 5: Consider the Consequences of Each Solution

"After evaluating the pros and cons of each solution, I think numbers 3 and 4 are the only viable options."

Step 6: Choose the Best One(s) to Try Out First

"After reading about techniques for defining relationships, I decided to assign each person in my group of friends a score according to the rating scale for closeness in Chapter 6. For comparison, I will also score some people at work that I know a little but consider casual acquaintances. I would expect friends to have higher scores—those who don't might not be friends. I will use the assertive statement formula to practicing saying "no" to people who are not my friends but who persistently ask for rides. I believe my honesty and *authenticity* will help me be assertive and my tendency to be *optimistic* will also help me implement this plan."

Step 7: Implement the Solution and Track Your Progress

"I will give myself 6 weeks to do the plan. I will measure success by the number of times I drove a person I consider a friend compared to the number of times I drove a person I do not consider a friend. As long as the rides with real friends exceed the rides with others, I consider it a success."

Step 8: Evaluate the Solution to See If It Met Your Goal

"After 6 weeks, I figured out that one person in the group is likely to be a genuine friend, but the other three are not. I have made an effort to make plans with the friend as much as possible and have tried to limit time out with the others. My friend is friends with the others, but she understands when I don't want to drive all the time. I have given a couple of rides to the others, but have said no three different times. I consider this plan 100% successful because I have given my friend a ride more often than the others. The others have used public transportation more often."

A Word about Modern Etiquette

One day a young man with an ASD whom I was working with raised an interesting question about making eye contact. While sitting with a group of people talking at a party, he was putting special effort into looking at the faces of the other people so he could better read their nonverbal communication and also convey that he was paying attention. But he noticed that nobody in the group was looking at anyone else; everyone was looking at his or her cell phone. They were talking to each other, but their eyes were on their phones, and they each seemed to be carrying on separate conversations through text messaging with people who were not even present. "How am I supposed to learn to make eye contact," he asked, "if nobody is making eye contact with anyone else?"

It was an excellent question. We're living in a time of great transition when it comes to the universal rules of social conduct and the treatment of our friends. Thanks to the explosion in communication technology, we each have access to more people more quickly in our day-to-day lives than ever before. This can be a great asset for friendship development because you can more easily keep in touch with people. It can also be helpful for the practical tasks of daily life. For example, if you are in the store and you forgot which brand of spaghetti sauce your spouse told you to pick up, just place a call while you're standing right there among the spaghetti sauce jars and you can have an instant answer. And if your spouse forgot the name also, but can recognize the label by sight, no problem! Just take a photo of the shelves and send it—better yet, a video tour of the whole spaghetti sauce aisle. You will no doubt leave that store with the right sauce. This is great for people who have problems with executive functions!

The downside to the instant access to dozens of people is that we are often failing to pay attention to the people we are with physically. If I am text messaging with my friend who lives halfway across the country while I am sitting at lunch with a local friend, I am more "with" the one who is hundreds of miles away than the one who is three feet away. Unfortunately, the universal rules of social conduct, which have traditionally been called "etiquette," have not caught up to the state of technology. At the moment, many neurotypical people are confused about social skills and what types of behaviors are considered "polite" or "rude" because there are so many more ways we can all communicate with one another.

Whether you're working on improving your social skills for the first time with this book or you have worked on it with a therapist, you can attest to how very complicated it is. Not only are the written "etiquette" rules in flux at the moment, but there are many "unwritten rules" about how one should act in various situations. How far away one should stand from another person while chatting at a cocktail party or how to act toward other people while riding in an elevator are things that neurotypical people just seem to know without reading a rule book, but they can cause problems for you if you have social differences because of an ASD. Typically, nobody receives formal instruction on these rules, and what is considered appropriate in one setting may be grossly inappropriate in another. Neurotypicals can infer such guidelines by observing others, but you may have difficulty with that.

You will never be able to find an absolute answer to every one of your social conduct questions with regard to making and keeping friends. The best you can do is to make sure you have resources on hand that can help you in many situations. I advise my patients to buy two books for this purpose. The first is any recent etiquette book. *Emily Post's Etiquette* (17th ed., HarperResource, 2004), is a comprehensive description of the "written rules" of social conduct intended for a wide audience. The second is *The Hidden Curriculum: Practical Solutions for Understanding Unstated Rules in Social Situations*, by Myles, Trautman, and Schelvan (Autism Asperger Publishing, 2004). This book was written specifically for people on the spectrum and can fill in the gaps left by a standard etiquette book. Between these two resources, you should be able to look up just about any question you have about the type of conduct expected by most people in a given situation. Keep in mind that you cannot expect everyone to follow these rules; not everyone has kept up to date on the latest etiquette. But taking the time to find out what *most* people would consider the "right" way to handle certain situations will increase your own confidence that you are doing the best you can.

Dating, Sex, and Marriage

Having a satisfying relationship with a romantic partner can be a great source of support and enrichment for any adult. Yet some people on the spectrum choose to stay single and/or celibate for a variety of reasons, and they are healthy and happy with that lifestyle. If you're among them, you probably don't need to read this chapter. However, the fact that you turned to this page suggests that you're still seeking clarity on this issue for yourself. This chapter will show you how to use the problem-solving approach to make a more definitive decision about your lifestyle, to find an intimate partner, or to improve your romantic life with someone. These struggles are among the most painful for my patients, and coming to a resolution may provide some emotional healing from troublesome social experiences you may have had.

Noel, introduced in Chapter 1, is 37, single, and lonely; he wants to date more often. He has had very little success using online dating services and has felt very *uncomfortable making conversation* with the few dates he did meet. He *persists with this strategy*, even though it is not bringing him the results he wants. He believes he is doing something to put off the women he meets, but he is not sure what it is.

George, age 29, has never felt comfortable talking to members of the opposite sex, although his social anxiety improved significantly when he worked with a behavioral therapist during college and made several friends. His desire to date is hindered by his belief that he would have to reveal that he is a virgin. He would like to go out with a woman with whom he worked on a project at their aerospace technology company but is terrified to ask her out because of *embarrassment about his sexual history*.

Carla, another person introduced in Chapter 1, sometimes avoids her husband because she *does not like to be hugged*, even though she enjoys sexual activity. Carla's husband has told her he feels hurt by her behavior, and now he is beginning to resent her because she hasn't been able to explain why she reacts this way due to her *difficulty communicating how she feels to others*.

In Chapter 1, your clock worksheet may have indicated that you are stressed at a particular time of day because of an issue related to dating, sex, or committed partnership. If so, some of the items on Worksheets 35–37 may look familiar since they were in the checklists in Chapter 1. Each sheet lists problems common to people on the spectrum but also leaves blank spaces at the bottom for you to fill in any other problems you have.

Problem Solving

If you identified more than one problem with intimate relationships, you will need to choose one to address first; you can then repeat the problem-solving steps for each of the other problems at a later time. As mentioned in Chapter 6, it makes sense to start working on the issue that is causing the most distress for you and/

WORKSHEET 35

My Problems with Dating

Check off (✓) the statements below that sound familiar to you or reflect your experiences with dating. If you have a problem with going on dates that does not appear on this list, fill it in on one of the blanks at the bottom of the list.

☐ I don't know where to meet people to date.

☐ I don't know when/how to approach someone I want to ask for a date.

☐ I don't like to go to crowded places, like parties or bars.

☐ I can't seem to make "small talk"—I can't keep a conversation going.

☐ I don't understand different gender roles or customs that apply on a date (e.g., how the woman should act, how the man should act, who should pick up the tab on a date).

☐ I want to meet someone to marry, but I have never had a girlfriend/boyfriend in my life—I don't know where to begin.

☐ I have joined several online dating services over the past few years, and I never got a date.

☐ I have had several relationships on the Internet, but they have all been with people who live far away, and we never seem to get to meet.

☐ I have had several relationships on the Internet, but things always seem to fall apart after we meet in person.

☐ _____

☐ _____

My Problems with Sex

Check off (✓) the statements below that sound familiar to you or reflect your experiences with sexuality. If your problem does not appear on this list, fill it in on one of the blanks at the bottom of the list.

☐ I feel very uncertain about how to handle sex.

☐ I am embarrassed about being a virgin at my age.

☐ I am very uncomfortable with my own sexuality.

☐ I don't enjoy sexual activity.

☐ I do not like to be touched.

☐ I have had some unpleasant sexual experiences in the past, and I am afraid to be sexual again.

☐ I doubt I can trust another person enough to become intimate.

☐ I am afraid another person will not understand or accept what arouses me (e.g., specific types of touch or particular fantasies I might have).

☐ _____

☐ _____

My Problems with Marriage/ Committed Partnership

If you are in a long-term relationship with a spouse or domestic partner, check off (✓) the statements below that sound familiar or reflect your experiences. If your problem does not appear on this list, fill it in on one of the blanks at the bottom of the list.

☐ I don't know what to do when there is a disagreement with my partner.

☐ My partner is unhappy with the amount of time I spend with him/her.

☐ My behavior sometimes embarrasses my partner at parties.

☐ I get so upset when my partner is upset, but I freeze and don't know what to do.

☐ My partner tells me I am insensitive.

☐ My partner embarrasses me when he/she corrects me in front of other people.

☐ My partner gets annoyed at me for not doing more chores around the house.

☐ My partner blames all of our problems on my ASD, and it makes me feel guilty.

☐ _____

☐ _____

or the people around you. The exercise on Worksheet 38 can help you figure out which one that is. Rate the level of distress caused by each problem and then pick the one with the highest score to tackle first. You can return to the others later, in order of most to least distress. It can also be helpful to talk over this prioritizing with a trusted person in your life.

The next few pages will guide you through the steps of solving the problem you just identified. For each step you will be asked to write your answers in the question boxes. Each box will give you instructions, and then I'll show you how *Noel* filled in the box.

Step 1: Identify and Define Your Problem with Your Romantic Life

What is bothering you about either meeting or getting along with romantic partners? You've already done this first step if you filled out Worksheets 35–38. Write the problem you have chosen to work on first below.

Choosing Which Problem to Work on First

If you checked off only one problem on Worksheets 35–37, you need not fill out this question box. Otherwise, list the problems you checked in the first column below. Then use this rating scale to estimate the amount of stress the issue is causing you and/or the people around you.

How much distress is this problem causing in my life?

Almost None	Some	Moderate Amount	A Lot	Extreme
1	2	3	4	5

Problem   **Distress Rating**

_____   _____

_____   _____

_____   _____

_____   _____

Step 1: Identify and Define Your Problem with Your Romantic Life

What is bothering you about your romantic life?

The problem that is bothering me most about my romantic life is:

_____

_____

_____

*Example. **Noel** had identified more than one problem and used Worksheet 38 to figure out which one to work on first.

Example from Noel

WORKSHEET 38

Choosing Which Problem to Work on First

How much distress is this problem causing in my life?

Almost None	Some	Moderate Amount	A Lot	Extreme
1	2	3	4	5

Problem	**Distress Rating**
I've spent a lot of time & money on dating services for nothing	5
I have difficulty making conversation with new people	4

> ### *Step 1: Identify and Define Your Problem with Your Romantic Life*
>
> The problem that is bothering me most about my romantic life is:
>
> *I have spent a lot of time and money on dating services and I have not gotten anything out of it—I did not enjoy my time, and I do not have a relationship after 3 years of trying.*

Step 2: Define Your Goal

What would you like to see change to minimize the problem you identified with your romantic life? What would need to be different for you to feel less bothered by the problem? The goal you lay out is simply the opposite of the problem you listed. List your goal in the box below, and if you need an example, look at Noel's box.

> ### Step 2: Define Your Goal
>
> *What would you like to see change to minimize the problem you identified with your romantic life?* The goal you lay out is simply the opposite of the problem you listed.
>
> To feel less stressed by this problem, I would like to:
>
> _____
>
> _____

Example. Noel's goal is shown below.

> ### *Step 2: Define Your Goal*
>
> To feel less stressed by this problem, I would like to:
>
> *Find a way to meet women that will not cost so much and will be less stressful*

Notice how he stated the goal as the opposite of his problem. Stating the goal in the affirmative gives Noel something to work toward and also lends itself to measuring success.

Step 3: Identify the Obstacles in the Way of Your Achieving the Goal

What is getting in the way of your goal? Here it is particularly important to consider your ASD characteristics as key players in your problem. As you go through this step, you may rely on the information you were given in Part I of this book about your ASD differences. As you think about the problem you listed above, look at the chart on page 304 called "ASD Differences That Can Contribute to Problems with Your Romantic Life." Read through that chart with your own problem in mind and also consider the following questions.

Thinking Differences

How might my *executive functioning* issues be contributing to my problems with dating, sex, or committed relationships? For example, do I have attention problems that make it hard for me to focus on conversations or to keep up with what is going on during a social outing? Do I have difficulty organizing information, which makes it hard for me to keep track of my obligations and responsibilities to my partner? Do I persist too long, repeating a strategy for dating that is clearly not working because I have difficulty shifting to new strategies? How might my *negative self-talk* be contributing to my problems with my romantic life? What am I saying to myself that is putting more pressure on me? Is it possible that I am engaging in perfectionistic thinking, all-or-nothing thinking, or catastrophic thinking that makes it hard to set realistic expectations for myself, my dates, or partners? For example, do I assume the worst will happen before a date or a sexual encounter? Do I expect perfection from myself and/or my partner?

Social Differences

How might my *social perception* be contributing to my problems making connections with dates or getting along with my partner? Could I sometimes be misunderstanding what my dates or partners are trying to tell me? For example, do I still feel uncertain about what a date expects of me? Is it hard to tell if someone is trying to flirt with me? Am I still uncertain about how I should handle conversations with acquaintances or friends who could potentially become dates? How might my *social/communication skills* be contributing to problems with dating, sex, or committed relationships? Is it possible that dates or partners are not communicating clearly enough about what they expect and I don't know how to seek clarification? For example, I feel uncertain about when and how to suggest getting together with someone for a date. Is my problem due in part to my not knowing what to say or do when dealing with someone who is already my spouse or partner? For example, I don't know how I should handle it if my spouse is annoyed with me or vice versa. Or I don't know what to say if a person I am not interested in is trying to go out with me or is making sexual advances toward me.

Emotional Differences

How might my emotional reactions to things be affecting my problems with dating, sex, or committed relationships? Do I have difficulty *regulating* my emotions? Do I take too long to calm down after an upsetting incident? Am I overreacting or underreacting to things that happen while I'm with my partner? Do I have difficulty *identifying* my feelings or *asking for help* when I am upset? Do I tend to avoid situations that cause me to feel too much anxiety or worry, such as initiating a date? Am I overwhelmed by anxiety that is related to a past traumatic experience with dating or sex?

Sensory and Movement Differences

How might my sensory issues be contributing to my problems in my romantic life? Am I *oversensitive* or *undersensitive* to certain types of light, sound, smell, taste, or touch? For example, I can't hear what my date is saying when we meet in bars or clubs because I can't screen out the background noise. Or I don't like to be touched in certain ways, which interferes with sex or physical intimacy. Or wardrobe choices that I make to accommodate my tactile sensitivities may look odd or make me stand out. How might my *movement* and *coordination* issues be contributing to my problems with dating or with romantic partners? For example, I avoid certain types of leisure activities (sports, games) with dates or partners because I don't want to appear clumsy. Is it possible that my hygiene is not acceptable to some people because my sensory/movement problems interfere with bathing or grooming?

Now fill out the question box below, trying not to think about problems besides the one you chose for this exercise.

Step 3: Identify the Obstacles in the Way of Your Achieving the Goal

What is getting in your way of your goal? Remember to focus *only* on the problem and goal you wrote down in Steps 1 and 2. First circle the category(ies) of ASD differences you suspect are involved in this problem:

Thinking   **Social**   **Emotional**   **Sensory/Movement**

I believe these differences are contributing in this way:

_____

_____

_____

Differences →	Thinking	Social	Emotional	Sensory/Movement
Problems with Dating	• *Attention regulation difficulties* may contribute to problems following conversations • *Catastrophic thinking* can lead you to assume the worst will happen if you ask for or go on a date • *All-or-nothing thinking* can lead you to hold unrealistic expectations for yourself or your date (e.g., perfect harmony) • Difficulties with *shifting attention* may lead you to persist with strategies that are not working	• You may have difficulty judging when an acquaintance or friend is a potential date • You may not notice or interpret cues or mind-read, making it difficult to know what others expect from you on a date or what the "unwritten rules" are • You may not notice or interpret cues or mind-read, making it difficult to know when others have negative intentions toward you; you may be overly trusting	• Your difficulty recognizing and *identifying negative emotions* can contribute to an inability to address anxiety you may feel around potential dating partners • Your difficulty *regulating your negative emotions* can contribute to anger toward others when you experience rejection • Your attempts to regulate strong emotions may appear as behaviors that others would deem odd (movements, gestures)	• *Hypersensitivity* to noise, light, smell, taste, or touch can cause discomfort in some social settings (e.g., parties, bars, clubs) • *Hyper- or hyposensitivity* (underresponsive sense) to temperature can contribute to wearing clothes not appropriate for the weather—can make you stand out to others • *Hypersensitivity or fine motor* problems can lead to poor hygiene and possible rejection by others
Problems with Sex	• *Attention regulation difficulties* can make it hard to coordinate your focus on a sexual partner • *All-or-nothing thinking* can make it difficult to interpret the "rules" of a sexual interaction • *Catastrophic thinking* can lead you to assume the worst will happen during a sexual encounter	• The unique way you process and express language can make it difficult to communicate with a sexual partner • The unique way you express language can make it hard to assert yourself when facing an unwanted sexual advance by another person • You may not notice or interpret cues or mind-read, making it difficult to know what a sexual partner expects from you	• Your difficulty recognizing and *identifying negative emotions* can prevent you from addressing the anxiety around sexual interactions • If you have a history of traumatic sexual experiences, you are more likely to have difficulty *regulating anxiety* surrounding sexual activity	• *Hypersensitivity* to noise, light, smell, taste, or touch can cause discomfort during sexual interactions • *Hypersensitivity or fine motor* problems can lead to poor hygiene and possible rejection by a sexual partner
Problems with Marriage or Committed Partnership	• *Attention regulation difficulties* contribute to problems following conversations • Difficulties *organizing information* may make it hard to follow through on commitments to your partner • *All-or-nothing thinking* can lead you to hold unrealistic expectations for yourself or your partner • *Catastrophic thinking* can lead you to assume the worst when there are disagreements or when your partner is angry	• The unique way you process and express language can make it difficult to communicate with your partner about your needs • You may not notice or interpret cues or mind-read, making it difficult to know what your partner expects from you	• Your difficulty *regulating your negative emotions* can contribute to anger outbursts that are frightening to your partner • Your difficulty *regulating your negative emotions* can contribute to extreme anxiety • Your methods of regulating your anger or anxiety may appear as maladaptive attempts to control your partner • You may become overwhelmed by anxiety if your partner appears upset	• *Hypersensitivity* to noise, light, smell, taste, or touch can cause discomfort during various aspects of family life with your partner

ASD differences that can contribute to problems with your romantic life.

Example. *Noel* filled out his Step 3 question box in this way:

Step 3: Identify the Obstacles in the Way of Your Achieving the Goal

(**Thinking**)   (**Social**)   **Emotional**   **Sensory/Movement**

I believe these differences are contributing in this way:

  My thinking differences have perhaps contributed to my inability to switch

gears and try a different approach to meeting women. My social differences

make me uncomfortable making conversations with strangers.

Did you circle more than one area of ASD differences? Noel's problem does have two potential sources of difficulty; his thinking (rigid, all-or-nothing thinking about dating strategies) and social (difficulty making conversation) differences are playing a role in his repeated disappointments with dating, illustrating that a single issue can have more than one cause.

Step 4: List Several Possible Solutions to Address the Obstacle(s)

What are the possible solutions for the obstacles? Try to list as many ideas as possible. Remember that this is the step some people call "brainstorming." Generate as many possibilities as come to mind, without inhibition. Don't judge or evaluate any solution that comes to mind—just write it down no matter how weird or silly it seems. In Step 5 you will weed through them and discard any that are not useful, so no harm can be done.

Start by looking at the Cheat Sheet at the end of Chapter 6. Find the ASD differences that you circled on the top row of the Cheat Sheet. Then look along the column underneath each and find the dots. Each dot marks the row in which you will find a solution in the far left column of the chart. Those approaches should be considered first for your problem, and Chapter 6 provides you with the instructions and tools for each of those solutions. Also, try to consider your *strengths* as you complete this step because they also play an important role in your solutions. Refer back to Worksheets 3 and 4 in Chapter 1. Write your primary strengths in the blanks here so you can keep them in mind while you are generating solutions.

My strengths are: _____, _____, and _____.

Step 4: List Several Possible Solutions to Address the Obstacle(s)

What are the possible solutions for the obstacles? Now, considering all of the solutions that you saw on the Cheat Sheet, and some you may think of on your own, list all the possibilities you can imagine to address the ASD differences involved in the problem you listed in Step 1. For the moment, ignore the score columns on the right.

I could try to:

List strategies below	Pro (+) score	Con (−) score	Total pro–con

Example. *Noel* filled out his question box this way:

Step 4: List Several Possible Solutions to Address the Obstacle(s)

I could try to:

List strategies below	Pro (+) score	Con (−) score	Total pro–con
1) keep joining dating services			
2) use thinking techniques to change strategies			
3) practice conversations w/women I know			
4) ask my friend who is married for advice			
5) give up on dating and stay single			

Noel listed everything that came to mind, even things that don't seem appropriate (e.g., give up on dating). He looked at the Cheat Sheet, which gave him ideas 2 and 3. This is an example of "brainstorming." He cannot possibly do all the things on this list but will use the next step to figure out what is most useful to him.

Step 5: Consider the Consequences of Each Solution

What are the pros and cons of each solution? Now you will take each item on your list and put it to the test of how feasible it is or how helpful it will be toward the goal you wrote down during Step 2. Use the question box below to give each item a score.

Step 5: Consider the Consequences of Each Solution

What are the pros and cons of each solution? Look back at each item you wrote down in Step 4. Then assign each one a score. Score the benefit (Pro +) in terms of how likely that strategy is to get you closer to your goal. Score the disadvantage (Con –) in terms of the effort, cost, or damage involved in implementing it.

Pro (+) Scale

How likely is it to get me closer to my goal?

Very Unlikely	Pretty Unlikely	Hard to Tell	Somewhat Likely	Very Likely
0	1	2	3	4

Con (–) Scale

How much effort, cost, or damage would this strategy involve?

None	Almost None	Some	A Lot	Extreme
0	1	2	3	4

Example. Noel's answers appear below. He carried out Step 5 and rated each one of his solutions from Step 4.

Step 4: List Several Possible Solutions to Address the Obstacle(s)

I could try to:

List strategies below	Pro (+) score	Con (−) score	Total pro−con
1) keep joining dating services	0	4	−4
2) use thinking techniques to change strategies	4	2	2
3) practice conversations w/women I know	3	1	2
4) ask my friend who is married for advice	3	0	3
5) give up on dating and stay single	0	4	−4

Step 6: Choose the Best One(s) to Try Out First

Which solutions should you try first? Now that you have scored all of your options, choosing the one or two strategies to start with should be easy. Which of your options had the highest total score? According to your own rating, the highest score has the most benefit compared to the cost, effort, or damage it could involve. Noel ended up with three solutions that seemed worthwhile to him. Notice that none of the ones he chose had a perfect 4 pro−con score. After reading about each strategy in Chapter 6, he believed that he needed to switch strategies but also knew it would be hard for him to break his old habit. That's why he assigned a "con" rating to all of his ideas, even the best ones. You may have some of the same feelings. In the end, you need not expect a "perfect" pro−con score of 4 to consider an option; you need only pick the ones with the highest score.

Step 6: Choose the Best One(s) to Try Out First

Which solutions should you try first? Which of the strategies in Step 5 had the highest score? Pick the top one or two and write them down below:

_____

_____

_____

Example. Noel filled out his question box in the following way, combining his solutions 2, 3, and 4.

Step 6: Choose the Best One(s) to Try First

Use thinking techniques to help myself switch strategies for dating, use communication techniques to talk to my friend about my problem, and also practice conversation with women who are not strangers (not dates)

Step 7: Implement the Solution and Track Your Progress

Now try the solution and track your progress. Use the next question box to map out your plan.

Step 7: Implement the Solution and Track Your Progress

Now try the solution and track your progress. Here is how:

_____

Where will I do it?

_____

When will I do it?

_____

What do I need to do it?

_____

How will I do it?

_____

_____

Who can help me, if needed?

_____

⇨

> How will I keep track of my success? (Look at your goal and then pick a way to track it—either a running count or a rating scale.)
>
> _____
>
> _____
>
> _____
>
> _____

Example. Noel studied the ***thinking techniques*** described in Chapter 6 and realized on some level he had been saying to himself for several years: "The only way I can meet a woman is through a dating service. I must keep trying this." Noel observed that this self-talk resulted from all-or-nothing thinking and an inability to shift his attention to a new strategy.

He also became aware that his sense of awkwardness in conversation tends to occur most with people he does not know, but he feels comfortable conversing with people he does know, like coworkers and friends. He even has some friendly acquaintanceships with some female coworkers. He then focused more on his ***communication*** in two ways. First he asked a married friend from college, Mike, what he thought. Together they came up with the idea of trying to meet women in places where things are more familiar or to get to know women as acquaintances and friends before asking them out. Mike had met his wife at a cycling club (which he had joined not to find a wife but just because he enjoyed cycling), and because Noel loves hiking, he and Mike agreed he should join various hiking clubs and go on their planned trips. Doing so would allow him to get to know people with a common interest, without the pressure of conversing with a stranger that comes with formal dates. His passion for the outdoors was what he considered a strength (***capacity for pleasure***), and he looked forward to being able to use that toward his goal. He could become friends with women he liked and then think about dating later. If he didn't meet someone right away, at least he'd be doing something he enjoys and finds relaxing.

> ## Step 7: Implement the Solution and Track Your Progress
>
> Where will I do it?
>
> _Some at work, and some at hiking locations._
>
> When will I do it?

During work hours and also during hikes.

What do I need to do it?

One or more hiking clubs to join. Stress Rating Scale.

How will I do it?

Practice chatting more with women I already know because I am not nervous around them. Join at least one hiking club and go on some hikes. Chat with people there and try to get to know them the same way I did with my coworkers—without pressure.

Who can help me, if needed?

My friend Mike.

How will I keep track of my success? (Look at your goal and then pick a way to track it—either a running count or a rating scale.)

My goal is to find a way to meet women that will not cost so much and will be less stressful. I will compare the money and time spent on my new strategy compared to the old. I will also compare my stress level after each hike with the stress involved in my previous activities w/dating services. I will try for 3 months.

Noel stopped participating in dating services and joined two different hiking clubs. He used the rating scale below to rate the stress he remembers feeling each time he participated in a dating service activity, which he estimated to be an average of 9. Then he rated how he felt about each hike he went on. He treated the other members of the club the same way he remembers treating his coworkers as he got to know them. Because he feels like he is well liked at work, he hoped the same result would occur in his clubs.

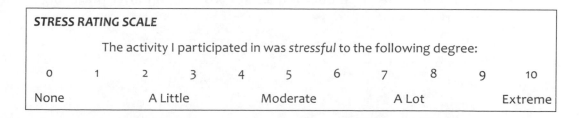

STRESS RATING SCALE

The activity I participated in was *stressful* to the following degree:

0	1	2	3	4	5	6	7	8	9	10
None		A Little			Moderate			A Lot		Extreme

Step 8: Evaluate the Solution to See If It Met Your Goal

Did the solution meet your goal, or do you need to use a different solution? At this point you've tried out your new solution and are ready to see if it helped you meet your goal. Use the question box below to evaluate your progress.

Step 8: Evaluate the Solution to See If It Met Your Goal

Did the solution meet your goal, or do you need to use a different solution? Answer the following questions to figure this out:

What was my goal? (Copy this from Step 2.)

_____

How did I measure my progress? (data, log, or record)

_____

What do the data show with regard to my goal?

_____

How would I rate my success, on a scale of 0–100% success for meeting my goal?

I was _____% successful.

0	10	20	30	40	50	60	70	80	90	100
None		A Little			Moderate			A Lot		Total

What should I do based on this success rate? (fill in the box next to the best choice)

☐ **Celebrate and keep doing what I am doing!**

☐ **Celebrate success and also modify the plan toward further improvement.**

Example. Noel filled out his question box this way after practicing his plan for 3 months.

Step 8: Evaluate the Solution to See If It Met Your Goal

What was my goal? (Copy this from Step 2.)

Find a way to meet women that will not cost so much and will be less stressful.

How did I measure my progress? (data, log, or record)

I rated my stress after each hike and compared it to the average of 9 I had for dating service activities in the past. I also tracked the cost in money and time.

What do the data show with regard to my goal?

I went on 7 hikes in 3 months. I had an average rating of 5 for stress level after hikes. I had higher ratings for the first few because I did not know anyone. After the 4th and 5th hikes the stress went down. For cost, I spent about $60/month on hikes (gas, food, fees) and about 15 hours each month. With the dating services, I was spending sometimes >$100/month and countless hours on my computer reading profiles and looking for messages of interest.

How would I rate my success, on a scale of 0–100% success for meeting my goal?

I was ___100___ % successful   *Less cost, less stress, and there are women in the club*

0	10	20	30	40	50	60	70	80	90	100
None			A Little		Moderate		A Lot			Total

What should I do based on this success rate? (fill in the box next to the best choice)

☒ **Celebrate and keep doing what I am doing!**

☐ **Celebrate success and also modify the plan toward further improvement.**

Noel was 100% successful in his goals of spending less, having less stress, and meeting some women. Notice he did not measure success by whether he got a date or started a romantic relationship. Instead, starting off with a realistic goal enabled him to break away from an unproductive strategy, which reduced his stress and increased his chances of meeting a woman and being in a relaxed and happy state when conversing with her.

George, as described at the beginning of this chapter, is ready to start dating and has become more comfortable talking to women since he started working, but he has never had sex before and believes he must reveal this to any woman he dates. The steps of his problem-solving sheet are presented below.

Step 1: Identify and Define Your Problem with Your Romantic Life

The problem that is bothering me most about my romantic life is:

I'm ashamed of being a virgin, and it is making me afraid to ask a woman on a date.

Step 2: Define Your Goal

To feel less stressed by this problem, I would like to:

Feel less inhibited because of the shame I have about my history and ask a woman on a date.

Step 3: Identify the Obstacles in the Way of Your Achieving the Goal

(**Thinking**)   (**Social**)   **Emotional**   **Sensory/Movement**

I believe these differences are contributing in this way:

My thinking differences are causing most of the problem—my all-or-nothing thinking and catastrophic thinking are both making me overly anxious about my past and what it means for dating now. My social differences may be leading me to get confused about how much or what type of information to share with a date or a person I do not know well.

Because he had seen a therapist for help with his social anxiety, George already had a lot of experience with examining and challenging negative self-talk. He used the Chapter 6 Cheat Sheet to come up with some solutions and remembered some of the strategies he had learned in therapy. He used the rating scale to weigh the pros and cons of each solution. The results of Steps 4 and 5 can be found in the box below.

Step 4: List Several Possible Solutions to Address the Obstacle(s)

I could try to:

List strategies below	Pro (+) score	Con (−) score	Total pro−con
1) forget dating and resolve to stay single	0	4	−4
2) use thinking techniques to address beliefs	4	1	3
3) rehearse ways to tell my dates I'm a virgin	2	4	−2
4) use techniques to understand others	4	1	3
5) ask out someone I am already friendly with	4	2	2
6) approach an attractive stranger at the mall	0	4	−4

In Step 6, George used the results of his evaluation to pick the three options with the highest pro−con score, which are highlighted in the Step 4 box. While it seemed logical at first to rehearse ways to tell dates he is a virgin, he realized from what he had learned in Chapter 6 that revealing this information might not be suitable for the relationship he had with a person he was just dating for the first time. In contrast, he had a lot of confidence in choices 2, 4, and 5 because of his previous therapy experience. He considered his *insight* a strength that he could benefit from now. His implementation plan appears below.

Step 7: Implement the Solution and Track Your Progress

Where will I do it?

   I will study and practice the thinking and social techniques at home, then practice at work.

When will I do it?

   During any free time at home and lunch time at work

⇨

> **What do I need to do it?**
>
> _Closeness Rating Scale, Shame and Inhibition Rating Scale_
>
> **How will I do it?**
>
> _Look at the diagrams about Closeness. Consider them as guides for the type of information I should be sharing with people I may be dating. Then practice thinking techniques to challenge my beliefs about my past history and current situation. Then ask my coworker to go to lunch._
>
> **Who can help me, if needed?**
>
> _My previous therapist_
>
> **How will I keep track of my success? (Look at your goal and then pick a way to track it—either a running count or a rating scale.)**
>
> _My goal is to feel less inhibited because of my history and ask a woman on a date. Use the Shame Rating Scale before and after I do my thinking techniques. See if I can then ask my coworker to lunch._

George realized he was engaging in **all-or-nothing thinking** with regard to his belief that he must tell any person he dates that he is a virgin. He realized his self-talk involved this statement: "Every woman I date will know I am a virgin, so I must tell each one as soon as possible." He was also engaging in **catastrophic thinking**, which involved statements such as: "It is absolutely unacceptable to be a virgin at the age of 30—it is a disaster that only gets worse the older I get."

George remembered from his therapy sessions that he could challenge those types of beliefs by examining evidence to the contrary. Using some of the **social techniques** in Chapter 6, he realized that his first dates would be with a woman he knew a little bit, which made the two of them acquaintances. According to the Closeness chart, that meant George shouldn't ask this woman about her personal or private life. Reversing what the chart said about how to seek and store information about another person to apply the same rule to *sharing* information about himself, as shown in the chart below, George understood that he probably shouldn't immediately share information about his personal or private life. He also read the section on disclosure at the end of Chapter 8, which gave him more guidelines about sharing personal things about himself (including his ASD diagnosis). The shame rating scale George used to monitor his feelings about his virginity helped him reach the conclusion that he need not and should not share his sexual history with someone he barely knows; he should wait until he knows and trusts someone before discussing that.

CLOSENESS	WHEN **SHARING** INFORMATION ABOUT MYSELF: 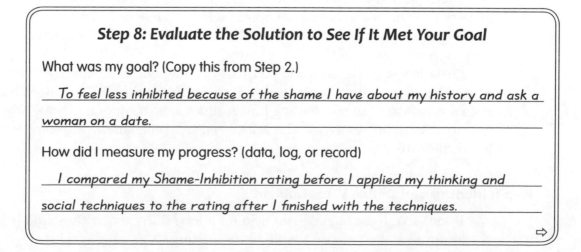
Not Close at All	*The immediate shared situation:* Share things related to the place you are both in and the reasons you are there. What brought you both there and what is going on in the moment? Don't share anything personal or private.
	Your superficial facts: Share things about your interests, hobbies, work, or school and keep it brief. Don't share anything personal or private.
	Your personal life: Share things about your home life or background, such as your family makeup (children, siblings) or where you grew up. Don't share facts that could possibly bring up painful emotions for you (e.g., family conflicts, divorce, deaths).
Extremely Close	*Your private life:* Share personal things that you may have discussed before or which you feel you can trust this person to understand (e.g., concerns, worries, personal dreams and hopes).

SHAME AND INHIBITION RATING SCALE

My *shame* interferes with asking someone for a date to the following degree:

0	1	2	3	4	5	6	7	8	9	10
None		A Little			Moderate			A Lot		Extreme

Here is the evaluation George did after he implemented his plan.

Step 8: Evaluate the Solution to See If It Met Your Goal

What was my goal? (Copy this from Step 2.)

To feel less inhibited because of the shame I have about my history and ask a woman on a date.

How did I measure my progress? (data, log, or record)

I compared my Shame-Inhibition rating before I applied my thinking and social techniques to the rating after I finished with the techniques.

⇨

What do the data show with regard to my goal?

My shame rating before doing this exercise was a 10—I felt extremely ashamed and it stopped me from asking anyone on a date. After my thinking and social exercises, my rating went down to a 5. I still feel embarrassed, but I am so relieved that I don't have to share that information with anyone until I know them really well. So I was not afraid to ask my coworker to have lunch with me one day. She agreed. It is not really a "date," but by having lunch with her I can get to know her better and decide later if I will ask her to get together after work.

How would I rate my success, on a scale of 0–100% success for meeting my goal?

I was ___80___ % successful   _My shame is less and I asked a woman to spend a little more time with me, even though it is not a traditional date yet._

0	10	20	30	40	50	60	70	80	90	100
None		A Little			Moderate			A Lot		Total

What should I do based on this success rate? (fill in the box next to the best choice)

☐ **Celebrate and keep doing what I am doing!**

☑ **Celebrate success and also modify the plan toward further improvement.**

George considered his strategies 80% successful. He did reduce his shame and inhibition, and he also asked his coworker to eat lunch with him. It is not a "real date" yet, but he figured he could decide on whether to ask her for a date outside of work after he got a chance to know her. He also decided that he would go back for a couple of therapy sessions to help him through that process. He felt proud of his progress.

Carla is struggling with the fact that her husband has expressed annoyance toward her and has told her he feels rejected because she seems to avoid him. She does not deny that she is avoiding him at times, but she does not know how to tell him why. Without displaying the worksheet, her problem-solving steps follow, in her own words.

Step 1: Identify and Define Your Problem

"I don't like to be hugged and held for a long time, and my husband is getting annoyed at me because I avoid him sometimes."

Step 2: Define Your Goal

"I would like to find a way to explain to my husband why I don't like long hugs, so I don't hurt his feelings anymore."

Step 3: Identify the Obstacles in the Way of Your Achieving the Goal

"I believe my *sensory* differences are causing the problem because I am extra sensitive to some types of touch (but not others). I also have *social* differences that are getting in the way of my communication with my husband about this."

Step 4: List Several Possible Solutions to Address the Obstacle(s)

1. "Get a divorce."
2. "Use communication techniques to explain things to my husband (got this idea from Cheat Sheet)."
3. "Find a therapist to help us."
4. "Have separate bedrooms for me and my husband."

Step 5: Consider the Consequences of Each Solution

"After evaluating the pros and cons of each solution, I think number 2 is the best solution, and 3 if needed."

Step 6: Choose the Best One(s) to Try Out First

"I read about the communication techniques that could help in a situation like this. My husband was with me when I was diagnosed with Asperger syndrome, so he already knows a little bit about it. I will tell him that I have sensory issues that make long hugs uncomfortable. I consider my *realism* and *authenticity* to be strengths that will help me in this situation."

Step 7: Implement the Solution and Track Your Progress

"I will use the Assertive Statement Formula from Chapter 6 to approach my husband about this issue. I will also tell him that I am not rejecting him. I will ask him not to try to hold me for a long time at once. I will consider myself successful if I am able to approach my husband about this. I am willing to go to a therapist if we cannot resolve this on our own."

Step 8: Evaluate the Solution to See If It Met Your Goal

"I approached my husband, and he was willing to listen. He agreed not to try to hug me for a long time at once. But he also said he felt unsure about how he can touch me. I am not sure how to answer him, so we are going to find a marriage counselor who is familiar with ASDs who can help us. I consider myself 90% successful because I talked to my husband about it and we agreed to work on it more with a therapist."

A Word about Online Dating

Patients and family members have asked me many times whether I think "online dating" or using Internet-based dating services is a good idea for people on the spectrum. Here's how I answer:

Using any kind of dating service, including newspaper classified advertisements, has both risks and benefits. It increases the number of people you're exposed to without having to rely only on friends and family to introduce you to potential dating partners. You can try to screen people by knowing something about them before meeting face to face. On the other hand, you can't be sure that participants are being truthful about themselves. And essentially, each time you arrange a first date you're going out with a total stranger, not an acquaintance you may have started to get to know elsewhere or who is known to someone you trust. Therefore, it's difficult to discriminate between people who are well meaning and those who have unkind motives.

For people on the spectrum, using the Internet to meet people can be advantageous because you can communicate through multiple modalities—text, voice, photos, videos. If you have difficulty reading nonverbal cues during face-to-face conversations, let's say, then using e-mail or instant messaging may be an easier way to get to know someone. At the same time, people on the spectrum may be more vulnerable than neurotypical people to the risks of "casting a wide net" on the Internet to meet dating partners. If you have thinking or social differences that make it difficult for you to judge the intentions of another person, you may be deceived by a person with malicious intentions. Also, the inevitable face-to-face meetings (assuming someone you find on the Internet is someone you actually want to date) can be a source of overwhelming anxiety for some people on the spectrum. With these factors in mind, here is a list of tips to consider when searching for people to date online (or even through newspaper personal ads):

- Consider all people "strangers" or "acquaintances" until you have met them numerous times in person without any negative experiences.
- Never give a stranger or an acquaintance your address.

- When meeting someone in person, always meet in a public place (e.g., diner, coffee shop, restaurant). Travel to and from that place on your own (e.g., do not have the person pick you up at your house or drive you home).
- When meeting someone in person, always make sure a trusted friend or family member knows where you are going and what time you expect to be home.
- Never give a stranger or an acquaintance any money for any reason whatsoever. Even if your acquaintance promises to pay you back, consider that the person may not really have the means to do so.
- Don't consider any person your "girlfriend" or "boyfriend" if you have never met that person face to face.

13

Health

Most of this book has focused on taking care of your mental and emotional well-being, but ASD differences can pose challenges for your physical health too. Some of my patients have problems following healthy lifestyle practices, while others have difficulty accessing medical treatment. Both types of problems can cause a lot of stress. Fortunately, whether you're free of serious health problems or struggling with a chronic medical condition, the problem-solving approach can help you overcome difficulties with managing your physical health.

Do you remember 51-year-old *Dan* from Chapter 1? Dan has been told that he has to lose 60 pounds to reduce his risk of heart disease, especially because he has a strong family history of cardiovascular problems. He wants to go on a diet but is *apprehensive about the idea of changing* his lifestyle and is overwhelmed by the prospect of getting started; he has no idea where to begin. In the meantime, he feels *guilty about eating* unhealthy foods.

Meredith was introduced in Chapter 1 and then revisited in Chapter 8, where her problems with multitasking at her garden center job were discussed. Problems with *multitasking* are affecting her health as well, as she finds it very stressful to keep track of everything she needs to do to care for her diabetes. She also feels *depressed* about the fact that she has never been able to use her education for a career in law and attributes this to the fact that she is consumed by the rigors of taking care of her chronic health problem.

Mark is 33, married, and a certified public accountant. He just got a new job working for a company that requires all employees to have an annual physical exam. Mark does not have any known medical problems, but he has not been to a doctor in over 7 years. The last time he had a physical, he had great difficulty following the doctor's fast speech and many questions and ended up feeling quite intimidated by the doctor's impatience with him. The whole experience provoked so much anxiety in him that he never went back. He is now very *nervous about having a physical exam* as required by his new employer because he is afraid he will not be able to *process what the doctor is saying* during the appointment.

In Chapter 1, your most stressful time of day as indicated by the clock worksheet may have been related to your healthcare. If so, the items on Worksheets 39 and 40 may look familiar, because they were listed first in Chapter 1. Each sheet lists problems common to people on the spectrum but also leaves blank spaces at the bottom for you to fill in any other problems you have.

WORKSHEET 39

My Problems with My Healthcare
Managing Personal Care

Check off (✓) the statements below that sound familiar or reflect your experiences with trying to manage the tasks of self-care. This includes personal hygiene and health-related responsibilities. If you have a problem with self-care that does not appear on this list, fill it in on one of the blanks at the bottom.

☐ I have a chronic medical condition, and I feel overwhelmed by it.

☐ I am afraid I will never be able to take care of health on my own—I need help from my parents for everything.

☐ I forget to take my medicine on some days.

☐ I always forget to renew my prescriptions until it is too late.

☐ My shower routine takes so long that I prefer to skip it.

☐ I will wear dirty clothes because I can't get to the laundry.

☐ I don't remember to brush my teeth every day.

☐ I am overweight, and I can't seem to follow a diet.

☐ I am a picky eater, and my diet is not balanced; I have been told I am underweight.

☐ I hate to shave but don't like a beard either.

☐ I sleep at odd hours, sleep too little, or sleep too much.

☐ I get so focused on my diet or exercise routine that I have been told I am overdoing it or that I am "obsessed" with it.

☐ I find it hard to tolerate medication side effects, so I don't always comply with prescription instructions.

☐ I can't find the time to exercise regularly.

☐ _____

☐ _____

WORKSHEET 40

My Problems with My Healthcare
Accessing Healthcare Services

Check off (✓) the statements below that sound familiar or reflect your experiences with using healthcare services. This includes making and keeping appointments with physicians, dentists, or other clinical providers. It also involves interfacing with the office and pharmacy staff. If your problem does not appear on this list, fill it in on one of the blanks at the bottom.

☐ I don't trust doctors, so I hate going to appointments.

☐ I can't keep track of all my appointments.

☐ Doctors talk too fast, and I can't follow what they say.

☐ I constantly worry that something is wrong with me, but I am afraid to be examined by a doctor.

☐ I am afraid to go to the dentist.

☐ I get nervous when I have to talk to receptionists to schedule appointments.

☐ I am afraid to ask questions when I don't understand what my doctor says.

☐ I get confused when the pharmacy staff asks me about my insurance.

☐ I become very angry if the office staff talks to me in a rude way.

☐ I have difficulty describing my symptoms to a doctor during a visit.

☐ I have been told I have a high pain threshold or I don't feel pain until a condition gets out of control (e.g., infected tooth), so I don't get help when I should.

☐ I have been told I have a low pain threshold or I feel pain almost all the time, even when the doctors can't find anything wrong.

☐ I never know whether to go to the doctor when I don't feel well because I have been told my pain is "psychosomatic" or that I am a "hypochondriac."

☐ _____

☐ _____

Problem Solving

If you checked off more than one healthcare problem, you will need to choose one to address first; then you can repeat the problem-solving steps for each of the other problems at a later time. As mentioned in Chapter 6, it makes sense to start working on the issue that is causing the most distress for you and/or the people around you. The exercise below can help you to figure out which one that is. Rate the level of distress caused by each problem and then pick the one with the highest score to tackle first. You can return to the others later, in order of most to least distress. It can also be helpful to talk over this prioritizing with a trusted person in your life.

WORKSHEET 41

Choosing Which Problem to Work on First

If you checked off only one problem on Worksheets 39 and 40, you need not fill out this question box. Otherwise, list the problems you checked in the first column below. Then use this rating scale to estimate the amount of stress the issue is causing you and/or the people around you.

How much distress is this problem causing in my life?

Almost None	Some	Moderate Amount	A Lot	Extreme
1	2	3	4	5

Problem   **Distress Rating**

_____   _____

_____   _____

_____   _____

_____   _____

From *Living Well on the Spectrum* by Valerie L. Gaus. Copyright 2011 by The Guilford Press.

The next few pages will guide you through the steps of solving the problem you just identified. For each step you will be asked to write your answers in the question box. Each box will give you instructions, and then I'll show you how **Dan** filled in the box.

Step 1: Identify and Define Your Healthcare Problem

What is bothering you about your healthcare? If you filled in Worksheets 39–41, you've already done this first step. Write the problem you've chosen to work on first below.

Step 1: Identify and Define Your Problem with Your Healthcare

What is bothering you about your healthcare?

The problem that is bothering me most about my healthcare is:

_____

_____

Example. **Dan** filled out his Step 1 question box this way:

Step 1: Identify and Define Your Problem with Your Healthcare

The problem that is bothering me most about my healthcare is:

I am very overweight, but I don't know how to start a diet or find time to

exercise.

Step 2: Define Your Goal

What would you like to see change to minimize the problem you identified with your healthcare? What would need to be different for you to feel less bothered by the problem you identified? The goal you lay out is simply the opposite of the problem you listed. List your goal in the box below, and if you need an example, look at Dan's box.

Step 2: Define Your Goal

What would you like to see change to minimize the problem you identified with your healthcare? The goal you lay out is simply the opposite of the problem you listed.

To feel less stressed by this problem, I would like to:

_____

_____

Example. **Dan's** goal is listed next.

> ### *Step 2: Define Your Goal*
>
> To feel less stressed by this problem, I would like to:
>
> *Make and start a weight-loss plan and feel confident that I can stick with it*
>
> *for a prolonged period of time.*

Notice how he stated the goal as the opposite of his problem. Stating the goal in the affirmative gives Dan something to work toward and also lends itself to measuring success. Also notice that Dan's goal is not too overzealous. Rather than saying "I will lose 60 pounds immediately," he decided he would be satisfied with simply having a plan to get started; his anxiety was being caused by the fact that he felt so lost in terms of how to begin.

Step 3: Identify the Obstacles in the Way of Your Achieving the Goal

What is getting in the way of your goal? Here it is particularly important to consider your ASD characteristics as hidden players in your problem. As you go through this step, you may rely on the information you were given in Part I of this book about your ASD differences. As you think about the problem you listed above, look at the chart on page 330 called "ASD Differences That Can Contribute to Problems with My Healthcare." Read through that chart with your own problem in mind and also consider the following questions.

Thinking Differences

How might my *executive functioning* issues be contributing to my problems with my healthcare? For example, do I have difficulty organizing information, which makes it hard for me to keep track of my grooming or self-care tasks? Do I have difficulty keeping up with my prescription renewals? Do I forget to do important things to stay healthy, like brush my teeth or take my medicine or vitamins? Do I find it hard to plan my medical appointments? Does my focus and concentration difficulty cause me to have problems concentrating during medical appointments? Do I become so hyperfocused on a lifestyle practice that others tell me I am "obsessed" (e.g., excessive exercise, preoccupation with diet, vitamins, supplements)? Do I persist too long, repeating a strategy that is clearly not helping me because I have difficulty shifting to new strategies (e.g., diet or exercise routines)? How might my *negative self-talk* be contributing to my problems taking care of my health? What am I saying to myself that is putting more pressure on me? Is it possible I am engaging in perfectionistic thinking, all-or-nothing thinking, or catastrophic thinking that makes it harder for me to carry out healthy lifestyle practices? For example, do I assume the worst will happen before an appointment? Do I expect perfection from myself when following a diet or exercise routine?

Social Differences

How might my *social perception* be contributing to my problems with taking care of my health? Is it possible I sometimes misunderstand what medical professionals or their staff are trying to tell me? For example, do I still feel uncertain about what I'm expected to do when I show up for a medical appointment? How might my *social/communication skills* be contributing to problems with my healthcare? Is it possible that medical professionals or their staff are not communicating clearly enough about what they expect and I don't know how to seek clarification? For example, I feel uncertain about what to say to a receptionist when I call to make an appointment. Or, I am still not sure how I should handle questions at the pharmacy. I am unsure how to handle it if a patient in a waiting room tries to strike up a conversation with me.

Emotional Differences

How might my emotional reactions to things be affecting my problems taking care of my health? Do I have difficulty *regulating* my emotions? Do I take too long to calm down after an upsetting incident? Do I have difficulty *identifying* my feelings or *asking for help* when I am upset? Am I overreacting or underreacting to things that happen at the doctor's office, dentist's office, or pharmacy? Do I tend to avoid situations that cause me to feel too much anxiety or worry, such as calling to make an appointment? Did I have some traumatic experience in the past related to my healthcare that is causing anxiety that stops me from taking care of a current health concern?

Sensory and Movement Differences

How might my sensory issues be contributing to my problems taking care of my health? Am I *oversensitive* or *undersensitive* to certain types of light, sound, smell, taste, or touch? For example, my sensitivity to touch makes it unbearable for me to sit through a physical exam. Or my high pain tolerance makes me miss important cues that I have a problem (e.g., an infection). Or I have very particular food preferences that restrict my diet to one that is not balanced. How might my *movement* and *coordination* issues be contributing to my problems with my healthcare? For example, I feel very clumsy when I try to exercise at the gym, and it's embarrassing to me. Or my coordination problems make it hard for me to shave properly or brush my teeth thoroughly.

Now fill out the question box below, but try not to think about other problems you have besides the one you chose for this exercise.

Step 3: Identify the Obstacles in the Way of Your Achieving the Goal

What is getting in the way of your goal? Remember to focus *only* on the problem and goal you wrote down in Steps 1 and 2. First circle the category(ies) of ASD differences you suspect are involved in this problem:

Thinking   **Social**   **Emotional**   **Sensory/Movement**

I believe these differences are contributing in this way:

_____

_____

_____

_____

_____

_____

Example. **Dan** filled out his Step 3 question box in this way:

Step 3: Identify the Obstacles in the Way of Your Achieving the Goal

(**Thinking**)   **Social**   (**Emotional**)   **Sensory/Movement**

I believe these differences are contributing in this way:

My thinking differences make it hard for me to organize myself enough to start to change my lifestyle. I have trouble shifting gears to change my habits. My all-or-nothing thinking makes me think I have to find the "perfect" weight-loss plan before I can start. My emotional differences involve my anxiety about change and my guilt about poor eating habits, which is so intense that it paralyzes me.

Differences →	Thinking	Social	Emotional	Sensory/Movement
Problems Managing Personal Care	• Difficulties organizing information make it hard to organize your personal spaces for grooming, meds, or diet • Difficulties organizing information make it hard to plan your tasks and schedule medical appointments • Working memory difficulties make it hard to do more than one task at a time • Focusing on detail but ignoring the "big picture" may cause you to overlook important aspects of grooming • Dichotomous, all-or-nothing thinking can cause undue pressure and anxiety around completing tasks • Intense focus on certain exercise or diet practices becomes "obsessive"	• Your difficulty initiating conversations may interfere with your ability to ask for help on tasks you do not understand or find difficult to complete • Any of your social differences can interfere with taking advantage of group exercise activities	• Your difficulty recognizing and identifying negative emotions that you are feeling can interfere with your awareness that you are struggling with your daily self-care and may need to change something (e.g., anxiety, anger) • Your difficulty regulating your negative emotions related to self-care can contribute to your experience of getting extremely overwhelmed by the pressures involved	• Hypersensitivity to noise, light, smell, taste, or touch can interfere with grooming and self-care • Hypersensitivity to taste can cause you to have a very restricted diet. • Hypersensitivity to discomfort can make it hard to tolerate medication side effects • Hyposensitivity (underresponsive sense) can interfere with picking up on important cues about your need for grooming or first aid (e.g., noticing a soiled garment, noticing a cut or bruise) • Fine motor problems (coordinated handwork) could affect tasks like brushing teeth, shaving, bathing • Gross motor (coordinated whole-body movement) problems could affect your ability to participate in some types of exercise
Problems Accessing Healthcare Services	• Attention regulation difficulties can make it hard to coordinate your focus during appointments with healthcare providers • All-or-nothing thinking or catastrophic thinking can lead you to expect the worst before an office visit	• Your difficulty initiating conversations may interfere with your ability to ask for clarification if you do not understand medical instructions • The unique way you process and express language can contribute to misunderstandings with medical professionals or their staff • The unique way you express language can make it hard to report your symptoms or assert yourself with medical professionals • You may not notice or interpret cues or mind-read, making it difficult to know what others expect from you during an office visit	• Your difficulty recognizing and identifying negative emotions can prevent you from addressing the anxiety you may feel around medical professionals and their staff • Your difficulty regulating your negative emotions can contribute to anger with medical professionals or their staff • Your difficulty regulating anxiety related to past traumatic experiences with medical problems can interfere with accessing needed services in the present	• Hypersensitivity to pain or touch can interfere with medical or dental exams • Hypersensitivity to pain can affect the accuracy of your symptom descriptions during exams • Hyposensitivity to pain can cause underreporting of important symptoms to physicians or dentists

ASD differences that can contribute to problems with healthcare.

Did you circle more than one area of ASD differences? In the example, Dan's problem has two potential sources of difficulty; his thinking (difficulty organizing himself and shifting gears, and perfectionistic thinking) and emotional (anxiety) differences are playing a role in his problem getting started on a weight-loss plan. This illustrates that often a single issue can have several causes.

Step 4: List Several Possible Solutions to Address the Obstacle(s)

What are the possible solutions for the obstacles? Try to list as many ideas as possible. Remember that this is the step some people call "brainstorming." Generate as many possibilities as come to mind, without inhibition. Don't judge or evaluate any solution that comes to mind—just write it down no matter how weird or silly it seems. In Step 5 you will weed through them and discard any that are not useful, so no harm can be done.

Start by looking at the Cheat Sheet at the end of Chapter 6. Find the ASD differences that you circled on the top row of the Cheat Sheet. Then look along the column underneath each and find the dots. Each dot marks the row in which you will find a solution in the far left column of the chart. Those approaches should be considered first for your problem, and Chapter 6 provides you with the instructions and tools for each of those solutions. Also, try to consider your *strengths* as you complete this step because they also play an important role in your solutions. Refer back to Worksheets 3 and 4 in Chapter 1. Write your primary strengths in the blanks here so you can keep them in mind while you are generating solutions.

My strengths are: _____, _____, and _____.

Step 4: List Several Possible Solutions to Address the Obstacle(s)

What are the possible solutions for the obstacles? Now, considering all the solutions you saw on the Cheat Sheet, and some you may think of on your own, list all the possibilities you can imagine to address the ASD differences involved in the problem you listed in Step 1. For the moment, ignore the score columns on the right.

I could try to:

List strategies below	Pro (+) score	Con (−) score	Total pro–con

*Example. **Dan** filled out his question box this way:*

Step 4: List Several Possible Solutions to Address the Obstacle(s)

I could try to:

List strategies below	Pro (+) score	Con (−) score	Total pro−con
1) ignore the people telling me to lose weight			
2) use scheduling techniques for diet and exercise			
3) ask my girlfriend to help organize the plan			
4) join a gym			
5) go on a crash diet and get it over with quick			
6) use thinking techniques for anxiety			

Notice that Dan listed everything that came to mind, even things that don't seem appropriate (e.g., ignore signs that he needs to lose weight). The Cheat Sheet gave him ideas 2, 3, and 6. This is an example of "brainstorming." He won't be able to do all the things on this list but will use the next step to figure out what is most useful to him.

Step 5: Consider the Consequences of Each Solution

What are the pros and cons of each solution? Now you will put each item on your list to the test of how feasible it is or how helpful it will be toward the goal you wrote down during Step 2. Use the question box to give each item a score.

Step 5: Consider the Consequences of Each Solution

What are the pros and cons of each solution? Look back at each item you wrote down in Step 4. Then assign each one a score. Score the benefit (Pro +) in terms of how likely that strategy is to get you closer to your goal. Score the disadvantage (Con -) in terms of the effort, cost, or damage involved in implementing it.

Pro (+) Scale

How likely is it to get me closer to my goal?

Very Unlikely	Pretty Unlikely	Hard to Tell	Somewhat Likely	Very Likely
0	1	2	3	4

Con (–) Scale

How much effort, cost, or damage would this strategy involve?

None	Almost None	Some	A Lot	Extreme
0	1	2	3	4

*Example. **Dan's** answers appear below. He carried out Step 5 and rated each one of his solutions from Step 4.*

Step 4: List Several Possible Solutions to Address the Obstacle(s)

I could try to:

List strategies below	Pro (+) score	Con (–) score	Total pro–con
1) ignore the people telling me to lose weight	0	4	–4
2) use scheduling techniques for diet and exercise	4	3	1
3) ask my girlfriend to help organize the plan	4	2	2
4) join a gym	3	3	0
5) go on a crash diet and get it over with quick	2	4	–2
6) use thinking techniques for anxiety	3	1	2

Step 6: Choose the Best One(s) to Try Out First

Which solutions should you try first? Now that you have scored all of your options, choosing the one or two strategies to start with should be easy. Which of your options had the highest total score? According to your own rating, the highest score has the most benefit compared to the cost, effort, or damage it could involve. Notice that Dan ended up with three solutions that seemed worthwhile to him, even though none of them had high pro-con scores. He believed his strategies had some promise, but he was nervous about changing his habits. Also he knew he would have to put a lot of effort into his changes and was worried that he wouldn't be able to keep up with the new plan. That's why he assigned a "con" rating even to ideas he had chosen after looking at the strategies in Chapter 6. Having doubt is natural; don't be surprised if you have some of those same feelings yourself. In the end, you need not expect a "perfect" pro-con score of 4 to consider an option; you need only pick the ones with the highest score.

Step 6: Choose the Best One(s) to Try Out First

Which solutions should I try first? Which of the strategies in Step 5 had the highest score? Pick the top one or two and write them down below:

_____

_____

_____

Example. **Dan** filled out his question box as follows, choosing ideas 2, 3, and 6.

Step 6: Choose the Best One(s) to Try Out First

Use scheduling techniques to figure out how to make lifestyle changes

Use thinking techniques to help anxiety

Ask girlfriend to help me make my plan (communication)

Step 7: Implement the Solution and Track Your Progress

Now try the solution and track your progress. Use the next question box to map out your plan.

Step 7: Implement the Solution and Track Your Progress

Now try the solution and track your progress. Here is how:

_____

Where will I do it?

_____

When will I do it?

_____

What do I need to do it?

_____

How will I do it?

_____

_____

Who can help me, if needed?

_____

How will I keep track of my success? (Look at your goal and then pick a way to track it—either a running count or a rating scale.)

_____

_____

_____

*Example. **Dan** ruled out the ideas of joining a gym and going on a crash diet when he evaluated them. He had previously thought he had to do those things and they were so intimidating that it contributed to his anxiety. But logical examination of all his options led him to conclude that those approaches were probably not right for him. He read about the **scheduling techniques** presented in Chapter 6 and started off by making a log of his typical day as it goes before starting any plan. He wanted to see how much time he has in the day and how he is currently using it. By reading about the ***communication techniques*** he realized he never thought to ask his girlfriend to help. She is a very organized person and he trusted her to be helpful and not judge him, so he decided she could help him put together a good plan. Then he studied the ***thinking techniques*** to figure out a way to address his all-or-nothing, perfectionistic thinking, as well as his anxiety about making changes. Dan's tendency to stick to one thing without changing was indeed an obstacle to getting started, but also contributes to his ***perseverance***, which is likely to be an asset once he starts a new plan.

Step 7: Implement the Solution and Track Your Progress

Where will I do it?

At home

When will I do it?

Discuss with girlfriend and make plan this Sunday, then practice plan every day afterward

What do I need to do it?

My Schedule and my Confidence Rating scale

How will I do it?

Keep log of my time starting today, meet with girlfriend on Sunday to go over it, make plan, and start the following week.

Who can help me, if needed?

My girlfriend

How will I keep track of my success? (Look at your goal and then pick a way to track it—either a running count or a rating scale.)

My goal is to start a weight-loss plan and to feel confident that I can stick with it for a prolonged period of time. I will consider myself successful if I map out plan with my girlfriend, start it, and can rate my confidence to be higher than it was before I started to address this.

As Dan examined his own thinking, he realized he was saying several things in his self-talk that were putting pressure on him in a nonproductive way. They were:

"I must do something drastic and extremely unpleasant in order to lose weight."

"I must be 100% compliant with any diet I go on to be successful."

"I must lose a lot of weight fast because I am facing an urgent situation."

Dan decided that he needed to explore the validity of these statements, so he did some research about the types of weight-loss strategies that seem to work best according to scientists who study healthy behaviors. He found out that people tend to lose weight and keep it off when they don't practice such rigid thinking—flexibility and goals for gradual lifestyle changes seem to work best. He used this information to challenge the three beliefs listed above. He made a daily schedule sheet that was inspired by his reading of Chapter 6 to get some data about the way he spends a typical day so he could show it to his girlfriend when he asked her to help him make a plan.

Daily Schedule	Day _Tuesday_ Date _April 13_
Time Blocks	Activities
7–8	Get up and make breakfast/ read paper
8–9	Watch the news/drive to work
9–10	Work
10–11	Work, 15-minute break with snack
11–12	Work
12–1	Go out to lunch
1–2	Work
2–3	Work, 15-minute break with snack
3–4	Work
4–5	Work
5–6	Drive home/pick up take-out dinner
6–7	Eat/ watch news
7–8	Watch TV
8–9	Watch TV/ Call girlfriend
9–10	Go on computer
10–11	Get ready for bed/read in bed/go to sleep

CONFIDENCE RATING

I feel *confident* that I will start and maintain a weight-loss program to the following degree:

0	1	2	3	4	5	6	7	8	9	10
None		A Little			Moderate			A Lot		Extreme

Step 8: Evaluate the Solution to See If It Met Your Goal

Did the solution meet your goal, or do you need to use a different solution? At this point you've tried out your new solution and are ready to see if it helped you meet your goal. Use the question box below to evaluate your progress.

Step 8: Evaluate the Solution to See If It Met Your Goal

Did the solution meet your goal, or do you need to use a different solution? Answer the following questions to figure this out:

What was my goal? (Copy this from Step 2.)

_____

How did I measure my progress? (data, log, or record)

_____

What do the data show with regard to my goal?

_____

How would I rate my success, on a scale of 0–100% success for meeting my goal?

I was _____% successful.

0	10	20	30	40	50	60	70	80	90	100
None		A Little			Moderate			A Lot		Total

What should I do based on this success rate? (fill in the box next to the best choice)

☐ **Celebrate and keep doing what I am doing!**

☐ **Celebrate success and also modify the plan toward further improvement.**

*Example. **Dan*** filled out his question box this way after he made his plan with his girlfriend.

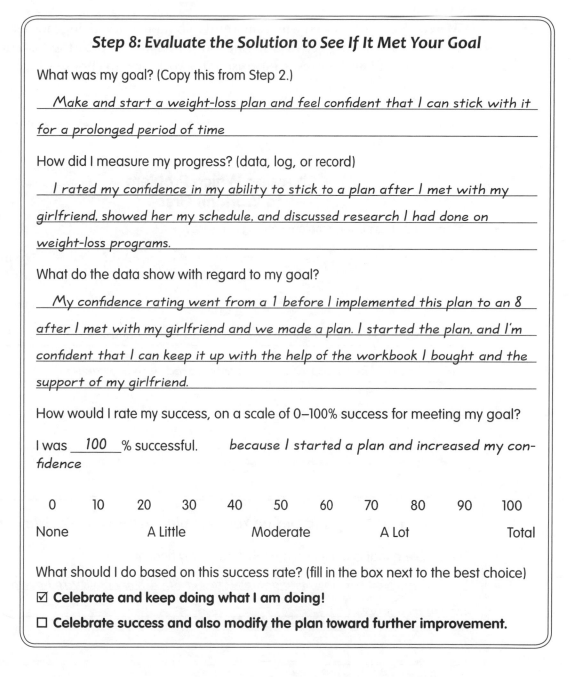

Step 8: Evaluate the Solution to See If It Met Your Goal

What was my goal? (Copy this from Step 2.)

  Make and start a weight-loss plan and feel confident that I can stick with it for a prolonged period of time

How did I measure my progress? (data, log, or record)

  I rated my confidence in my ability to stick to a plan after I met with my girlfriend, showed her my schedule, and discussed research I had done on weight-loss programs.

What do the data show with regard to my goal?

  My confidence rating went from a 1 before I implemented this plan to an 8 after I met with my girlfriend and we made a plan. I started the plan, and I'm confident that I can keep it up with the help of the workbook I bought and the support of my girlfriend.

How would I rate my success, on a scale of 0–100% success for meeting my goal?

I was __100__% successful.   *because I started a plan and increased my confidence*

0	10	20	30	40	50	60	70	80	90	100
None			A Little		Moderate			A Lot		Total

What should I do based on this success rate? (fill in the box next to the best choice)

☑ **Celebrate and keep doing what I am doing!**

☐ **Celebrate success and also modify the plan toward further improvement.**

Dan was very relieved and proud of himself because he was able to ask for help. He and his girlfriend took the information about his schedule as well as the research he had done about weight-loss programs and found a workbook called *The Learn Program for Weight Management* by Kelly Brownell (American Health, 2004). Dan decided to buy that and follow it because, among other things, it shows the reader how to make gradual lifestyle changes and how to practice thinking techniques to change health behaviors. Starting something that seemed realistic dispelled his original self-talk statements and boosted his confidence that he could stick with it.

Meredith gets depressed when she thinks about not practicing law because she has difficulty managing her health. She's also overwhelmed by the tasks involved in taking care of her diabetes, so she used the worksheet to choose which problem to work on first.

Example from Meredith

WORKSHEET 41

Choosing Which Problem to Work on First

How much distress is this problem causing in my life?

Almost None	Some	Moderate Amount	A Lot	Extreme
1	2	3	4	5

Problem	Distress Rating
I am overwhelmed with what I have to do for my diabetes	4
I am depressed because my diabetes interfered with my career	5

Step 1: Identify and Define Your Problem with Your Healthcare

The problem that is bothering me most about my healthcare is:

I'm depressed because my diabetes interfered with my ability to have a career as a lawyer.

Step 2: Define Your Goal

To feel less stressed by this problem, I would like to:

Feel less depressed about my diabetes and my career

Step 3: Identify the Obstacles in the Way of Achieving Your Goal

(Thinking)   Social   (Emotional)   Sensory/Movement

I believe these differences are contributing in this way:

My thinking differences (executive functioning) make it hard for me to
multitask. Also I do negative self-talk and judge myself harshly for this.
My emotional differences contribute to my strong feelings of sadness and
depression, which I can't seem to control.

For the next step, Meredith thought of as many solutions as she could, even ones that didn't seem feasible. She used the Cheat Sheet from Chapter 6 and also made up some solutions of her own. After listing them, she used the rating scale from the Step 4 problem-solving question box to weigh the pros and cons of each solution. The results of Steps 4 and 5 can be found in the box below.

Step 4: List Several Possible Solutions to Address the Obstacle(s)

I could try to:

List strategies below	Pro (+) score	Con (−) score	Total pro–con
1) take the bar exam and look for a law job	4	4	0
2) use thinking techniques for depression	4	3	1
3) use organizational techniques to multitask	3	3	0
4) find a therapist to help with my goal	4	2	2

In Step 6, Meredith used the results of this evaluation to pick the two options with the highest pro–con score, which are highlighted in the Step 4 box. Notice that the total scores are not a "perfect 4." Meredith believed she would need to put a lot of effort into her plan to help herself with depression. She found the prospect so intimidating that she felt discouraged by this exercise until it occurred to her that she could go to therapy for help. That's why she added option number 4 to her list. She read about the *thinking techniques* in Chapter 6 and was interested in the *mindfulness* and *acceptance* strategies that she saw but did not think she could practice them without some help. She did believe that her long-standing trait of *perseverance* would be helpful to her in this situation. Her implementation plan appears in the next box.

Step 7: Implement the Solution and Track Your Progress

Where will I do it?

    In a therapist's office and at home

When will I do it?

    Whenever I can get an appointment with a therapist

What do I need to do it?

    My own Depression Rating Scale and a cognitive-behavioral therapist

How will I do it?

    Look for a therapist with a cognitive-behavioral approach to help me address the depression I feel about my diabetes and career.

Who can help me, if needed?

    I will check CBT referral lists and also check with local ASD organizations for referrals.

How will I keep track of my success? (Look at your goal and then pick a way to track it—either a running count or a rating scale.)

    After I complete some sessions with my therapist I will measure my level of depression using my own rating scale and also considering therapist's input. My own rating right now, before therapy, is 8.

Meredith's depression rating scale appears below.

DEPRESSION RATING

I feel *depressed* about my diabetes interfering with my law career to the following degree:

0	1	2	3	4	5	6	7	8	9	10
None		A little		Moderate			A Lot			Extreme

Meredith did find a therapist through a local ASD organization. While that person had never worked specifically with diabetes before, he did have a lot of experience using cognitive-behavioral therapy for depression and also had experience with ASDs. Here is the evaluation Meredith did after she completed eight sessions of therapy with him.

Step 8: Evaluate the Solution to See If It Met Your Goal

What was my goal? (Copy this from Step 2.)

Feel less depressed about my diabetes and my career.

How did I measure my progress? (data, log, or record)

I rated my depression before and after my eight sessions of therapy.

What do the data show with regard to my goal?

My therapist helped me apply thinking techniques and also led me to resources for managing the emotional aspects of coping with diabetes. He assessed my depression and told me it is improved. Also, my own rating was an 8 before therapy and is now about 4. I am still a little depressed, but I have more hope that I can feel better and continue to work on other goals.

How would I rate my success, on a scale of 0–100% success for meeting my goal?

I was __85__ % successful   *because my goal was to become less depressed*

0	10	20	30	40	50	60	70	80	90	100
None		A Little		Moderate			A Lot			Total

What should I do based on this success rate? (fill in the box next to the best choice)

☑ **Celebrate and keep doing what I am doing!**

☐ **Celebrate success and also modify the plan toward further improvement.**

Mark needs to get a routine physical exam for his new employer but feels anxious about going because he was intimidated by the doctor during his last checkup, 7 years ago. Without showing his worksheet, here are his problem-solving steps, in his own words:

Step 1: Identify and Define Your Problem

"I am afraid to go to my doctor for a physical because I cannot keep up with what he tells me and asks me."

Step 2: Define Your Goal

"I would like to make an appointment with my doctor and communicate with my doctor during the appointment."

Step 3: Identify the Obstacles in the Way of Your Achieving the Goal

"I believe my *social* differences are causing the problem, particularly communication. I've always had difficulty following what people say when they talk fast, and I am afraid to ask them to slow down. I also have *thinking* differences, that involve negative self-talk and all-or-nothing thinking."

Step 4: List Several Possible Solutions to Address the Obstacle(s)

1. "Quit the new job so I don't have to get a physical."
2. "Use communication techniques to ask the doctor to slow down and clarify (got this idea from Cheat Sheet)."
3. "Use thinking techniques to reconsider my beliefs about my role as a patient (also got this idea from Cheat Sheet)."
4. "Try a new doctor."

Step 5: Consider the Consequences of Each Solution

"After evaluating the pros and cons of each solution, I think numbers 2, 3, and 4 are all reasonable to try out."

Step 6: Choose the Best One(s) to Try Out First

"After reading about communication techniques, I believe I can ask the doctor to repeat, slow down, or clarify when I am not following. The thinking techniques I read about made me realize I'm saying this irrational thing to myself about my role as a patient: 'I will look stupid if I stop the doctor and ask him to repeat or slow down.' Finally, I can go to a different doctor because it has been so long since I went to mine it will not matter. After discussing this with my wife, I realize I have traits that will be assets here; one is my sense of *personal responsibility* for my new job and obligations, and the other is my *rationality* and tendency to use logic to solve problems."

Step 7: Implement the Solution and Track Your Progress

"I'm going to make up an assertive statement (similar to the one in Chapter 6) to prepare for asking the doctor to either slow down or repeat. Here are two things I am prepared to say: 'Excuse me, but I did not catch what you just said. Can you please repeat that?' or 'I'm going to take a moment to write down what you just said.' I'll also take a pad and pen with me to write down important things the doctor might tell me during the visit. I now realize that it *is expected* for a patient to ask a doctor for clarification or to repeat things that are not understood. My wife likes her doctor, and she told me that she is very friendly and patient. I will make an appointment with her. I'll consider myself successful if I can make the appointment and then communicate with the doctor effectively."

Step 8: Evaluate the Solution to See If It Met Your Goal

"I made an appointment with my wife's doctor. She was very friendly and did not talk that fast, but I did ask her twice to repeat different questions. I consider myself 100% successful on my goal."

A Word about Routine Health Monitoring

Many people on the spectrum report difficulty keeping track of their medical information and also communicating it effectively to professionals. Here are a few tips to make that part of your life more manageable. Consider sharing these guidelines with the neurotypical people in your life as well, since they have universal value in today's confusing world of healthcare.

- Take a note pad and pen with you to all appointments with medical professionals and therapists (physicians, physician's assistants, nurse practitioners, mental health practitioners, physical therapists, speech therapists, occupational therapists, nutritionists).
- Carry with you a single current list of *all your medications and vitamins and nutritional supplements* (including natural remedies that come in pill, powder, or liquid form). Make sure your list includes the daily dose or quantity you consume of each item. Show this list to *each and every practitioner* you have contact with, whether they seem interested or not.
- Do not leave the office of any practitioner until you are clear on what you have been

instructed to do in terms of follow-up or self-care. Make sure it gets written on your note pad.

- Keep a medical log in which you list, in chronological order, all the significant health events and tests you have had in your adult life. If you have a health problem that has been with you since birth or childhood, make sure your log includes that information as well. If you have a history of mental health diagnosis and treatment, make a separate log for that. Limit each entry to one line. Show this log to all practitioners you are visiting for an initial consultation. Respectfully request that they read it, even if they do not seem interested. A sample blank log appears on the facing page, and some sample entries are presented after that.

PERSONAL MEDICAL LOG

Beginning with your birth date, list in chronological order all the significant medical events in your history as follows:

Date	Event (illness, injury, surgery, or test)	Doctor/Hospital	Results or Diagnosis

From *Living Well on the Spectrum* by Valerie L. Gaus. Copyright 2011 by The Guilford Press.

PERSONAL MEDICAL LOG

EXAMPLE

Beginning with your birth date, list in chronological order all the significant medical events in your history as follows:

Date	Event (illness, injury, surgery, or test)	Doctor/Hospital	Results or Diagnosis
10/21/1978	Birth	Dr. Smith St. Mary's	C-section, no complications
6/14/1989	Appendix removed, emergency surgery. 4 days in hospital	Dr. Jones St. Mary's	Appendicitis
9/27/1997	Broke right arm in biking accident—wore cast for 2 months	Dr. Ames	Broken forearm
3/7/2008	CAT scan of abdomen because of pain	Dr. Singh	Gallstones and inflamed gallbladder
4/24/2008	Gallbladder removed—laparoscopic surgery	Dr. Singh	Inflamed gallbladder

From *Living Well on the Spectrum* by Valerie L. Gaus. Copyright 2011 by The Guilford Press.

14

Putting Yourself in Charge of Your Life and Finding Help When You Need It

By now I hope you've gained a better understanding of the specific ways an ASD has given you both strengths and vulnerabilities and how you can apply that knowledge to problem solving that will help you reduce daily stress and meet your life goals. Reading this book and filling out some of the boxes as you read is a good start. But if you adopt the problem-solving approach as a lifelong resource, you'll have the means to identify and apply positive solutions for years to come. The full problem-solving worksheet at the back of the book is available for you to photocopy whenever you need it.

Defining Success Your Way

The key to your success is to *know yourself*. Taking an honest, objective look at your unique strengths and weaknesses will help you design the best plans for reaching your goals. I hope the chapters you read helped you do that. By embracing the way your mind operates, including what is strong as well as what is vulnerable, you can always find a way to capitalize on the strengths and compensate for the weaknesses. As stated at the beginning of this book, if you ignore part of that picture, you will be hindered. Focusing only on areas of weakness will leave you immobilized by an identity defined by impairment and disability. Focusing only on strengths puts you at risk for repeating ineffective strategies because you are failing to build in plans and solutions that can help you compensate. Looking squarely at the strengths you can capitalize on *and* the weaknesses you'll have to compensate for will free you to be yourself, take charge of your life goals, and make big strides toward achieving them. This idea could not have been expressed any better than by Eustacia Cutler, mother of the famous autistic scientist Temple Grandin. In a recent note to me she wrote: "True character strength comes from looking the devil in the eye."

When you do, I believe you'll find that you're better off than you might have feared. I do some consulting work at a school for students with mild learning disabilities, ADHD, and ASDs. The school has a long tradition of providing a supportive environment that nurtures strengths and bolsters students' self-esteem. When a new self-advocacy program was launched, part of the curriculum involved helping the middle and high school students examine their own learning style, which included understanding strengths *and* weaknesses. At first, some of the staff were worried that involving students in frank discussions about their "weaknesses" might be hurtful—it seemed counter to the strong commitment the school has toward fostering healthy self-esteem. But once the program got under way, the students were grateful to receive specific information about the best and worst ways they learn. Some were relieved, saying "You mean that's the only problem I have? I always thought it was much worse than that!" Others expressed gratitude for learning specific ways they could take control of their studying environment by making changes to suit their style and asking others to accommodate them where needed. It felt good to them to be able to speak for themselves rather than to rely on parents and teachers speaking *for* them and *about* them. The empowerment they gained was totally consistent with the supportive mission of the school after all.

You may not have had the benefit of a self-advocacy program when you were a teenager. Hopefully, this book has helped you become better equipped to harness your strengths, identify your weaknesses, and communicate with others effectively about the types of help or accommodations you need from them.

Finding Help

As I've mentioned in this book, some of my patients have expressed the belief that being truly independent means never asking for help. I tell them that it may seem like a paradox, but any successful independent adult can stay that way only by *knowing when and how to ask for help*. Knowing how to get help is a strong sign of *independence* because the help you get is actually going to *support your self-sufficiency*.

You may have noticed that a number of the people I introduced in earlier chapters to illustrate the problem-solving process were utilizing other people in their solutions. There are two primary ways you can do this in your life. One is by reaching out to people in your immediate surroundings to give you *social support*. The other is to get *professional support* by going to a practitioner and essentially hiring that person to provide you an evaluation or treatment based on special training and expertise. Most people need to do both at one time or another in their lives.

Social Support

People who are in your life because they are family members, friends, or romantic partners can be great sources of help and reinforcement. For that matter, you are often providing help to others, even if you do not realize it, because you are part of the natural support systems of each of your loved ones and friends. Providers of social support (also called *natural support*) are not paid professionals, but can often be more powerful helpers than anyone you will hire. Here are some examples of people who may be in your social support network.

Family and Friends

Think about each relative (parent, sibling, grandparent, uncle, aunt, adult child), friend, or romantic partner you have in your life. Now list the ones who you believe take a genuine interest in your welfare and whom you find trustworthy. List them here:

_____

_____

_____

_____

_____

_____

Now think about the things each one of these people already does to support you. Worksheet 42 can be used to help you cover all the possible sources of support from each person.

After you fill out the checklist, look over it again, but ask yourself if there are areas that you did not check off where you wish that person would help you more. Then consider which things you did check off where you *don't* think you need help from that person. If you would like to see more or less support in different areas, you can initiate a conversation to discuss it with that person. One tool you can use to initiate can be found in the next question box. Look at Worksheet 43. Fill your name in the blank, and ask the supporter you have in mind to fill out that sheet, but don't reveal what you wrote on yours. After the person is done, invite him or her to sit down with you to compare sheets. Did your answers match? If so, then you each have a similar perspective on how that person is supporting you. If your answers are very different, you can express how you *would like* that person to help you. Whether your answers match a lot or not, be sure to express gratitude to that person for being in your life. You would be surprised at how often people are not aware of how helpful they are really being. Finding out that their support is noticed and appreciated can be very encouraging to them and will also enrich the relationship you have with that person.

My Natural Supports

Check off (✓) the ways in which _____ (fill in the name of a trusted person in your life) provides you with support. Support can take all of the forms listed below.

☐ **Emotional Support**

  ☐ listening

  ☐ validating

  ☐ encouraging

  ☐ advising

☐ **Basic Daily Living Support**

  ☐ meal preparation

  ☐ living space

  ☐ laundry

  ☐ housecleaning

  ☐ shopping

  ☐ transportation

☐ **Financial Support**

  ☐ money supply

  ☐ banking tasks

  ☐ financial management/planning

☐ **Health Support**

  ☐ filling prescriptions

  ☐ administering medication

  ☐ making appointments with health providers

☐ **Recreation (hobbies, interests, social activities)**

  ☐ joining with me in participating in activities

  ☐ arranging for activities

  ☐ paying for activities

☐ **Resource Coordination**

  ☐ researching special services

  ☐ filling out applications

  ☐ telephone connections with specialists

WORKSHEET 43

How I Support _____

Check off (✓) the ways in which you support your loved one or friend. Support can take all of the forms listed below.

- ☐ **Emotional Support**
    - ☐ listening
    - ☐ validating
    - ☐ encouraging
    - ☐ advising
- ☐ **Basic Daily Living Support**
    - ☐ meal preparation
    - ☐ living space
    - ☐ laundry
    - ☐ housecleaning
    - ☐ shopping
    - ☐ transportation
- ☐ **Financial Support**
    - ☐ money supply
    - ☐ banking tasks
    - ☐ financial management/planning
- ☐ **Health Support**
    - ☐ filling prescriptions
    - ☐ administering medication
    - ☐ making appointments with health providers
- ☐ **Recreation (hobbies, interests, social activities)**
    - ☐ joining with him/her in participating in activities
    - ☐ arranging for activities
    - ☐ paying for activities
- ☐ **Resource Coordination**
    - ☐ researching special services
    - ☐ filling out applications
    - ☐ telephone connections with specialists

Support Groups

The other type of social support that can be invaluable comes from support groups. In contrast to treatment or therapy groups (described in the next section), support groups are usually organized by people (not necessarily professionals) who have been affected by a particular diagnosis (medical or mental health). The purpose is to gather with a group of affected people so that support can be shared in several forms. Factual information about the conditions can be disseminated, resources and referrals can be exchanged, and emotional support can be mutually provided among the participants. You can find a support group for just about any medical or mental health problem you can think of, but the type that is most relevant here are those that serve adults on the spectrum. Associations that organize such groups may also have groups set aside for the family members of diagnosed individuals. The resource list at the back of the book includes several organizations that may have local chapters in your geographical region.

Professional Support

For many people, the reliance on social support along with self-help techniques like the ones you read about in this book is enough to address obstacles and work toward goals. However, at one time or another, people can hit points in their lives when some professional help is warranted. Here are some questions you can ask yourself to help you figure that out for yourself.

- "Is my problem persisting even after I attempted to address it using the self-help techniques described in this book?"
- "Am I suffering from depressed or irritable mood that lasts for several weeks without remission?"
- "Am I feeling so hopeless that I think about suicide?"
- "Am I suffering from anxiety that is so severe that I cannot even attempt the self-help strategies recommended to me?"
- "Am I bothered by vivid memories or images of traumatic experiences, even those that happened many years ago (e.g., bullying, physical or sexual assault)?"
- "Is my anger causing intense outbursts that are resulting in property damage, injury, or threat of injury to myself and/or other people?"
- "Am I engaging in compulsive rituals that consume a large portion of my time and which I have attempted to control but cannot?"
- "Am I engaging in eating habits that involve extreme dietary restrictions and significant weight loss, repeated purging (forced vomiting or use of laxatives), and/or excessive bingeing episodes that feel out of control?"
- "Am I using alcohol or nonprescribed drugs to cope even though I would prefer not to?"

If you answered "yes" to one or more of these questions, you would benefit from consulting a professional about your problem. But how should you choose? Following is a list of professional disciplines whose members can offer expert help for people on the spectrum. You can also use the Cheat Sheet on page 359 to guide you to the appropriate professional according to the type of ASD differences that are causing the most difficulty for you. Keep in mind that this sheet is only a rough guide, intended to give you hints about what you might want to try first if you are having a significant problem with one type of ASD difference (e.g., sensory movement differences might be best served by an occupational therapist first).

Before you think about consulting a specific professional, however, make sure you have a good ***primary care physician***. Before addressing any ASD difference that may be causing distress for you, it's important to rule out an underlying medical condition or medication side effect as the cause of the problem. Countless medical conditions can, if undiagnosed, manifest as behavioral or emotional problems. Likewise, emotional turmoil and chronic stress can exacerbate many preexisting medical conditions (e.g., stomach ulcers, cardiovascular disease, irritable bowel syndrome). You need a primary care physician who understands ASDs, is familiar with your particular ASD symptoms, and is willing to consider your health with a holistic perspective that includes all the relevant factors. If you are not sure how to find someone like that, ask a trusted friend or family member to help you do a search and/or contact one of your local ASD organizations for referral information.

Psychologists

Psychologists who treat patients are practitioners who have been trained in the science of human behavior as well as the best techniques to use to help people change behavior and alleviate distress. They can have the following degrees: PhD, PsyD, EdD, MS, or MA. The licensing and certification rules are different in each state, so it is best to check with your state's licensing board to be sure a particular psychologist is qualified to practice independently in your state. You may go to a psychologist for two possible reasons: to get an *evaluation* and/or to participate in *psychotherapy*.

Evaluations are formal assessments done using various tests and tools designed to answer questions about a person's cognitive, behavioral, or emotional functioning. They can help you understand specific areas of strength, weakness, or emotional distress. Psychologists trained in different subspecialties can carry out these specific types of evaluations:

■ **Neuropsychological evaluation**—an extensive battery of tests designed to pinpoint the specific areas of brain function and information processing that are either strengths or weaknesses/deficits. These tests can be conducted only by neuropsychologists—psychologists who have received specialized training in these techniques. They are very valuable in helping people on the spectrum find out about their own executive functions and attention/focus issues.

- ■ **Functional behavioral assessment**—a systematic evaluation of a specific behavior or set of behaviors that involves observation and careful collection of data on the occurrences of the behavior and circumstances surrounding those occurrences. These are best conducted by behavioral psychologists who have been certified in applied behavior analysis (ABA). The results give you information about the function of your maladaptive behavior (the behavior you wish to change) and important clues about the types of behavioral interventions that are likely to be most effective.

- ■ **Psychoeducational evaluation**—a battery of tests that usually includes an IQ test plus other tests of academic aptitude. These can be conducted by clinical or school psychologists and can guide educational programming for an individual.

- ■ **Psychological evaluation**—a battery of tests aimed at assessing the presence of psychiatric or mental health symptoms. These can be conducted by clinical psychologists and can inform mental health diagnosis and treatment.

Psychotherapy is a process in which a patient and therapist meet regularly and work toward a mutually agreed upon goal. The therapist uses intervention techniques that are based on his or her training and are tailor made to alleviate various behavioral or mental health problems. There are many different philosophies that may be driving a particular therapist's work, and that is called an "orientation." The most commonly practiced types are psychodynamic, humanistic, behavioral, and cognitive. Research on the therapy techniques that are most effective in alleviating problems reported by people on the spectrum supports the use of behavioral and cognitive-behavioral approaches.

Psychotherapy can be conducted individually (one on one with patient), in family therapy (in which the whole family is the "patient" and the therapist intervenes in their interactions), couple therapy (where two partners work together on improving their relationship), and group therapy (where a group of patients makes a commitment to meet regularly with a therapist to work on goals through their interactions with each other).

Social Workers

Social workers have been trained to intervene in human problems with a focus on understanding the systems in which people are functioning. They can have the following credentials: MSW, CSW, LCSW, each indicating a different level of training and certification. Again, check with your state licensing board to determine eligibility to practice in your state. Social workers can be particularly helpful in educating you about *systems and resources* and how to access them. Many also practice *psychotherapy* in the same ways that were described in the previous section.

Mental Health Counselors

Mental health counselors have been trained to carry out psychotherapy and counseling techniques to treat a variety of behavioral, emotional, and mental health problems. They may have a MA, MS, or MEd degree. Check with your state licensing board to find out if a particular practitioner has been licensed and certified to practice *psychotherapy* in your state.

Psychiatrists

A psychiatrist is a physician whose training has been specialized in the treatment of mental health disorders. Psychiatrists may have a MD or DO degree. They can offer *psychiatric medication evaluations and treatment*, as well as *psychotherapy* as described above. While there is no medication that has been shown to treat ASDs per se, many pharmacological agents can reduce some symptoms of anger, anxiety, and depression that often accompany ASD. You may consider getting a psychiatric evaluation when nonpharmacological approaches have not brought you any relief and/or you want to use a medication regimen as part of a comprehensive treatment plan that includes both medication and psychotherapy.

Speech–Language Pathologists

Speech–language pathologists are trained in the science of human language and communication, as well as the techniques to remediate problems with speech, language, or, in some cases, feeding and swallowing. They often have MA, MS, or PhD degrees and then, to verify certification, CCC-SLP (Certification of Clinical Competence in Speech–Language Pathology) as part of their credentials. As always, check with your state licensing board. For people with AS and HFA, speech–language pathologists can be most helpful with *pragmatics*, the social use of language. People with ASDs often have no problem with speech or diction, so my patients are sometimes puzzled when I refer to an SLP. But pragmatics are a different issue as they relate only to *how* language is used to participate effectively in a social interaction. This might include a focus on conversation skills, nonverbal communication, and reading the subtle cues of a communication partner. SLPs may work one on one with patients or may conduct communication groups that involve several patients.

Occupational Therapists

Occupational therapists are trained to help people improve performance on a vast array of daily activities and self-care tasks. It is a large field, and the types of problems they help people with vary greatly depending on a practitioner's area of specialty. While some may be involved in helping someone improve daily functioning after an injury or stroke, others are working with toddlers with developmental disabilities and still others are working with the elderly to improve cognitive functioning. They usually must have an MS or PhD degree to be licensed to practice independently. For people with ASDs, the field of occupational therapy has proved to be very helpful in alleviating the distress that can come from the sensory and motor problems described in this book. After assessing your current functioning using specialized tools and tests, an occupational therapist can devise a treatment plan and work with you on improving sensory and movement problems so that you more easily function from day to day.

Vocational Counselors

Vocational counselors, who can also be called *rehabilitation counselors*, have received specialized training in helping people with disabilities prepare for and find meaningful work. Usually possessing an MA, MS, or PhD degree, vocational counselors can be tremendously helpful in determining what your specific obstacles are to finding and keeping the type of job you want.

When considering using any of the professionals listed here, make sure the person meets the following criteria:

- Should be licensed and certified to practice the stated discipline in your state. Most states have a website you can use to look up any professional by name to find out if the person has the appropriate credentials.
- Should be experienced with ASDs in adults. If the person has only a little experience (e.g., has worked with children with ASDs only), but is willing to learn more about it and is receptive to reading material you provide about it, I would still consider trying out the person for a brief time. It is better to use someone who is receptive to learning about you as an individual than someone who claims to have knowledge about ASDs but is uninterested in your individual characteristics.
- Should address you in a respectful way with a tone and pace that makes you feel comfortable. If your practitioner has an interpersonal style that makes you feel very uncomfortable, it is not likely to be a successful partnership.

Also remember that you can always try someone out for a short time and then switch to a different provider if you are not happy. Many people on the spectrum have difficulty being assertive about this, but you will only be wasting your time and resources if you persist in going to someone for help who is clearly not making things any better for you.

In conclusion, the tools you practiced using in this book can become permanent parts of your bag of tricks, for you to come back to again and again when you hit various obstacles in your life. As you know, living with an ASD is both a gift and a source of stress. By taking charge of your life and defining success on your own terms, you are empowered to create and enjoy the lifestyle that you want. I wish you success on your journey!

Locate the ASD difference that is affecting you the most on the top of the chart. Then look down that column to find the dots, which lead you to corresponding practitioners to help you address that problem.

PROFESSIONALS	Thinking	Social	Emotional	Sensory/ Movement
Psychologist	*	*	*	
Social Worker	*	*	*	
Mental Health Counselor	*	*	*	
Psychiatrist	*	*	*	*
Speech–Language Pathologist	*	*		
Occupational Therapist	*			*
Vocational Counselor	*	*		

Cheat sheet of professional help for ASD differences.

Appendix

Problem-Solving Worksheet

Photocopy this form as many times as you want, to use the problem-solving steps in addressing different problems as they arise.

Step 1: Identify and Define Your Problem

What is bothering you most?

The problem that is bothering me most is:

_____

_____

_____

Step 2: Define Your Goal

What would you like to see change to minimize the problem you identified? The goal you lay out is simply the opposite of the problem you listed.

To feel less stressed by this problem, I would like to:

_____

_____

_____

Step 3: Identify the Obstacles in the Way of Your Achieving the Goal

What is getting in the way of your goal? Remember to focus *only* on the problem and goal you wrote down in Steps 1 and 2. First circle the category(ies) of ASD differences you suspect are involved in this problem:

Thinking   **Social**   **Emotional**   **Sensory/Movement**

I believe these differences are contributing in this way:

_____

_____

_____

_____

_____

_____

Step 4: List Several Possible Solutions to Address the Obstacle(s)

What are the possible solutions for the obstacles? Now, considering all the solutions that you saw on the Cheat Sheet, and some you may think of on your own, list all the possibilities you can imagine to address the ASD differences involved in the problem you listed in Step 1. Remember to consider your strengths. For the moment, ignore the score columns on the right.

I could try to:

List strategies below	Pro (+) score	Con (−) score	Total pro−con

Step 5: Consider the Consequences of Each Solution

What are the pros and cons of each solution? Look back at each item you wrote down in Step 4. Then assign each one a score. Score the benefit (Pro +) in terms of how likely that strategy is to get you closer to your goal. Score the disadvantage (Con –) in terms of the effort, cost, or damage involved in implementing it.

Pro (+) Scale

How likely is it to get me closer to my goal?

Very Unlikely	Pretty Unlikely	Hard to Tell	Somewhat Likely	Very Likely
0	1	2	3	4

Con (–) Scale

How much effort, cost, or damage would this strategy involve?

None	Almost None	Some	A Lot	Extreme
0	1	2	3	4

Step 6: Choose the Best One(s) to Try First

Which solutions should you try first? Which of the strategies in Step 5 had the highest score? Pick the top one or two and write them down below:

_____

_____

Step 7: Implement the Solution and Track Your Progress

Now try the solution and track your progress. Here is how:

Where will I do it?

_____

When will I do it?

_____

What do I need to do it?

_____

How will I do it?

_____

Who can help me, if needed?

_____

How will I keep track of my success? (Look at your goal and then pick a way to track it—either a running count or a rating scale.)

_____

_____

_____

Step 8: Evaluate the Solution to See If It Met Your Goal

Did the solution meet your goal, or do you need to use a different solution? Answer the following questions to figure this out:

What was my goal? (Copy this from Step 2.)

_____

How did I measure my progress? (data, log, or record)

_____

What do the data show with regard to my goal?

_____

How would I rate my success, on a scale of 0–100% success for meeting my goal?

I was _____% successful.

0	10	20	30	40	50	60	70	80	90	100
None		A Little			Moderate		A Lot			Total

What should I do based on this success rate? (fill in the box next to the best choice)

☐ **Celebrate and keep doing what I am doing!**

☐ **Celebrate success and also modify the plan toward further improvement.**

Resources

Positive Psychology and Problem Solving

Nezu, A. M., Nezu, C. M., & D'Zurilla, T. J. (2006). *Solving life's problems: A 5-step guide to enhanced well-being*. New York: Springer.

Positive Psychology Center, University of Pennsylvania: *www.ppc.sas.upenn.edu/publications. htm*

  ▪ Readings, information, and resources related to positive psychology and happiness.

Seligman, M. E. P. (2002). *Authentic happiness: Using the new positive psychology to realize your potential for lasting fulfillment*. New York: Free Press.

Seligman, M. E. P. (2011). *Flourish: A visionary new understanding of happiness and well-being*. New York: Free Press.

Descriptions of ASDs

American Psychiatric Association. (2000). *Diagnostic and statistical manual of mental disorders* (4th ed., text revision). Washington, DC: Author.

American Psychiatric Association. (2013). *Diagnostic and statistical manual of mental disorders* (5th ed.). Washington, DC: Author.

Attwood, T. (2006). *The complete guide to Asperger's syndrome*. London: Jessica Kingsley.

Baron-Cohen, S. (2008). *Autism and Asperger syndrome: The facts*. London: Oxford University Press.

McPartland, J. C., Klin, A., & Volkmar, F. R. (Eds.). (2014). *Asperger syndrome* (2nd ed.). New York: Guilford Press.

Shore, S. M., & Rastelli, L. G. (2006). *Understanding autism for dummies*. Hoboken, NJ: Wiley.

Autobiographical Accounts of ASD

Carley, M. J. (2008). *Aspergers from the inside out: A supportive and practical guide for anyone with Asperger's syndrome*. New York: Penguin.

Finch, D. (2012). *The journal of best practices: A memoir of marriage, Asperger syndrome, and one man's quest to be a better husband*. New York: Scribner.

Grandin, T. (1995). *Thinking in pictures and other reports from my life with autism*. New York: Doubleday.

Grandin, T. (2004). *Developing talents: Careers for individuals with Asperger's syndrome and high-functioning autism*. Shawnee Mission, KS: Autism Asperger.

Newport, J. (2001). *Your life is not a label: A guide to living fully with autism and Asperger's syndrome*. Arlington, TX: Future Horizons.

Newport, J., & Newport, M. (2002). *Autism-Asperger's and sexuality: Puberty and beyond*. Arlington, TX: Future Horizons.

Newport, J., & Newport, M. (2007). *Mozart and the whale: An Asperger love story*. London: Jessica Kingsley.

Paradiz, V. (2002). *Elijah's cup: A family's journey into the community and culture of high-functioning autism and Asperger syndrome*. London: Jessica Kingsley.

Prince-Hughes, D. (2004). *Songs of the gorilla nation: My journey through autism*. New York: Harmony Books.

Robison, J. E. (2007). *Look me in the eye: My life with Asperger's*. New York: Crown.

Shore, S. (2003). *Beyond the wall: Personal experiences with autism and Asperger syndrome* (2nd ed.). Shawnee Mission, KS: Autism Asperger.

Slater-Walker, C., & Slater-Walker, G. (2002). *An asperger marriage*. London: Jessica Kingsley.

Wiley, L. H. (2001). *Asperger syndrome in the family: Redefining normal*. London: Jessica Kingsley.

Wiley, L. H. (2014). *Pretending to be normal: Living with Asperger's syndrome (Autism Spectrum Disorder)*. London: Jessica Kingsley.

Zaks, Z. (2006). *Life and love: Positive strategies for autistic adults*. Shawnee Mission, KS: Autism Asperger.

Social Cognition and Social Understanding

Baron-Cohen, S. (2004). *Mind reading: The interactive guide to emotions* [DVD and CD-ROM set]. London: Jessica Kingsley.

Cohen, M. R. (2011). *Social literacy: A social skills seminar for young adults with ASDs, NLDs, and social anxiety*. Baltimore: Brookes.

Fiske, S. T., & Taylor, S. E. (1984). *Social cognition*. New York: Random House.

Goleman, D. (2006). *Social intelligence: The new science of human relationships*. New York: Bantam.

Grandin, T., & Barron, S. (2004). *The unwritten rules of social relationships*. Arlington, TX: Future Horizons.

Myles, B., Trautman, M., & Schelvan, R. (2004). *The hidden curriculum: Practical solutions for understanding unstated rules in social situations*. Shawnee Mission, KS: Autism Asperger.

Post, P., Post, A., Post, L., & Senning, D. P. (2011). *Emily Post's etiquette: Manners for a new world* (18th ed.). New York: William Morrow.

Shore, S. (Ed.). (2004). *Ask and tell: Self-advocacy and disclosure for people on the autism spectrum*. Shawnee Mission, KS: Autism Asperger.

Winner, M. G., & Crooke, P. (2009). *Socially curious and curiously social: A social thinking guidebook for teens and young adults with Asperger's, ADHD, PDD-NOS, NVLD, or other murky undiagnosed social learning issues.* San Jose, CA: Think Social.

Winner, M. G., & Crooke, P. (2011). *Social thinking at work: Why should I care?* San Jose, CA: Think Social; Great Barrington, MA: North River Press.

Brain Anatomy and Function

Beaumont, J. G. (2008). *Introduction to neuropsychology* (2nd ed.). New York: Guilford Press.

Carter, R. (2009). *The human brain book.* New York: Darling Kindersley.

Therapy Approaches

Applied Behavior Analysis (ABA)

Kearney, A. J. (2007). *Understanding applied behavior analysis: An introduction to ABA for parents, teachers, and other professionals.* London: Jessica Kingsley.

Cognitive-Behavioral Therapy (CBT)—General

Beck, A. T. (1976). *Cognitive therapy and the emotional disorders.* New York: International Universities Press.

Beck, J. S. (1995). *Cognitive therapy: Basics and beyond.* New York: Guilford Press.

Burns, D. (2008). *Feeling good: The new mood therapy.* New York: HarperCollins.

Moodgym: *www.moodgym.anu.edu.au*

 ▪ A free self-help program to teach cognitive-behavioral therapy skills to people vulnerable to depression and anxiety.

Cognitive-Behavioral Therapy (CBT)—For ASDs

Gaus, V. (2007). *Cognitive-behavioral therapy for adult Asperger syndrome.* New York: Guilford Press.

Scarpa, A., White, S. W., & Attwood, T. (Eds.). (2013). *CBT for children and adolescents with high-functioning autism spectrum disorders.* New York: Guilford Press.

Cognitive-Behavioral Therapy (CBT)—For Co-Occurring Anxiety

Attwood, T. (2004a). *Exploring feelings: Cognitive behaviour therapy to manage anxiety.* Arlington, TX: Future Horizons.

Knaus, W. J. (2008). *The cognitive behavioral workbook for anxiety: A step-by-step guide.* Oakland, CA: New Harbinger.

Cognitive-Behavioral Therapy (CBT)—For Co-Occurring Depression and Anger

Attwood, T. (2004b). *Exploring feelings: Cognitive behavior therapy to manage anger.* Arlington, TX: Future Horizons.

Greenberger, D., & Padesky, C. (1995). *Mind over mood: Change the way you feel by changing the way you think*. New York: Guilford Press.

Knaus, W. J. (2006). *The cognitive behavioral workbook for depression: A step-by-step program*. Oakland, CA: New Harbinger.

Mindfulness and Acceptance—General

Brach, T. (2003). *Radical acceptance: Embracing your life with the heart of a Buddha*. New York: Bantam.

Germer, C. (2009). *The mindful path to self-compassion: Freeing yourself from destructive thoughts and emotions*. New York: Guilford Press.

Guna, B. H. (2002). *Mindfulness in plain English*. Somerville, MA: Wisdom Publications.

Harris, R. (2008). *The happiness trap: How to stop struggling and start living*. Boston: Trumpeter.

Hayes, S. C., & Smith, S. (2005). *Get out of your mind and into your life*. Oakland, CA: New Harbinger.

Hayes, S. C., Strosahl, K., & Wilson, K. G. (1999). *Acceptance and commitment therapy: An experiential approach to behavior change*. New York: Guilford Press.

Mindfulness and Acceptance—For ASDs

Mitchell, C. (2008). *Asperger's syndrome and mindfulness: Taking refuge in the Buddha*. London: Jessica Kingsley.

Mitchell, C. (2014). *Mindful living with Asperger's syndrome: Everyday mindfulness practices to help you tune in to the present moment*. London: Jessica Kingsley.

Rubio, R. (2008) *Mind/body techniques for Asperger's syndrome: The way of the pathfinder*. London: Jessica Kingsley.

Mindfulness and Acceptance—For Co-Occurring Anxiety

Forsyth, J., & Eifert, G. (2008). *The mindfulness and acceptance workbook for anxiety: A guide to breaking free from anxiety, phobia, and worries using acceptance and commitment therapy*. Oakland, CA: New Harbinger.

Use of Companion/Service Animals

Assistance Dogs of America: *www.adai.org*
- General information about use of service dogs.

Autism Service Dogs of America: *www.autismservicedogsofamerica.org*
- Information about use of service dogs and how to apply.

Pavlides, M. (2008). *Animal-assisted interventions for individuals with autism*. London: Jessica Kingsley.

Pichot, T. (2012). *Animal-assisted brief therapy: A solution-focused approach* (2nd ed.). New York: Routledge.

Meditation, Relaxation, and Yoga

Benson-Henry Institute for Mind Body Medicine: *www.massgeneral.org/bhi*
- Information about managing stress, how to elicit the relaxation response, and relaxation CDs.

Cautela, J. R., & Groden, J. (1978). *Relaxation: A comprehensive manual for adults, children, and children with special needs*. Champaign, IL: Research Press.

George Washington University Counseling Center: *www.gwired.gwu.edu/counsel/asc/index. gw/Site_ID/46/Page_ID/14558*
- Podcasts about deep breathing, progressive muscle relaxation, and other relaxation techniques.

Sounds True: *www.soundstrue.com*
- Audiovisual materials for purchase related to meditation and yoga.

Tara Brach, PhD: *www.tarabrach.com*
- A variety of meditation resources including how to meditate, meditation CDs and MP3s, and audio talks.

The Meditation Mind: *www.themeditationmind.com*
- Articles about meditation and relaxation techniques and tips.

University of Massachusetts Medical School/The Center for Mindfulness: *www.umassmed. edu/cfm*
- Mindfulness-based stress reduction and links to books and CDs.

University of Michigan: *www.med.umich.edu/painresearch/patients/relaxation.pdf*
- A chapter from *The Relaxation Response* with text about breathing, progressive muscle relaxation, and visualization and a weekly tracking sheet.

Yoga.com: *www.yoga.com*
- Articles, a yoga studio locator by zip code, and yoga DVDs.

Yoga to the People: *www.yogatothepeople.com/tryOnlineClass.shtml*
- Free online yoga classes.

Other Self-Help Tools

Buron, K. D., & Curtis, M. (2012). *The incredible 5-point scale: The significantly improved and expanded second edition*. Shawnee Mission, KS: Autism Asperger.

Innovative Interactions. (2000). *Talk Blocks® for work*. Seattle, WA: Author.

Websites for Autism Spectrum Organizations

United States—National Sites

Autism Network International: *www.autreat.com*
- Self-help and advocacy site run by adults with autism. Annual retreat information.

Autism Society: *www.autism-society.org*
- Basic information about autism and Autism Society chapter locater by state for people who would like to be more involved.

Global and Regional Asperger Syndrome Partnership (GRASP): *www.grasp.org*
- An educational and advocacy organization serving and run by people on the autism spectrum. Offers articles and interviews, lists of support groups on- and off-line, and e-lists.

OASIS@MAAP (jointly operated by Online Asperger Syndrome Information and Support and MAAP Services for Autism and Asperger Syndrome: *www.aspergersyndrome. org*
- A resource for families, individuals, and medical professionals that provides articles, educational resources, links to local, national, and international support groups, sources of professional help, conference information, recommended reading, and moderated support message boards. Many materials can be accessed for free, but for a monthly or annual membership fee you can also get the newsletter and other information and support.

Organization for Autism Research (OAR): *www.researchautism.org*
- Science-based organization dedicated to funding research and distributing evidence-based materials for use by individuals, families, and educators.

Wrong Planet: *www.wrongplanet.net*
- A Web community designed for individuals with ASDs, ADHD, and other neurological differences, as well as their families, and professionals who work with them. This site has a discussion forum, articles section, a blogging feature, and a chat room.

United States—Regional Sites

The following organizations are headquartered in particular regions but offer information that is helpful for anyone and can be accessed by joining their e-mail lists.

Asperger's Association of New England (AANE): *www.aane.org*
- New England–based association whose website offers up-to-date information on resources, interventions, and conferences.

Asperger Syndrome and High Functioning Autism Association (AHA): *www.ahany.org*
- New York–based association whose website lists support groups, newsgroups, and listservs all devoted to disseminating up-to-date information on research, interventions, and conferences for people with AS or HFA.

Asperger Autism Spectrum Education Network (ASPEN): *www.aspennj.org*
- New Jersey–based association devoted to disseminating information on research and intervention as well as local conferences.

Penn Autism Network (PAN): *www.med.upenn.edu/pan*
- Philadelphia-based organization whose mission is to disseminate information and resources to help adults with ASDs and their families.

Australia

Autism Spectrum Australia: *www.aspect.org.au*
- National organization devoted to building confidence and capacity in people with an ASD, their families, and their communities by providing information, education, and other services.

Canada

Autism Today: *www.canadianautism.org*
- Large online resource center with easily accessible information about all aspects of ASDs.

United Kingdom

National Autistic Society: *www.autism.org.uk*
- This website includes information about autism and AS, the NAS, and its services and activities across the United Kingdom.

Websites for Mental Health Organizations

American Psychological Association: *www.apa.org*
- Provides information on a variety of topics, links to publications, and a consumer help center and psychologist locator by zip code.

Anxiety and Depression Association of America: *www.adaa.org*
- Provides consumer and professional information about anxiety disorders and maintains a searchable therapist referral directory.

Association for Behavioral and Cognitive Therapies: *www.abct.org*
- Provides consumer information about behavioral and cognitive-behavioral therapies and maintains an international therapist referral directory of cognitive-behavioral therapists.

Association for Behavioral Contextual Science: *www.contextualpsychology.org*
- Provides consumer information about mindfulness-based versions of cognitive-behavioral therapy and maintains an international therapist referral directory of therapists trained in these techniques.

Mental Health America (formerly National Mental Health Association): *www.nmha.org*
- Provides free information on specific disorders, referral directory to mental health providers, national directory of local mental health associations;1-800-969-6642 (M–F, 9–5 EST).

National Alliance on Mental Illness: *www.nami.org*
- Provides consumer information about mental illness and contacts and referral sources for mental health care around the United States.

National Association for Dual Diagnosis: *www.thenadd.org*
- Provides information and resources regarding co-occurring mental illness and intellectual, learning, or autism spectrum disorders.

Substance Abuse and Mental Health Services Administration: *www.samhsa.gov*
- Referrals to wide range of mental health treatment providers and facilities including those offering sliding scale fees; 1-800-789-2647.

Index

About the Author

Valerie L. Gaus, PhD, is a clinical psychologist in private practice in Long Island, New York. She has provided mental health services to people with autism spectrum disorder since receiving her doctorate in 1992. Dr. Gaus serves on the advisory board of the Asperger Syndrome and High Functioning Autism Association and on the grant review committee of the Organization for Autism Research, and has lectured internationally on Asperger syndrome and related topics. She is the author of an acclaimed book for therapists on conducting cognitive-behavioral therapy with people on the spectrum.